DUKE UNIVERSITY HOSPITAL
NURSING SERVICES
Durham, North Carolina

Quality Assurance: Guidelines for Nursing Care

J.B. LIPPINCOTT COMPANY

Philadelphia • *Toronto*

Library of Congress Cataloging in Publication Data

Duke University, Durham, N. C. Duke Hospital. Nursing
    Services.
    Quality assurance: guidelines for nursing care.

    Includes index.
    1. Nursing—Standards.   2. Nursing audit.
I. Title. [DNLM: 1. Nursing care—Standards.
2. Quality assurance. Health care—North Carolina—
Nursing texts. WY16 D877q]
RT85.5.D84 1980   610.73′02′18   80-12185
ISBN 0-397-54315-8

1 3 5 6 4 2

The authors and publisher have exerted every effort to ensure that drug selection and
dosage set forth in this text are in accord with current recommendations and practice at the
time of publication. However, in view of ongoing research, changes in government
regulations, and the constant flow of information relating to drug therapy and drug
reactions, the reader is urged to check the package insert for each drug for any change in
indications and dosage and for added warnings and precautions. This is particularly
important when the recommended agent is a new or infrequently employed drug.

Quality Assurance: Guidelines for Nursing Care is written for nurses who intend to be explicit about and accountable for the quality of care they provide. Quality assurance programs provide the means by which groups of nurses and their employers can reasonably assure the public that the services rendered in their institution are equivalent to agreed upon standards of care for similar patients in other locations.

It is not desirable nor is it economically feasible for each nurse and every institution to develop a unique system of quality control. It is appropriate, however, for institutions that have invested large amounts of personnel time and energy in developing such programs to share their information and experience. The net result should be to stimulate the development of better approaches more rapidly and to pass on measurable benefits to the patients the institution exists to serve.

The purpose of this book is to state in distinct terms the agreed upon nursing standards of care and the beginning of an evaluation system for one institution. It may bring nursing a step closer to establishing nationally recognized standards of care, and to defining viable operational methods for evaluating the quality and the impact of nursing interventions on the outcome of health care.

To some this may sound premature and presumptuous since program strategies selected for one institution may not be acceptable to another. Each organization is obligated to consider the needs of specific patient populations, the setting in which the care takes place, and the unique perspectives and talents represented by the cadre of health care personnel.

By sharing how both the program and this book came into being and how they are applied, others may find it easier to consider thoughtfully their own practices and their institution's commitment to quality assurance.

It should be noted that all of the written standards included in this book, hereafter called Guidelines of Care, have been critically reviewed by nurses from different parts of the country who are considered by the publisher to be expert practitioners in their respective fields of nursing. We anticipated and received notes that reflect differing regional and institutional medical and nursing practices. However, there were far fewer of these comments than expected, indicating that nurses and others can benefit from focusing on their similar approaches to patient care rather than on their differences.

PROGRAM DEVELOPMENT

In the Fall of 1972, the administrative leadership group of the Nursing Services confronted the question of accountability: Can we define and measure nursing care well enough to offer a promise to our consumers? It wasn't until a year later that a project director was recruited to coordinate initial efforts. We believed that the primary purpose of any evaluation is not to justify what exists, but to place a value on the services provided in order to retain what is worthwhile and to make improvements where they are needed. Administratively, we needed a comprehensive data base to assist in solving problems, making sound decisions, and charting future plans.

In its direct care application, we wanted a program that would let every nurse know the nature and extent of patient outcomes to strive for, and the related care patients should receive. At the same time we thought that nurses could benefit from an objective way to determine how they measure up to established criteria. We believed that In-service Education programming should be coordinated in support of the competencies described. In summary, we wanted a broad-based system of evaluation that would meet the purposes of the care giver, the educator, and the manager.

The result is our Quality Assurance Program in Nursing (QAPN), which is a relatively simple and straightforward strategy designed to improve patient care, increase nursing skills and confidence, and enhance the total patient care program of the institution. More than 5 years of development and testing have produced results indicating the overall success of the plan, as well as revealing areas where modifications and improvements are necessary.

Basically, the program involves (1) setting explicit, desirable *patient outcomes* or end results in terms of alteration of health status and patient satisfaction; (2) identifying the significant nursing activites or *nursing process* directed to achieving the outcomes; and (3) simultaneously measuring the extent to which outcome and process criteria are met to determine the effectiveness of nursing care. Although we are aware of the lack of tested evaluation methods and the need for research data to link specifically certain nursing process and patient outcomes, we are confident that careful pursuit of this method will eventually provide nurses with better information than any other approach.

A basic premise of our program is the need for the involvement of as many members of the nursing staff, at as many levels as possible, throughout the development process. Often, however, it is impractical to expect full participation, particularly in the time-consuming job of writing clinical guidelines. Long delays can result owing to patient load and fluctuating needs for staffing. The foundation of the program is formed by the written guidelines. If the staff agrees that the guidelines accurately reflect their accountability for patient care, then construction of evaluation tools and the subsequent steps of securing and interpreting measurements and taking steps to alter care become a natural progression of events.

Coordination among different components of the health care system is important. Although nurses are expected to collaborate during each phase of program development with physicians and other members of the team who contribute to the patient's care, the guidelines reflect a separate, yet interdependent, contribution of nursing to the patient's total care. Recognition of this accountability in helping patients reach certain health outcomes is an important step for the profession.

The motivation to continue striving for excellence means that the guidelines cannot be set at a minimum acceptable level, but rather one that is optimal for the patient and achievable by the nurses within the institution. As time progresses, data are needed to consider the economic factor; guidelines should also reflect the level of nursing service for which consumers are willing to pay.

Outcome and process data provide clues to corrective action and cost effectiveness. Measurement criteria should meet at least four theoretical and practical considerations to be used for evaluation:

1. They should be explicit in terms of what will be measured, at what level of performance, and at what critical times.
2. They should distinguish differences in quality of care.
3. The institution should possess the techniques needed for their measurement.
4. Costs involved in the evaluation should be justified.

It was agreed that data should be gathered from a variety of sources: hospital charts, records, direct observation, and patient, family, and practitioner interviews. While the patient's chart has been regarded as the major data source for most health care evaluations, it is not sufficient for a quality assurance program. The patient's chart may record *what* was performed, but it does not consistently tell *how* it was performed, nor what happened to the patient as a result. It is expected, however, that this program will encourage more accurate and clearly stated documentation.

It was further determined that peer review would be the major assessment method. This was consistent with the overall belief in staff involvement and self-motivation, and was also the most verifiable method, since nurses have the special knowledge of patient care not readily perceptible to those who are not experts in the field. The pressure to measure evidence objectively in unique human situations where complexities, exceptions, and abstractions abound has lead us to the conclusion that concurrent nursing judgments are essential and in fact are a primary component of the program. Certainly, careful preparation of reviewers and attention to their tools and techniques are critical.

WRITING THE GUIDELINES

Once these principles were established, the first task of the QAPN committee was to write an operational definition of delivering nursing care that was consistent with the goals of the program and was described from the patient's perspective. Next, it was decided to set two types of guidelines: General Guidelines, covering a broad range of desirable patient outcomes for which nurses are accountable, and specific patient population guidelines, addressing the particular needs of patients in areas such as medicine, surgery, obstetrics, pediatrics, critical care, and rehabilitation.

Nurses representing all of the traditional services pooled their expertise to describe General Guidelines. Many of these are concerned with the "four C's": courtesy, compassion, comfort, and caring. These were considered to be central issues, especially in a complex institution missions of which include teaching and research in addition to the provision of patient care. Nurses met for 2 hours every 2 weeks for nearly a year in order to complete the General Guidelines.

After this intensive effort, the committee was eager to build the assessment tool with which to measure their newly developed guidelines. This presented an ideal opportunity to proceed directly to patients and ascertain the degree to which certain personal and environmental needs had been met. At the same time, it enabled the nurses to ask questions aimed at determining the patients' satisfaction with their care.

The General Guidelines assessment tool was developed, tested, and revised until it met with the approval of the entire committee. This was followed by a 3-month trial period of peer review. Each member of the QAPN committee was responsible for orientation of one or two nursing units, and all nursing personnel received full orientation before any evaluation took place.

The positive reception and interest generated by the initial review phase were followed by a more permanent system of peer review which included every non-intensive care inpatient unit. Three reviewers representing each unit were trained for their responsibilities. They were assigned evaluations on other units that they conducted and logged for 3-month periods. As numerous assessments were completed by different reviewers, patterns of care became clearly apparent. The peer review was not intended to focus on a particular nurse's performance, nor has it tended in that direction.

After each review period, every unit conducted a Unit Review Meeting in which cumulative results were analyzed and reviewed by as many members of the nursing staff who could attend. These meetings were found to be an effective way to exchange ideas and clear any possible misinterpretation of written data. The meetings also afforded a time for reflection, a time for feeling proud of goals attained and jobs well done, and also a time to set goals for improvement. During the most recent fiscal year, 1977 to 1978, 1058 General Guidelines evaluations were conducted and results reported to the responsible nursing staffs. The evaluation tool used to collect this data can be found in the Appendix.

At the same time that these General Guidelines were being developed, other groups, formed because of their particular clinical knowledge and experience, were writing specific patient population guidelines. The subjects for the guidelines were chosen by the clinical groups based on what they considered their most important patient populations. Some were based upon nursing problems, medical diagnoses, phases of hospitalization, and treatment modalities. Each guideline first describes the desired patient outcomes, which are usually related to a "critical episode of care" according to the defined problem or illness. For example, in the case of myocardial infarction, the time of admission is expected to be a critical episode. In this instance the guidelines center on patient outcomes and important aspects of the nursing process related to it. Guidelines have now been developed for 11 areas of clinical practice, and 157 of these are included in this text.

Included in the Appendix are several examples of evaluation tools that were designed and tested for use in determining the extent to which desired patient outcomes are achieved and selected elements of nursing process are accomplished. Data can be collected concurrently by peer review through the methods of chart review, patient interview, and direct observation.

AREAS OF CONCERN

In developing the Quality Assurance Program, the biggest problem has been time. Because of the patient imperative, clinical groups occasionally have had to defer planned periods of work on guidelines and evaluation tools. In addition, each aspect of peer review takes preparation time. A hurried assessment loses a great deal of its value. Moreover, each aspect of the program must be carefully explained to all involved since the keystone of the program is staff awareness and commitment. Making the guidelines come alive for the long-term staff members who have lived without them for years, as well as for new staff members, is the difficult task of implementation. Planned as a part of orientation of new personnel, the introduction of the clinical guidelines must be strategically spaced so that expectations become clear but not overwhelming.

Money is, of course, another area of concern. Time, materials, and resources are valuable assets. Although the current program involves only one salary of the QAPN Director and part-time secretarial support, the other costs are inherent in the working time spent by the nursing staff. We believe that the cost of not having the program, although impossible to calculate, would be greater than the nurses or their patients would want to bear.

A third area of concern is the readiness of an institution to undertake a pervasive program. It requires the firm backing of the administrative staff and sufficient personnel to organize and implement it. If, for example, there is a serious staffing deficit that prevents consistent delivery of a basic minimum level of nursing care, it is folly to spend time and money to measure unattainable standards.

BENEFITS

The success of the Duke Quality Assurance Program in Nursing relates largely to the presence of three factors: (1) the administrative expectation was clear—we will have a quality assurance program; (2) the nursing practitioners were given freedom and opportunity to express their finest efforts in the kind of system they wanted; (3) the Director of QAPN focused the program and connected the component parts to create a coherent whole.

The program receives priority attention from the administrative leadership so that its mandates are taken seriously. Nurses at the care delivery level have a program directed toward the impact of their care on the patient. Anticipating change, staff members constantly reviewed the guidelines for possible revision and improvement to keep abreast of current practice. It is a logical step to link program goals with other functions of the nursing department and the institution, including recruitment, staffing, supervision, continuing education, and research.

The benefits to the patient are obvious. All patients have a better chance of reaching desired health outcomes if they are clearly stated. From the patient's viewpoint, the nursing processes are goal-oriented. Nurses benefit from improved planning, accurate evaluations, strengthened self-confidence, and the concomitant increase in the body of nursing knowledge. The institution benefits from having a better data base upon which to make plans and decisions, and has the satisfaction of providing patients with a high quality of care.

Finally, the actual process of program development improves both patient care and staff satisfaction. Nurse practitioners have seldom been encouraged to take time to explore the specific effects of nursing care on patients. The "giving" of care has always occurred; the planning and evaluation aspects have been underdeveloped. According to one of the nursing staff members in the Duke program, "You don't have to be a head nurse or even an R.N. to feel as if you've contributed something to it. I think the program has given people who really love nursing the way I do a reason to feel good about themselves." We may well discover that the "journey" we are taking in creating the program is just as important as arriving at the "destination."

Mary Ann Peter, R.N., M.S.N.
Director of Quality Assurance Program in Nursing
October 1973 to July 1978

It has been said that one of nursing's greatest shortcomings has been its failure to clearly define and specifically delineate its functions and unique contributions. Five hundred nurses in one acute care setting have undertaken the challenge to define the essence of their nursing practice in precise language and to begin to evaluate its effectiveness.

This manual is written by practicing nurses for other practicing nurses, nursing students, nurse educators, and nurse managers. It is not intended to replace nursing texts or procedure manuals. Its purpose—to raise the general quality of patient care delivered by nurses—is focused in three directions:

1. To describe the clinical essentials of nursing care related to specific patient populations through an outcome-process model
2. To promote the basic and continued education of nurses by stating requisite nursing knowledge and skills
3. To permit the systematic evaluation of nursing care through tools designed and tested at the bedside.

This manual may be used as a resource for students to enable them to establish basic care plans in defining the most appropriate nursing intervention related to the management of specific patient/client populations. It can also serve as a reference for nurses practicing in an institutional setting whether on an inpatient or outpatient basis in the interest of providing the highest standards of direct nursing care, pre– and postoperative managment, discharge planning and patient teaching.

The nurses involved in preparing these guidelines generously and anonymously contributed to this written work by making their nursing interventions explicit so that others could learn from them. In that sense, this manual should be used as a catalyst—a means of comparison with actual nursing practice and professional expectations. Of course there are regional as well as individual differences based on the multidisciplinary practices in each clinical setting.

It may be of interest to note that the approach taken in developing a comprehensive, integrated Quality Assurance Program is entirely consistent with goals stated by the Joint Commission on Accreditation of Hospitals in their 1980 manual. It is significant when a program developed out of the strong beliefs of nursing personnel also satisfies the mandates of an external regulatory agency.

To briefly summarize the contents, the Introduction describes the evolution of the Duke University Quality Assurance Program in Nursing and the development of this manual. The table of contents lists the eleven sections of guidelines grouped according to clinical categories. In the Appendix are three evaulation tools designed to collect data concurrently through patient observation, patient interview, and chart review.

We recommend that the reader peruse the material carefully before establishing a care plan in order to contrast the patient's specific needs and the desired outcomes with those listed. Since many patients fit into several populations, more than one guideline may apply. In order to avoid redundancy, the guidelines are cross-referenced when there is any overlapping.

We invite you to share this material which represents a point of progress in a dynamic process. We expect it to continue to change in response to the needs of patients and to the knowledge and experience of the nursing staff.

When a multimillion dollar outer space mission was aborted at the last minute for the lack of a 50-cent piece of equipment, it was relatively easy to establish the fault. The news media provided thorough coverage of the 50-cent error. For the most part, the great performance and incredible synchronization of literally millions of parts and people went unheralded. As always, it is so much easier to condemn or commend one, two, or three persons than it is to acknowledge adequately the contributions of the very many. That represents the dilemma of this assignment.

Hundreds of heroines and heroes who contributed to the Quality Assurance Program in Nursing (QAPN) must remain unnamed. There were those who worked a little harder to see that nursing care was delivered while their colleagues were in a conference room defining patient outcomes and nursing processes. There were the nursing supervisors who strongly believed that the program would measurably improve the quality of patient care, and they consciously directed their administrative leadership and decision-making in support of the project. Then there were approximately 500 nursing staff members who deliberated in small work groups, and they are, in fact, the authors of this publication. Head nurses, staff nurses, licensed practical nurses, in-service instructors, and nurse clinicians shared their wisdom, argued about details, agonized over accuracy, laughed away some tense moments, and shared pride in their finished products. The leadership of the nurse clinician group deserves extra commendation. They demonstrated a special interest in and a special talent for making nursing care explicit as a basis for measurement and training.

As always, there were a few "spark plugs" that kept the big engine humming. Dorothy J. Danielson, the first project director, built a sound chassis during her 12 months of service. Mary Ann Peter, her successor, was the catalyst, the editor, the arbitrator, and the "professional's professional" in the work groups for 4½ years. Her vision and implementation of this project as a management strategy for improving patient care were outstanding. In July of 1978, when she became the Director of Nursing Services for Duke University Hospital—North Division, Norma Harris, Renal Transplant Nurse Clinician, took a 5-month "mini-sabbatical" to be the project director for QAPN. She guided all of us through the many facets of getting a manuscript to the publisher on time, as well as continuing to assist ongoing work groups write new guidelines. Gwendolyn Fortune read every guideline and made the work of many nurses consistent in form, format, and grammar. And last but not least, nothing of this magnitude can be accomplished without good secretaries and reams and reams of paper. Betsy Wagner, who did the largest portion of the typing and retyping, not only did that exceptionally well, but also always with a smile.

Wilma A. Minniear, R.N., M.S.N.
Executive Director of Nursing Services
May 15, 1979

Acknowledgment is also given to Aspen Systems Corporation, Germantown, MD, for permission to use some of the material from an article which appeared in the Spring 1977 issue of Nursing Administration Quarterly devoted to quality assurance and peer review.

Contents

CHAPTER I
Guidelines for general care

INTRODUCTION: In this section guidelines are presented which describe the common nursing care needs of the ambulatory care patient and the hospitalized patient.

These general guidelines identify patient care outcomes and the related nursing process which are generally desirable and applicable to all patients regardless of age, health/illness status, therapy, or location within the health care facility. Consideration is given to key nursing activities directed toward meeting the individual's needs for safety, nutrition, rest and comfort, acceptance as a human being, personal identity, maintenance of vital body functions, and health knowledge related to self-care.

Special emphasis is given to the diagnostic, curative, and preventive aspects of care which are indicated for the patient using the ambulatory care services.

The described nursing process in these general guidelines reflects the basic nursing philosophy of courtesy, compassion, comfort, and caring for all patients.

Included in the appendix is an evaluation tool specifically designed and tested for use in determining the extent to which the desired outcomes are achieved for the hospitalized patient. The tool is designed to collect data concurrently by peer review through direct observation and interview of the patient. Data can then be analyzed in relation to the patient's satisfaction with hospital care and the degree to which selected individual and environmental needs are met.

Cumulative data are evaluated in ward peer review meetings with a focus towards identification of strengths and needs and selection of chosen courses of corrective action with regard to needs. Included in the appendix is a form used to summarize the content of a peer review meeting.

Patient Outcome	Process

A. *The patient is in a safe environment*	1. Provide a safe environment.
	   a. Identify patient and records accurately, including special information when necessary.
	     • Addressograph plate
	     • Arm band
	     • Door card
	     • Bed card
	     • Chart cover, including special precautions and allergies
	     • Special precautions and/or information posted on door or above bed
	   b. Plan room and unit environment so it is free from preventable hazards; take appropriate remedial action if needed.
	     • Plan patient's bed environment free from hazards.
	       Demonstrate and explain use of bed and safety aids.
	       Use siderails when indicated. Refer to hospital regulations.
	       Keep patient's bed in "low" position when unattended unless contraindicated.
	       Use restraints when indicated. Refer to hospital regulations.
	   c. Inform patient and family about room and unit as he will need to use it.
	   d. Maintain surveillance of room and unit (considerations: cleanliness, operating condition, physical arrangement).
	     • Floor
	     • Furniture
	     • Equipment
	     • Electrical connections
	     • Lighting
	     • Contaminated material
	     • Dangerous supplies, drugs, potentially hazardous objects
	     • Necessary items (bell cord, side rails, personal belongings, etc.)
	   e. Evaluate patient's capacity for safeguarding himself.
	     • Assess need for supervision of activities.
	     • Selectively provide for supervision and nursing assistance as needed.
	   f. Plan patient's physical care individually, taking into account his limitations and/or specific requirements in the following:
	     • Body alignment
	     • Positioning
	     • Transfer between bed and stretcher/chair
	     • Ambulation
	     • Bathing
	     • Eating
	     • Elimination of bowel and bladder
	     • Personal hygiene (mouth care, hair, beard, nails, etc.)
	     • Smoking
	     • Medications
	     • Diagnostic studies
	     • Treatments
	   g. Initiate and maintain isolation when necessary for patient protection.
	     • Wound and skin precautions
	     • Enteric precautions
	     • Needle precautions
	     • Respiratory isolation
	     • Protective isolation
	     • Strict isolation
	   h. Maintain alertness and ability to protect patients in the event of a fire or disaster.

B. *The patient has adequate periods of rest*	2. Assure adequate rest to prevent rest deprivation from occurring.
	   a. Evaluate sleep patterns.
	   b. Attempt to place patient in appropriate bed according to space available and rest needs of patient.
	   c. Plan giving of medications, treatment, etc. to allow for periods of rest.
	   d. Coordinate activities of health personnel providing services to patients to allow for periods of rest.
	   e. Attempt to restrict visitors to approved times and number.
	   f. Exercise control over unnecessary noise and lights.

Patient Outcome	Process

C. *The patient maintains desired nutritional status*	3. Provide for maintenance of nutritional status.
	   a. Check for proper diet order, tray distribution, and nourishment between meals.
	   b. Inform patient regarding dietary routine and specific diet.
	   c. Reinforce importance of proper nutrition as a part of patient's health status.
	   d. Observe patient's total nutritional intake including food ingestion and retention and administration of intravenous fluids.
	   e. Assess patient's changing nutritional needs and request diet modification accordingly.
	   f. Assist with food selection as needed.
	   g. Request dietary consultation as needed.
	   h. Assist with feedings as necessary.

D. *The patient has minimized pain and discomfort*	4. Plan intervention to minimize patient's physical discomfort.
	   a. Assess patient's changing needs for control of pain.
	    • Initiate appropriate nursing action through independent nursing judgment or nurse/physician collaboration.
	    • Inform patient of plan for dealing with discomfort.
	   b. Recognize individual responses and attitudes toward pain and therapeutically support the patient in coping with discomfort.
	    • Respond as promptly as possible to patient's need for pain relief.

E. *The patient has a sense of acceptance as a person and of value as a human being*	5. Approach patient with a consistently respectful and caring attitude.
	   a. Convey a sense of concern and warmth.
	   b. Identify oneself on initial contact with patient.
	   c. Respond as promptly as possible to any patient request.
	6. Be aware that patient's behavior is indicative of inner feelings, explore why patient is behaving a certain way, and encourage expression of feelings and constructive means of dealing with stress.
	7. Recognize that changes in physical appearance and functioning may affect patient's behavior.

F. *The patient has a sense of personal identity*	8. Assist patient to maintain sense of personal identity.
	   a. Communicate what patient can expect routinely and continue to explain health related procedures as they are scheduled.
	   b. Accept the patient's right to question and request additional information about procedures and treatments.
	   c. Individualize approach to patient care by encouraging patient's participation in planning and assessing care.
	   d. Avoid talking about patient in his presence unless he is included.
	   e. Avoid personal conversations among staff in patient area.
	   f. Use patient's proper name or name preference patient has stated when interacting with him.

G. *The patient is knowledgeable about nature of illness, procedures, treatments, and planned program directed toward health restoration and maintenance*	9. Teach patient about health-illness state and plan for health maintenance.
	   a. Begin at admission to plan teaching approach by assessing patient's:
	    • Level of understanding • Level of acceptance
	    • Ability to comprehend • Physical limitations
	   b. Collaborate with physician and other health team members to maintain a consistent approach regarding health-related teaching.
	   c. Consider cultural and religious influences, *e.g.,* food preferences.
	   d. Provide opportunities for patient participation in health teaching program.
	   e. Use appropriate available aids in teaching.
	    • Visual aids
	    • Written material
	    • Tapes
	    • Community resources
	   f. Inform patient of available community resources which can assist him in his continuity of care and maintenance of health care program.
	   g. Assess teaching/counseling needs throughout hospitalization.

H. *The patient is adjusting to health status limitations*	10. Assist patient in adjustment to health limitations.
	   a. Assess patient's perception of health status limitations.
	   b. Support appropriately patient's coping mechanisms.
	   c. Attempt to identify specific problems of patient's inability to cope with health status limitations.
	   d. Utilize resource people who can assist patient with his problems *e.g.,* family members, psychiatrist, chaplain, nurse clinician, social workers, public health nurse.
	   e. Assist patient to obtain and use necessary supplies, equipment, and resource people.

Patient Outcome	Process

I. *The patient has normal physiological function*
• *Bowel*
	11. Assist patient to maintain bowel function.
	    a. Assess bowel status from patient or family. Note pre-existing bowel problems.
	    b. Plan bowel program with patient, appropriate others, and physician to correlate as closely as possible with normal habits.
	      • Insure adequate fluid intake, which may include one glass of prune juice daily.
	      • Encourage fruit, vegetables, and bulk in diet as indicated.
	      • Encourage ambulation.
	      • Provide privacy and comfort during bowel evacuation.
	      • Consider patient's response to:
	         Immobilization
	         Stress
	         Medications
	         Fluid and food intake
	         Lack of privacy
	    c. Monitor bowel function.
	      • Keep record of amount, consistency, and color of stools.
	      • Check signs and symptoms of bowel complications such as distention, diarrhea, constipation, nausea and vomiting, and loss of appetite.
	    d. Evaluate daily the patient's bowel function and modify bowel program according to changing bowel needs.

• *Urinary*	12. Assist patient to maintain urinary function.
	    a. Assess patient's ability to void. Consider:
	      • Fluid intake
	      • Time since last voiding
	      • Bladder distention, discomfort
	      • Pain inhibiting voluntary response to void
	      • Normal voiding habit
	      • Privacy
	      • Position
	    b. Initiate nursing measures to stimulate voiding as needed.
	      • Provide privacy and comfort
	      • Offer fluids
	      • Use Credé's method, pour warm water over perineum, run water from faucet, elevate head of bed, tap lower abdomen, stroke inner thigh, etc.
	    c. Monitor urinary function.
	      • Record fluid intake and output.
	    d. Assure periurethral hygiene daily and p.r.n.

• *Cardiovascular*	13. Assist patient to maintain cardiovascular function.
	    a. Assess present status and pertinent past history. Consider:
	      • Routine vital signs: temperature (T), pulse (P), respiration (R), blood pressure (BP)
	      • Weight
	      • Peripheral circulation
	      • Condition of skin: color, temperature, lesions
	      • Complaints or history of:
	         Hypertension
	         Heart disease
	         Cerebral vascular disease
	         Peripheral vascular disease
	         Diabetes mellitus
	      • Drug therapy
	    b. Support normal circulation by:
	      • Support hose as ordered • Change of body position
	      • Appropriate exercises and activity • Skin care
	    c. Support normal fluid balance by:
	      • Monitoring intake and output
	      • Checking for signs of fluid overload or dehydration

• *Respiratory*	14. Assist patient to maintain respiratory function.
	    a. Assess present status and pertinent past history. Consider:
	      • Rate, depth and character of respirations

Patient Outcome	Process

	• Complaints or history of:
	    Dyspnea, orthopnea Production of sputum
	    Smoking Respiratory problems, *e.g.,* obstruction, infection
	    Coughing
	b. Support respiratory function by:
	  • Positioning for patient comfort and ease of respirations
	  • Turning, coughing, deep breathing patients who are confined to bed (frequency determined by patient needs)
	  • Assistive devices as ordered:
	    Incentive spirometry
	    Intermittent positive pressure breathing (IPPB)
	    Humidifer
	    Oxygen

• *Skin*	15. Maintain integrity of skin.
	  a. Assess present status and pertinent past history. Consider:
	    • Motor and sensory status
	    • Age
	    • Nutritional status
	    • Peripheral circulation
	    • History of decubitus, skin disorders, hypersensitive skin
	    • Bowel and bladder control
	    • Open wound or stoma
	    • Abrasions, lacerations, presence of hematoma, contusion, local edema, presence of pressure areas
	    • Poor skin hygiene
	  b. Plan generalized skin care program with patient.
	    • Bathe patient every day unless otherwise indicated.
	    • General skin care considerations:
	      Dry skin: mild soap to axilla, feet, perineum, oil in bath water, lotion to dry areas
	      Oily skin: frequent washing. (Follow patient preference in treatment)
	      Dry, scaly feet: soak in warm, soapy water q.i.d.; apply emollient
	    • Prevent prolonged periods of pressure to skin through frequent change of body position and massage to bony prominences.
	    • Use comfort devices as needed such as sheepskin, booties, alternating pressure mattresses.
	  c. Communicate plan of care to other personnel.

• *Sensory Perception*	16. Assist patient to maintain sensory perception.
	  a. Determine impairment of hearing, vision, touch, smell, and taste.
	  b. Assist and instruct patient in care of supportive aids and in protection from damage of aid or loss.
	  c. Observe patient's behavior to various amounts and kinds of sensory stimulation or deprivation. Consider:
	    • Verbal and nonverbal communication; need for reorientation
	    • Noise, light, odor
	    • Sleep, rest and activity patterns
	    • Medications
	  d. Modify sensory intake in relation to patient's needs.

• *Motor ability*	17. Maintain motor ability.
	  a. Assess present activity status and pertinent past history. Consider:
	    • Arthritis problems
	    • Orthopaedic, neurological limitations; prostheses
	    • Peripheral vascular problems
	    • Visual problems
	    • Pain
	    • Psychosocial factors
	  b. Consult with patient and physician regarding desirable patient activities and establish activity program.
	  c. Provide patient with assistance as necessary.
	    • Consider needs for physical therapy and/or supportive aids.
	  d. Evaluate effectiveness of activity program and readjust as necessary.

Ambulatory patient general care guidelines

Patient Outcome	Process

PREFACE: These guidelines are applicable to all ambulatory care patients. Specific patient outcomes with regard to health maintenance of the child and the legal aspects of pediatric care are included. Examples are given, where applicable.

A. *The patient and family are knowledgeable about health care facility as they need to use it*

1. Provide assistance to the patient in using the outpatient facility.
   a. Assess mental and physical capability of patient/family to take care of themselves.
   b. Allow patient as much responsibility as appropriate.
   c. Give explicit directions about area providing service.
   d. Assist patient to make arrangements to go to another facility when medically necessary:
      • Ambulance
      • Patient's vehicle
      • Public transportation
      • Institutional transportation
   e. Assist patient unable to manage independently, *e.g.,* wheelchairs, escort service, special instructions.

B. *The patient maintains personal identity and sense of value as a human being*

2. Assist the patient to maintain sense of personal identity and value as a human being.
   a. Listen and learn; provide opportunity for expression of needs and concerns, *e.g.,*
      • Physical well-being
      • Physical care needs in the clinic
      • Home/family situation
      • Personal problems
   b. Offer explanations and answer questions, *e.g.,* delays, diagnostic procedures.
   c. Respect patient's right to privacy; avoid unnecessary body exposure.
   d. Recognize and encourage patient's effective use of support person and/or family member. Include security object such as teddy bear, doll, and blanket, as indicated.

C. *The patient is in a safe environment*

3. Provide a safe environment.
   a. Identify patient and records accurately:
      • Clinic card and/or arm band
      • Clinic records
      • Data from source of referrals, *e.g.,* letters, radiographs, laboratory studies.
   b. Maintain surveillance of health care area.
      • Consider cleanliness, operating condition, physical arrangement and special precautions.
         Floor
         Furniture
         Equipment
         Electrical connections
         Lighting
      • Proper disposal of contaminated materials and waste
      • Proper storage of dangerous supplies, drugs, and potentially hazardous objects.
      • Have available:
         Necessary personal items, *e.g.,* intercom, bell cord, bed straps, personal belongings
         Necessary medical items, *e.g.,* emergency equipment: suction, O_2, padded tongue blades
      • Post necessary information in rooms and on doors, *e.g.,* ''no smoking, oxygen in use'', ''isolation precautions''.
   c. Assess patient's capacity for safeguarding himself and provide for supervision as necessary.
      • Remember to stay with patients who require supervision, *i.e.,* children, older persons.
      • Use siderails or restraints when indicated.
      • Demonstrate and explain use of intercom and/or bell cord and safety aids being used.
   d. Assess potentially dangerous situations and call security officer for assistance as needed, *e.g.,* violent patients, visitors requiring supervision.
   e. Initiate and maintain protection as necessary for patient and staff.
      • Wound and skin precautions
      • Enteric precautions
      • Needle precautions
      • Respiratory isolation
      • Protective isolation
      • Strict isolation
      • Psychological isolation, *i.e.,* disfigured and distraught patients
   f. Document important information related to safety of patients and staff.
      • Communicable diseases, *e.g.,* hepatitis

Patient Outcome	Process

	• Loss of possessions
	• Use of restraints
	• Hospital related injury with treatment and care provided
	• Medication errors
	• Evidence that might be used later for legal purposes
	
	g. Plan patient's physical care, taking into account his limitations and/or specific needs, such as:
	  • Ability to ambulate
	  • Transfers between bed, examination table, stretchers/wheel chairs
	  • Side rails, restraints as needed
	  • Body alignment, positioning
	  • Diet
	  • Medications
	  • Allergies
	  • Diagnostic studies
	  • Treatments
	
	h. Maintain alertness and ability to protect patients in the event of a fire or other disaster.

D. *The patient attains a relative state of comfort*	4. Provide for rest and comfort needs.
	  a. Assess physical and mental discomfort.
	    • Respond to needs for relief of discomfort.
	    • Give medications as ordered.
	    • Give information/clarification as needed.
	  b. Assess need for rest.
	    • Coordinate activities to provide periods of rest.

E. *The patient maintains nutritional status*	5. Assess patient's immediate nutritional needs and encourage patient to obtain nourishment as needed.

F. *The patient is knowledgeable about nature of illness, procedures, treatments and planned program directed toward health restoration and maintenance*	6. Teach patient about health-illness state and plan for health maintenance.
	  a. Plan approach by assessing patient's:
	    • Current level of understanding
	    • Ability to comprehend
	    • Physical limitations
	    • Level of acceptance of illness and prescribed treatment
	    • Home situation and financial status
	    • Ability to cope with illness, physical limitations, and other life responsibilities.
	  b. Collaborate with physician, patient/family, and other health team members in planning for health care. Encourage patient's participation in establishing an acceptable health care program.
	  c. Provide knowledge/skills related to:
	    • Health status
	    • Procedures and treatments performed
	    • Planned program directed toward health restoration and maintenance, including medications, diet, activity level
	    • Obtaining and using necessary supplies and equipment
	    • Coping with health status limitations
	    • Community resources
	  d. Use appropriate teaching techniques and aids:
	    • Return demonstration and explanations • Visual aids and models
	    • Written material • Role playing
	  e. Identify and utilize community resources/services as needed and initiate referrals.
	    • Public health agencies and programs
	    • Vocational rehabilitation agency
	    • Mental health clinics
	    • Community support groups
	  f. Utilize resource people who can assist in providing care: family members, social worker, public health nurse, dietician, nurse clinician.

G. *The patient maintains physiological functions. This includes:*	7. Identify patient care needs and institute measures accordingly.
	  a. Obtain a general nursing assessment through interview, observation, and chart review. Information may include:
	    • Reason for clinic visit (chief complaint)

Patient Outcome	Process

	• Acute needs, *e.g.*, pain, hemorrhage
	• Physical signs and symptoms, *e.g.*, vital signs, height, weight, skin color
	• Pertinent medical history. Include:
	    Age; stage of growth and development
	    Symptoms
	    Infections
	    Prior serious illness and/or hospitalization
	    Other health problems and physical handicaps/limitations
	    Medications: current and illicit
	    Allergies
	    Immunization record
	• Current emotional status, *e.g.*, patient/family interaction
	• Educational level
	• Occupation
	• Family situation
	    Home environment
	    Impact of illness on family
	    Finances
	• Perception of health status; include pertinent questions and concerns. Other sources of health care, *e.g.*, local physician, local clinics, public health nurse
	b. Establish with patient/family problems, needs, and goals.
	c. Provide nursing measures according to the patient's needs.
	    • Direct physical care
	    • Emotional support
	    • Teaching
	    • Referral: intrahospital or interagency
	d. Evaluate and document patient's progress and response to care.

• *Respiratory*	8. Assist patient to maintain respiratory function.
	a. Assess current respiratory status/needs and pertinent information of present and past history.
	    • Signs and symptoms:
	        Respiratory rate and depth
	        Skin: color, temperature, moisture, and turgor
	        Dyspnea, orthopnea
	        Coughing: production and color of sputum
	        Chills/fever
	    • Presence of chronic states, *e.g.*, cystic fibrosis, tuberculosis
	    • Allergies, *e.g.*, pollen, dust
	    • Smoking habits
	    • Current medications
	    • Previous surgery/radiographs
	b. Explain diagnostic procedures and provide care as needed.
	    • Chest radiographs • Pulmonary function test
	    • Bronchoscopy • Thoracocentesis
	c. Provide nursing measures according to the patient's priority needs.
	    • Position patient for comfort and ease of respirations.
	    • Provide emotional support.
	d. Teach techniques/knowledge needed for home care.
	    • Turn, cough, and deep breathing exercises
	    • Postural drainage
	    • Tracheostomy care
	    • Use of equipment, *e.g.*, oxygen, humidifier, nebulizer
	    • Diet prescriptions
	    • Medications
	e. Secure necessary supplies or instruct in obtaining supplies for home use.

• *Cardiovascular*	9. Assist patient to maintain cardiovascular function. a. Assess current cardiovascular status/needs and pertinent information of present and past history.

9

Patient Outcome	Process

* Signs and symptoms:
    Pulse rate, rhythm, and character
    Blood pressure (note postural changes)
    Respiratory rate and depth
    Condition of skin: color, temperature, moisture, lesions, turgor (include nail beds and mucous membranes)
    Extremities: numbness, tingling, edema
    Mental alertness
    Pain: location, sensation, possible causes, methods of relief.
* Current medications
* Chronic disease states, *e.g.,* hypertension, rheumatic heart disease, diabetes
* Risk factors, *e.g.,* diet, smoking habits, stress, exercise patterns
* Pacemaker, *e.g.,* problems, function, patient's knowledge

b. Explain diagnostic procedures and provide care as needed.
* Cardiac catheterization
* Arteriogram
* Electrocardiogram
* Chest radiograph

c. Provide nursing measures according to the patient's priority needs.
* Position patient for comfort.
* Observe patient for changes in cardiac status and provide emergency care if needed.
* Give emotional support.

d. Teach techniques/knowledge needed for home care.
* Diet prescriptions
* Medications
* Application of antiembolic hose
* Skin care
* Prescribed exercise routine
* Intake and output measurement and recording
* Precautions: avoid tight garments, cold weather conditions, and stressful situations
* Pacemaker care

e. Secure necessary supplies or instruct in obtaining supplies for home care.

* *Neurological* 10. Assist patient to maintain neurological function.
a. Assess present neurological status/needs and pertinent information of present and past history.
* Signs and symptoms:
    Headache: degree and description
    Nausea/vomiting
    Neck rigidity
    Pupil changes
    Confusion and disorientation (person, place, and time)
    Loss of motor and/or sensory function, *e.g.,* bowel and bladder, facial ptosis, speech, hearing and visual changes
* Behavioral changes, *e.g.,* mood, affect, thought processes, and overt behavior
* Chronic disease states, *e.g.,* multiple sclerosis, Parkinson's disease, seizure disorders (identify aura, patterns, frequency, duration, and post seizure state)
* Current medications: prescribed and illicit
* Previous psychiatric hospitalizations

b. Explain diagnostic procedures and provide care as needed.
* Electroencephalogram (EEG): awake and asleep
* Brain scan and skull films
* Lumbar puncture
* Blood levels, *e.g.,* alcohol, sugar

c. Provide nursing measures according to the patient's priority needs.
* Orient to surroundings.
* Use side rails/safety straps as appropriate.
* Monitor anesthesia and/or sleep EEG recovery.
* Observe for neurological changes.
* Establish seizure precautions.

Patient Outcome	Process

	d. Teach techniques/knowledge needed for home care.
	    • Skin care
	    • Prescribed exercise routine, gait training
	    • Diet prescription
	    • Medications
	    • Use of equipment, *e.g.,* walkers, trapeze, bedside commode
	    • Seizure precautions
	e. Secure necessary supplies or instruct in obtaining supplies for home use.

• *Urinary*	11. Assist the patient to maintain urinary function.
	a. Assess present urinary status/needs and pertinent information of present and past history.
	    • Signs and symptoms:
	        Vital signs
	        Frequency, nocturia, and urgency of urination; note volume
	        Burning and pain on urination
	        Changes in color, clarity, and odor
	        Hematuria
	        Pain: location, sensation, possible causes, methods of relief
	        Incontinence
	    • Chronic disease states, *e.g.,* calculi, cystitis, prostatitis, nephritis
	    • Allergies, *e.g.,* drugs, seafood, and iodine dye
	    • Previous radiographs and/or surgical procedures
	    • Current medications
	b. Explain diagnostic procedures and provide care as needed.
	    • Urine specimens: voided, clean catch, catheterization, and 24-hour urine collection
	    • Intravenous pyelogram
	    • Cystoscopy
	    • Cystometrogram
	    • Blood chemistries, *e.g.,* creatinine, blood urea nitrogen
	c. Provide nursing measures according to the patient's priority needs.
	    • Position patient for comfort.
	    • Provide emotional support.
	    • Assist with treatments and surgical procedures, *e.g.,* urethral dilation and hydraulic bladder dilation.
	d. Teach techniques/knowledge needed for home care.
	    • Foley catheter care
	    • Urostomy care
	    • Dressings
	    • Self catheterization and/or changing condom catheter
	    • Medications
	    • Importance of adequate fluid intake
	e. Secure necessary supplies or instruct in obtaining supplies for home use.

• *Gastrointestinal*	12. Assist patient to maintain gastrointestinal function.
	a. Assess present gastrointestinal status/needs and pertinent information of present and past history.
	    • Signs and symptoms:
	        Loss of appetite, food intolerance
	        Nausea and vomiting: note characteristics of vomitus
	        Difficulty swallowing
	        Weight loss
	        Flatus and belching
	        Pain: location, sensation, possible causes, methods of relief
	        Bowel changes: consistency, frequency, amount, color, presence of blood and mucus
	        Tremors and decreased mental function
	        Jaundice
	    • Body changes indicating poor nutritional status
	        Condition of mouth, gums, teeth, tongue, dentures
	        Dehydration
	        Muscle loss or weakness
	        Edema

Patient Outcome	Process

	• Chronic disease states, *e.g.,* ulcers, diverticulitis, cirrhosis, pancreatitis
	• Allergies
	• Previous radiographs and/or surgical procedures
	• Current medications
	• Risk factors, *e.g.,* alcohol intake, eating patterns, stress
	  d. Explain diagnostic procedures and provide care as needed.
	     • Radiographs, *e.g.,* upper gastrointestinal (GI) series with small bowel follow-through, barium enema and air contrast studies
	     • Ultrasound
	     • Rectal examination: anoscopy, proctoscopy
	     • Esophagoscopy, gastroscopy, colonoscopy
	     • IV cholangiogram, oral cholecystogram, T-tube cholangiogram
	  e. Provide nursing measures according to the patient's priority needs.
	     • Position patient for comfort.
	     • Provide emotional support.
	     • Observe patient for changes and provide emergency care as needed.
	     • Assist with treatments and surgical procedures, *e.g.,* esophageal dilation, removal of polyp, biopsy, foreign objects, fecal impactions.
	  f. Teach techniques/knowledge needed for home care.
	     • Use of laxatives or stool softeners for barium removal following GI series
	     • Bowel regimen to prevent or treat constipation
	     • Stoma care
	     • Dressing changes, wound care
	     • Signs and symptoms indicating GI problems
	     • Diet prescription
	     • Medications
	  g. Secure necessary supplies or instruct in obtaining supplies for home use.

• *Musculoskeletal*	13. Assist patient to maintain musculoskeletal function.
	  a. Assess present musculoskeletal status/needs and pertinent information of present and past history.
	     • Signs and symptoms:
	        Vital signs
	        Extremities: numbness, tingling, edema, and/or hematomas
	        Condition of skin: color, moisture, lesions, turgor (include nail beds and mucous membranes)
	        Pain: location, sensation, possible causes, methods of relief
	        Immobilization
	        Mental alertness
	        Chills/fever
	     • Current medications
	     • Congenital abnormalities
	        Hip dislocation
	        Club foot
	        Agenesis of limbs
	        Scoliosis, kyphosis, lordosis
	        Myelodysplasia
	        Cerebral palsy
	     • Traumatic injuries
	        Fractures, sprains, and dislocations
	        Replants
	        Spinal cord injuries
	     • Chronic disease states, *e.g.,* arthritis, osteomyelitis
	     • Tumors
	  b. Explain diagnostic procedures and provide care as needed.
	     • Radiographs
	     • Injections and aspirations
	     • Arthrogram
	     • Thermogram
	     • Electromyelogram

Patient Outcome	Process

	• Bone scan
	• Blood studies, *e.g.,* complete blood count (CBC), sedimentation rate, uric acid
	  c. Provide nursing measures according to the patient's priority needs.
	     • Position patient for comfort.
	     • Elevate injured extremity.
	     • Immobilize injured site, *e.g.,* cervical support, splint fracture.
	     • Apply ice packs if appropriate.
	     • Observe patient for changes.
	     • Assist with treatments as necessary, *e.g.,* cast application and removal, injections, aspirations, splint application, prosthetic and orthotic fittings.
	  d. Teach techniques/knowledge needed for home care.
	     • Gait training to include crutches, canes, walkers, and braces
	     • Cast care
	     • Stump care
	     • Body alignment
	     • Double diapering of infants with hip dislocations
	     • Medications
	     • Diet prescription
	     • Skin care
	     • Traction, including skin and skeletal
	     • Exercises: strengthening and range of motion
	     • Wound care
	     • Safety devices within home environment, *e.g.,* grasp bars in bathroom, commode chair
	     • Use of assistive equipment, *e.g.,* wheelchair with removable arms, walker, brace, cane
	  e. Secure necessary supplies and equipment or instruct in obtaining these for home use.

• *Skin*	14. Assist the patient to maintain skin integrity.
	  a. Assess present skin status/needs and pertinent information of present and past history.
	     • Signs and symptoms:
	       Condition of skin: color, temperature, moisture, turgor
	       Abrasions, lacerations, hematoma, contusion, local edema, pressure areas
	       Itching, burning
	       Rash, hives
	       Edema
	     • Skin disorders, *e.g.,* psoriasis, hypersensitive skin
	     • Infections, *e.g.,* chicken pox, impetigo, scabies, poison ivy
	     • Allergies, *e.g.,* drugs, foods, metal, cosmetics, plants
	     • Risk factors:
	       Diet
	       Medications
	       Stress
	       Overexposure to sun, wind, cold, and heat
	       Motor and/or sensory deficits
	     • Aging process
	  b. Explain diagnostic procedures and provide care as needed.
	     • Biopsy
	     • Skin tests
	     • Laboratory studies, *e.g.,* antibody titers, blood chemistry
	  c. Provide nursing measures according to the patient's priority needs.
	     • Give emotional support.
	     • Observe patient for change and provide emergency care as needed.
	     • Assist with treatments and surgical procedures, *e.g.,* cryosurgery, decubitus debridement, excision of skin lesions.
	  d. Teach techniques/knowledge needed for home care.
	     • Care of skin, hair, and scalp: stress importance of daily hygiene
	     • Application of topical medications, lotions, emollients
	     • Cleansing and proper dressings for open wounds, stomas, decubiti, and ulcers
	     • Preventive measures such as positioning to relieve pressure points, use of protective and appropriate clothing
	     • Diet prescription
	  e. Secure necessary supplies or instruct in obtaining supplies for home use.

Patient Outcome	Process

• *Reproductive*	15. Assist the patient to maintain reproductive function.
	    a. Assess present reproductive status/needs and pertinent information of present and past history.
	        • Signs and symptoms:
	            Vital signs, height, weight, age
	            Bleeding: frequency, duration, amount, color
	            Discharge: duration, amount, odor
	            Lesions
	            Pain: location, sensation, possible causes, methods of relief
	        • Congenital abnormalities
	        • Chronic disease states, *e.g.,* vaginitis, endometriosis, pelvic inflammatory disease, prostatitis, sexually transmitted diseases, tumors, lesions
	        • Menstrual cycle
	            Onset
	            Dysmenorrhea
	            Amenorrhea
	            Polymenorrhea
	        • Pregnancy
	        • Medications
	        • Previous radiographs and/or surgical procedures
	    b. Explain diagnostic procedures and provide care as needed.
	        • Blood, urine laboratory studies
	        • Pelvic examinations: Pap smear
	        • Semen analysis
	        • Urinary chorionic gonadotropin
	        • Ultrasound
	        • Hysterosalpingogram
	        • Endometrial biopsy and brush
	        • Culdoscopy
	        • Urethral smears and/or cultures for fungus, bacteria
	    c. Provide nursing measures according to the patient's priority needs.
	        • Give emotional support.
	        • Position patient for comfort.
	        • Observe patient for changes and provide emergency care as needed.
	        • Assist with treatments and surgical procedures; *e.g.,* cryosurgery, amniocentesis, saline injections for therapeutic abortions, chemotherapy.
	    d. Teach techniques/knowledge needed for home care.
	        • Family planning
	        • Prenatal care
	        • Diet prescription
	        • Medications
	        • Venereal disease prevention
	        • Self-breast examinations
	    e. Secure necessary supplies or instruct in obtaining supplies for home use.

• *Endocrine*	16. Assist the patient to maintain endocrine function.
	    a. Assess present endocrine status/needs and pertinent information of present and past history.
	        • Signs and symptoms:
	            Blood pressure
	            Excessive thirst
	            Increased appetite
	            Polyuria
	            Blurred vision
	            Physical appearance, *e.g.,* growth patterns, obesity, precocious puberty, moon face, hirsutism
	            Behavioral changes, *e.g.,* mental confusion, inappropriate responses to environment
	        • Current medications
	        • Chronic disease states, *e.g.,* diabetes, hypothyroidism, Cushing's disease
	        • Risk factors:
	            Family history
	            Diet

Patient Outcome	Process
	Activity level

Activity level
Stress
  b. Explain diagnostic procedures and provide care as needed.
  • Twenty-four-hour urine collection
  • Radiographs, *e.g.*, thyroid uptake
  • Laboratory studies: glucose tolerance tests, thyroid panel, fasting blood sugar
  • Indirect laryngoscopy
  c. Provide nursing measures according to the patient's priority needs.
  • Give emotional support.
  • Observe patient for changes and provide emergency care as needed.
  d. Teach techniques/knowledge needed for home care.
  • Management care of diabetes
    Urine testing
    Insulin injections
    Symptoms of hypo- and hyperglycemia
    Skin care
    Exercise
  • Diet prescriptions
  • Medications
  • Twenty-four-hour urine collection
  e. Secure necessary supplies or instruct in obtaining supplies for home use.

• *Blood and blood forming tissues*

17. Assist the patient to maintain hematologic function.
  a. Assess present hematologic status/needs and pertinent information of present and past history.
  • Signs and symptoms:
    Vital signs
    Jaundice
    Pallor
    Weight changes
    Nausea and vomiting
    Generalized or localized swelling
    Chronic fatigue and dyspnea
    Pain: location, sensation, possible causes, and methods of relief
    Hemorrhage, *e.g.*, easy bruising
    Condition of mucous membranes (oral, nasopharyngeal, vaginal, rectal) Note color, bleeding, exudates, lesions, and tenderness.
    Appetite changes
  • Current medications
  • Chronic disease states, *e.g.*, anemia, leukemia, hemophilia, sickle cell anemia.
  • Previous radiographs, and/or surgical procedures
  • Risk factors:
    Family history
    Activity level
    Smoking
    Exposure to infectious disease
  b. Explain diagnostic procedures and provide care as needed.
  • Laboratory studies, *e.g.*, CBC, platelet count, sedimentation rate, 24-hour urine, urinalysis, and stool specimens
  • Radiographs, *e.g.*, liver and spleen scans, skull films, skeletal surveys
  • Bone marrow
  • Lumbar puncture
  c. Provide nursing measures according to the patient's priority needs.
  • Give emotional support.
  • Position patient for comfort.
  • Observe patient for changes and provide emergency care as needed.
  • Assist with treatments as necessary, *e.g.*,
    Transfusions of blood, plasma
    Chemotherapy
    Radiation therapy

Patient Outcome	Process
	d. Teach techniques/knowledge needed for home care.
	• Mouth care, skin care, and general hygiene
	• Medications
	• Diet prescription
	• Precautionary measures, *e.g.,* reducing exposure to communicable diseases, avoiding trauma/injury
	• Measurement of temperature
	• Comfort measures
	• Signs and symptoms to report immediately, *e.g.,* unusual bleeding or swelling, sudden rise in temperature
	e. Secure necessary supplies or instruct in obtaining supplies for home use.

• Oral structure

18. Assist the patient to maintain oral structure function.
    a. Assess present oral status/needs and pertinent information of present and past history.
        • Signs and symptoms:
            Pain: location, sensation, possible causes, and methods of relief
            Caries
            Bleeding
            Occlusion or bite
            Swelling
            Lesions
            Inflammation of the mouth.
        • Current medications
        • Chronic disease states such as
            Infections, *e.g.,* trench mouth, thrush, herpes simplex
            Lesions, *e.g.,* cysts, ulcers, tumors
            Peridental disease
            Arthritis of temporal mandibular joint
        • Deformities such as
            Protruding mandible
            Cleft palate
            Oral/facial, *e.g.,* tongue tied, open bite.
        • Traumatic injuries such as fractures, dislocations, lacerations, loose teeth
    b. Explain diagnostic procedures and provide care as needed.
        • Radiographs
        • Impressions
        • Biopsy
    c. Provide nursing measures according to patient's priority needs.
        • Give emotional support.
        • Position patient for comfort.
        • Observe patient for changes.
        • Assist with treatments and surgical procedures.
            Extractions and impactions
            Excision of lesion
            Replantations or stabilization of teeth
            Closed reduction of fractured jaw
            Frenotomy: clipping of frenum under tongue
            Preparation of gum for dentures
            Gingivectomy: removal of excessive gum tissue
    d. Teach techniques/knowledge needed for home care.
        • Dental maintenance
            Brushing
            Use of dental floss
            Proper nutrition
            Importance of regular checkups
        • Medications
        • Diet prescription
        • Proper rinsing for postprocedure care
        • Dressing changes and pressure dressing maintenance

Patient Outcome	Process
	• Precautionary measures, *e.g.,* importance of having wire cutters available for patients with wired jaws
	• Signs and symptoms to report immediately, *e.g.,* excessive bleeding or swelling, excessive and prolonged pain
	e. Secure necessary supplies or instruct in obtaining supplies for home care.

• *Eye, Ear, Nose, Throat*

19. Assist the patient to maintain eye, ear, nose, and throat function.

a.   Assess present eye, ear, nose, and throat status/needs and pertinent information of present and past history.
 • Signs and symptoms:

Pain: location, sensation, possible causes and method of relief	Inflammation
	Hoarseness
Swelling	Mouth breathing
Lesions	Hypo- and hypernasality
Rash	Obstructions
Drainage: color, odor, and consistency	Hearing loss
Bleeding, *e.g.,* nose bleeds	Visual impairment

 • Current medications
 • Chronic disease states
    Infections, *e.g.,* rhinitis, otitis media, peritonsillar abscess, syphilis, tuberculosis
    Lesions, *e.g.,* cyst, ulcer, tumor, polyp
    Allergies, *e.g.,* hay fever
    Otosclerosis
    Glaucoma
 • Deformities

Deviated septum	Atresia of ear
Saddle nose	Keloid

 • Traumatic injuries

Cauliflower ear	Fractures
Foreign body	Lacerations
Dislocations	Esophageal strictures

b.   Explain diagnostic procedures and provide care as needed.
 • Evaluation of hearing and vision
 • Electronystagmogram
 • Balance disorder tests
 • Specialized radiographs, *e.g.,* mastoid films, tomograms for head and neck, and sinus films
 • Biopsies
 • Cultures
 • Skin tests for bacterial hypersensitivity
 • Central spinal fluid leakage test

c.   Provide nursing measures according to patient's priority needs.
 • Give emotional support.
 • Position patient for comfort.
 • Observe patient for changes.
 • Assist with treatments and surgical procedures.
    Irrigations
    Tracheostomy and stoma care
    Local anesthesia for office procedures
    Cryosurgery for removal of warts, moles
    Insertion and/or removal of packing
    Cauterization
    Esophageal dilations

d.   Teach techniques/knowledge needed for home care.
 • Tracheostomy and stoma care
 • Eye, ear, and nasal irrigations
 • Instillation of eye, ear, and nose solution/ointment
 • Wound and dressing care
 • Mouth care
 • Medications

17

Patient Outcome	Process
	• Diet prescriptions
	• Care of tympanoplasty
	e. Secure necessary supplies or instruct in obtaining supplies for home use.
H. *The patient maintains psychosocial function*	20. Assist the patient to maintain psychosocial function.
	a. Assess present psychosocial status/needs and pertinent information of present and past history.
	• Signs and symptoms:
	General behavior and appearance, *e.g.,* condition of hair, clothing, facial expression, verbal and nonverbal communications, and character of movements: slow and rapid
	Manner of speech, *e.g.,* spontaneous, relevant, coherent, undistracted
	Body movements, *e.g.,* gestures, tremors
	Affect
	Content of thinking, *e.g.,* rational, accuracy of thought, auditory and visual hallucinations, orientation: person, place, time
	Ability to understand instructions
	• Current medications: tobacco, alcohol, patent and illicit drugs
	• Cultural factors: social, geographical, religious
	• Stages of growth and development: birth to old age
	• Significant life events such as actual or potential losses of:
	Loved one Self esteem
	Body function and/or appearance Financial security
	• Previous psychiatric hospitalizations
	b. Explain diagnostic procedures and provide care as needed.
	• Psychological testing
	• Electroencephalogram: awake and asleep
	• Laboratory studies, *e.g.,* glucose tolerance test, blood level of bromides, amphetamines, etc.
	c. Provide nursing measures according to patient's priority needs.
	• Listen and learn: give patient and family opportunity for expression of needs and concerns about physical care needs, home/family situations, physical well-being, and personal problems.
	• Assess potentially dangerous situations and call security officer for assistance as needed, *e.g.,* violent patient.
	• Initiate and maintain protection for patient as necessary.
	• Observe patient for changes.
	• Give emotional support.
	• Collaborate with physician to refer patient with special psychiatric needs, *e.g.,* consider community mental health center.
	• Consult with resource people as needed, *e.g.,* physician, psychiatric nurse clinician, social worker.
	• Administer medications such as tranquilizers per physician's orders. Observe for desired effects and side effects.
	• Use restraints per physician's order.
	d. Teach techniques/knowledge needed for home care.
	• Medications
	• Diet prescription
	• Physical care, *e.g.,* attention to hygiene, safety, rest, elimination
	• Follow-up care, *e.g.,* referral to other social/health care agencies, regular therapy sessions, what to do in event of crisis/emergency
	e. Secure necessary supplies or instruct in obtaining supplies for home use.
I. *The child and parents are knowledgeable of health maintenance measures* **J.** *The child and parents recognize legal aspects of health agency care*	21. Teach techniques/knowledge needed for continuing health maintenance of the child such as:
	a. Normal growth and development d. Dental care
	b. Medication doses e. Immunization
	c. Nutrition f. Accident and poisoning prevention
	22. Consider legal requirements for care of the pediatric patient.
	a. Patient below age of 18 must be accompanied by parent or legal guardian in order to receive care. Exception: medical emergencies and special situations when written permission by legal guardian has been given for continuing care.
	b. A patient who has a legal document indicating emancipated minor status is treated as an adult.

CHAPTER II
Guidelines for basic care when there is deviation from normal

INTRODUCTION: Illness frequently involves alterations in the individual's capacity to maintain homeostasis. There are common features in the nursing care required by the patient who experiences such temporary or permanent deviations from normal function.

In these guidelines the described nursing intervention is directed towards helping the patient to adjust to or compensate for the imposed limitation or disability resulting in the deviation from normal.

Frequent reference to this section is made in many of the specific patient care guidelines to delineate desired outcomes and nursing process related to these critical episodes of care or patient care problems that require highly skilled nursing intervention.

Activity guidelines when there is deviation from normal

Patient Outcome	Process

A. *The patient functions at a maximum level of independent activity in relation to condition*	1. Refer to Chapter I Guidelines for General Care, to maximize patient's ability to maintain normal activity.
	 2. Assess activity limitation and consider present physical status and pertinent past history.
	   a. Motor and sensory deficits; patient with prosthesis
	   b. Arthritis problems
	   c. Peripheral vascular problems
	   d. Visual problem
	   e. Pain
	   f. Psychosocial factors
	   g. Medication effects, *e.g.*, steroid myopathy
	   h. Cardiovascular status
	   i. Age
	 3. Institute planned activity program with patient.
	   a. Initiate activity to increase muscle tone, joint mobility, and circulation according to nature of limitation.
	     • Depressed level of consciousness: Passive range of motion exercises
	     • Immobilized 48 hours: Active and passive range of motion exercises
	     • Motor and sensory neurodeficits: Active and passive range of motion exercises
	     • Problems with progressive activity: Active exercises and ambulation
	   b. Seek assistance of physical therapist for evaluation and follow-up.
	   c. Monitor patient's physiological and psychological responses.
	   d. Increase or adjust levels of activity according to patient's readiness and energy level.
	     • Consult with physician regarding realistic expectations of patient's capability.
	     • Provide adequate rest, fluid balance, and nutritional intake to promote energy level.
	   e. Communicate regularly with patient, family, physician, and physical therapist regarding progress and any needed goal adjustment.

B. *The patient is knowledgeable about activity program*	4. Establish postdischarge activity goals with patient.
	   a. Provide information about current level of activity (including restrictions) and ways in which family can participate.
	   b. Assess patient's ability to carry out goals within his home situation. Suggest appropriate modifications of home environment.
	   c. Collaborate with physical therapist in teaching and discharge planning.
	 5. Provide necessary assistive devices, *e.g.*, cane. Include written instructions about use.
	 6. Inform patient of health agencies which might provide assistance in his continuity of care.
	 7. Initiate interagency referral as needed.

Bladder care guidelines when there is deviation from normal bladder function

Patient Outcome	Process

A. *The patient is free of preventable urinary tract complications*	1. Refer to Chapter I Guidelines for General Care, p. 5 to maximize patient's ability to maintain normal urinary function.
	2. Manage indwelling catheter and urinary drainage system in a safe manner.
	   a. Use general measures to minimize chance of urinary tract infection:
	     • Wash hands thoroughly before and after providing care.
	     • Minimize trauma when inserting catheter.
	     • Force fluids unless contraindicated.
	     • Observe for signs of infection.
	     • Consult physician to remove catheter as soon as possible.
	   b. Use specific measures to minimize infection and promote drainage.
	     • Tape catheter securely to patient in a manner to prevent tension. Alternate tape site q 24 to 48 hours.
	     • Keep drainage tubing slack and coiled in bed.
	     • Hang bag below level of bladder.
	     • Prevent interruption of closed drainage system (aspirate tubing for specimen).
	     • Observe for obstruction, *e.g.,* kinks in tubing, plugged catheter.
	     • Use aseptic technique when disconnecting or reconnecting drainage system tubing.
	     • Consider restraining patient who pulls at catheter.
	     • Wash perineal areas and catheter q 8 hours using antimicrobial solution as indicated. Give special attention to foreskin if male patient.
	     • Change Foley catheter q 7 days or according to hospital policy.
	     • Change silastic catheter q 30 days or according to hospital policy.
	     • Collect specimens for urinalysis, culture, and sensitivity as ordered by physician (usually within 72 hours after insertion and then weekly).
	3. Manage external urinary drainage system in a safe manner.
	   a. Apply condom to penis and secure with foam adhesive strip.
	   b. Check penis and scrotum q 8 hours for edema and excoriation.
	   c. Change condom q 24 hours. Cleanse area thoroughly.
	   d. Consider restraining patient who pulls at condom.
	   e. Check for obstruction, e.g., twisted condom, kinks in tubing.

B. *The patient is knowledgeable about bladder drainage*	4. Plan goals with patient and family prior to and throughout urinary regimen.
	   a. Encourage patient to participate in care and monitoring of intake and output as appropriate.
	   b. Inform patient about any complication and treatment.
	5. Teach postdischarge management if indicated, i.e., teach technique of care and explain rationale.
	6. Provide:
	   a. Necessary equipment and aids including written instructions about care
	   b. Information about health care agencies which might provide assistance in continuity of care
	7. Initiate interagency referral as needed.

Bowel care guidelines when there is deviation from normal bowel function

Patient Outcome	Process
A. *The patient is free of preventable bowel complications*	1. Refer to Chapter I Guidelines for General Care, p. 5 to maximize patient's ability to maintain normal bowel function. 2. Assess the nature of the patient's abnormal bowel function. Consider special needs of patients who: 　a. Have history of bowel problems prior to or during hospitalization, *e.g.,* excessive use of laxatives 　b. Are immobilized, *e.g.,* in traction 　c. Are comatose or unable to communicate needs 　d. Are postoperative 　e. Are elderly 　f. Are neurologically impaired, *e.g.,* spinal cord dysfunction 3. Identify signs and symptoms of constipation/fecal impaction. 　a. Subjective symptoms as abdominal and rectal discomfort, diarrhea, nausea, and vomiting 　b. Objective signs as impaction, distention, flatus, liquid stool, elevated temperature 4. Institute therapeutic bowel program as indicated. 　a. Fecal impaction: 　　• Give oil retention enema followed by soap suds enema or as indicated. 　　• Manual extraction by physician or nurse followed by soap suds enema. 　　• Consult physician for oral laxative order. 　b. Painful hemorrhoids: 　　• Consult physician for appropriate orders. 　c. Diarrhea: 　　• Assess for probable causes such as antibiotics, tube feeding, impaction, emotional stress. 　　• Consult physician for appropriate orders. 　　• Provide special attention to surrounding skin areas.
B. *The patient is knowledgeable about bowel management*	5. Establish goals with patient and physician for normal bowel functioning program. Include appropriate dietary and fluid intake and activity modifications. 　a. Reevaluate considering patient's changing needs. 　b. Encourage patient to participate actively in achieving management goals. 6. Teach postdischarge management.

Pain

Patient Outcome	Process

A. *The patient achieves a relative state of comfort*

PREFACE: These guidelines are applicable to but not comprehensive for patients with intractable pain.

1. Assess the factors which denote the presence of pain.
   a. Objective symptoms:
      - Patient appearance: facial expression, affect, posture, muscular activity
      - Sympathetic nervous system indicators: pallor, flushing, diaphoresis, blood pressure, pulse, respiration, dilatation of pupils
      - Emotional responses: anger, withdrawal, frustration, sadness, denial, atypical behavior
   b. Subjective description:
      - Onset of pain
      - Location and radiation
      - Intensity
      - Duration (continuous or intermittent, occurring in relationship to other events)
      - Aggravating and relieving events
      - Associated symptoms, *e.g.,* nausea, anorexia
   c. Causes of pain and sources which affect pain perception:
      - Specific: tissue damage, *e.g.,* trauma, ischemia, incision; muscle spasm
      - Nonspecific: aspects of stress including psychological factors such as anxiety, fear; fatigue
      - No apparent cause
   d. Psychological influences:
      - Body image
      - Role
      - Attitude
      - Emotional resources
      - Perceived threat to life
   e. Socio-cultural influences:
      - Role: in family, in society
      - Age
      - Sex
      - Nationality
      - Religion
   f. Patient's previous experience and helpful measures in dealing with pain
2. Formulate and implement individualized plan for dealing with patient experiencing pain. Consider such nursing actions as:
   a. Be present, listen to patient, answer questions, attempt to dispel fears. Recognize need to express pain, *e.g.,* through talking, crying, yelling, withdrawal.
   b. Value suggestions from patient about possible effective measures.
   c. Learn of usual pain levels (as related to patient's disease process and probable effective measures).
   d. Use pain-relieving measures appropriate to specific patient.
      - Analgesics: type, dose, route, frequency dependent upon intensity of pain, patient size, patient's reaction to drug.
      - Antiemetics: nausea may accompany pain and/or analgesics.
      - Heat or cold applications
      - Change of position
      - Modification of the room environment, *e.g.,* amount of light, humidity, privacy, noise, temperature
      - Relaxation techniques, *e.g.,* breathing, massage
      - Distraction: drawing attention away from pain, *e.g.,* conversation, music, games, reading, TV
      - Substitute stimulation, *e.g.,* rocking, rubbing, patting
   e. Be aware that patient may not ask for pain relief measures
   f. Be aware of own feelings about pain and management of pain

B. *The patient is free of or has minimal complications associated with treatment of pain*

3. Observe for signs and symptoms indicative of complications associated with the treatment of pain.
   a. Compromised systemic functions: inadequate pulmonary toilet, inability to void adequately, inadequate intake
   b. Change in vital signs:
      undertreatment—increase pulse and blood pressure, respirations short or shallow
      overtreatment—decrease pulse and blood pressure, slow respirations, periods of apnea

27

Patient Outcome	Process
	c. Pain not relieved: restlessness, sleeplessness, irritability, anorexia
	d. Delay in return to normal those physiologic functions which may produce pain
	e. Effects of prolonged undertreatment: fears of future pain, psychoneurosis, intractable pain states
	f. Effects of prolonged overtreatments: drug abuse, *e.g.,* habituations/addictions
	4. Be aware that many analgesics are potentiated by anesthetics and other medications. Consider:
	a. Appropriate time interval of pain-relieving drugs and patient's reaction to pain-relieving drugs.
	b. Combination of synergistic drugs: analgesic and tranquilizer
	5. Collaborate with physician and significant others to revise treatment plan for dealing with pain.
C. *The patient is knowledgeable about pain management*	6. Plan management goals with patient and family throughout hospitalization.
	7. Teach patient about medications.
	a. Provide patient with information regarding pain medications prescribed at discharge: Form, dosage, side effects, timing with activities, use of prescription.
	b. Give patient a written list of medications that were ineffective or to which he developed an idiosyncratic response.
	8. Teach symptoms of pain which should be reported immediately:
	a. Increase in intensity or pattern of pain
	b. Increase in incisional discomfort with tenderness, redness, heat, swelling
	9. Reassure patient that incisional pain will gradually lessen. (Increase in activity may temporarily increase soreness.)

Pulmonary care guidelines when there is deviation from normal function

Patient Outcome	Process

A. *The patient is free of preventable pulmonary complications*	1. Refer to Chapter I Guidelines for General Care, p. 5 to maximize patient's ability to maintain normal pulmonary function.
	2. Determine the basis of patient's abnormal pulmonary function.
	  a. Assess signs and symptoms of pulmonary problems.
	    • Quality of respirations:
	      Ease of respirations: Examples of abnormal:
	        Dyspnea: subjective assessment of difficulty breathing, "short of breath" (SOB)
	        Use of accessory muscles: scalenus, sternocleidomastoids, retraction of intercostal spaces
	        Orthopnea: SOB in recumbent position, relieved by raising trunk to sitting position
	      Rate and depth of respirations:
	        Normal range: 12 to 20 per minute (adult)
	        Tachypnea: 30 to 60 per minute (adult), rapid shallow
	      Ratio of inspiration to exhalation:
	        Normal: 1:2
	      Breathing pattern: examples of abnormal
	        Cheyne-Stokes: periods of apnea followed by gradually increasing depth of respirations and then gradually decreasing depth of respirations
	        Kussmaul: deep respirations, similar to a normal sigh (seen in metabolic acidosis, *i.e.*, diabetic ketoacidosis)
	    • Adequacy of respiration (PO_2 and PCO_2)
	      Oxygenation:
	        PO_2, normal range: 85 to 100 mm. Hg.
	        O_2 saturation normal range: 90 to 100 mm. Hg.
	        Hemoglobin normal range: 14 to 18 gms per 100 ml
	        Hypoxemia: range of symptoms including pallor, cyanosis (may be confined to nail beds, lips, or may be generalized), flaring of nares, tachycardia, hypotension, unconsciousness, confusion, delirium, impaired judgment and motor function, headache
	      Ventilation:
	        PCO_2 normal range 35 to 40 mm. Hg.
	        pH normal range 7.35 to 7.47
	        Respiratory alkalosis decreased $PaCO_2$
	        Respiratory acidosis increased $PaCO_2$
	        Hypercaenia: confusion, hypertension, unconsciousness, dizziness, suspiciousness, sweating, headache, asterixis (periodic, repetitive flapping of hands when arms are outstretched)
	    • Other associated findings
	      Sputum: quantity, consistency, color
	      Coughing: frequency, duration, time of occurrence, character (*e.g.*, hacking, productive)
	      Temperature
	  b. Assess risk factors.
	    • Previous history of respiratory problems, *e.g.*, COPD, tuberculosis (TB), pneumonia, asthma
	    • Immobilization, *e.g.*, CVA, spinal cord injury
	3. Provide nursing measures to improve pulmonary function. Sequentially institute measures from the following:
	  a. Bronchodilator therapy
	  b. Humidification
	  c. Repositioning
	  d. Postural drainage with percussion and vibration
	  e. Deep breathing using incentive spirometry and diaphragmatic breathing exercises
	  f. Coughing and/or ET suctioning
	4. Evaluate effectiveness of treatment plan and readjust components as needed.
	  a. Monitor sputum quantity and character in relation to culture reports and antibiotics.

Patient Outcome	Process
	b. Chest radiograph findings
	c. Blood gases
	5. Inform patient regarding condition and treatment for any pulmonary complication.
B. *The patient is knowledgeable about pulmonary care*	6. Plan with patient and teach postdischarge management of care.
	a. Assess patient's ability to care for self.
	b. Provide necessary equipment and aids, *i.e.,* written instructions.
	7. Inform patient of health agencies which might assist in continuity of care.
	8. Initiate interagency referral as needed.

Skin care guidelines when there is deviation from normal skin condition

Patient Outcome	Process

A. *The patient is free of preventable skin complications*	1. Refer to Chapter I Guidelines for General Care, p. 6 to maximize patient's ability to maintain normal integrity of skin.
	2. Determine the basis of the patient's abnormal skin condition and consider:
	   a. Motor and sensory status
	   b. Age
	   c. Nutritional status
	   d. Peripheral circulation
	   e. Bowel and bladder control
	   f. Poor skin hygiene
	   g. Prolonged immobilization
	3. Assess the degree of skin involvement and institute nursing measures accordingly:
	   a. Reddened skin areas that do not disappear after repositioning:
	     • Keep clean and dry.
	     • Keep area pressure free by repositioning q 2 hours.
	     • Massage area frequently with lotion. Use gentle circular motion.
	   b. Excoriated skin areas:
	     • Wash gently, rinse and pat dry q 8 hours and after each incontinence.
	     • Keep area pressure free by repositioning q 2 hours.
	     • Apply hair dryer on "cool" setting to area for 15 minutes q 4 hours.
	     • Apply Karaya powder lightly as indicated after removal of previous application.
	   c. Skin breakdown-decubitus:
	     • Wash gently, rinse, and pat dry q 8 hours and p.r.n.
	     • Keep area pressure free by repositioning q 2 hours. If possible position patient on abdomen frequently.
	     • Massage surrounding area every 2 to 4 hours with lotion. Use gentle circular motion.
	     • Keep area open to air.
	     • Apply heat lamp at 24 inches from wound for 15 minutes q 4 hours.
	     • Apply soothing, drying agent to area q 8 hours, *e.g.,* Karaya powder.
	     • Check with physician if irrigation is indicated.
	     • Record observation of wound size, depth, drainage, and color q 48 hours.
	     • Report to physician signs of infection or extension.
	     • Observe other body areas for potential breakdown.
	   d. Communicate plan of care to all nursing personnel.
	4. Consider use of assistive devices as sheepskin, air mattress.
	5. Institute measures to improve nutritional status, activity status, and bowel and bladder control, if indicated.
	6. Evaluate effectiveness of treatment plan and readjust components as needed.

B. *The patient is knowledgeable about preventive and therapeutic skin care*	7. Teach patient and family the value and methods of preventing and/or treating skin problems. 8. Delegate responsibility of skin care program to patient and family and provide assistance as necessary. 9. Arrange assistance for continuity of care of skin problems when needed. • Initiate interagency referral if needed.

CHAPTER III
Guidelines for the patient undergoing diagnostic studies

INTRODUCTION: Consideration should be given to the Diagnostic Studies General Care Guidelines for each patient who undergoes *any* diagnostic procedure. Due to the nature of certain diagnostic studies, it is essential to provide nursing interventions based on the specific needs of patients experiencing these special procedures. The following guidelines highlight the patient's needs and key nursing activities based on the specifics of the diagnostic study and the desirable patient outcome of a comfortable, safe, and expedient study.

Often reference is made in other sections of this manual to these guidelines to delineate desired outcomes and process related to patient problems that require highly skilled nursing interventions.

The guidelines can serve as an important detailed resource for the nurse in providing information for the patient undergoing diagnostic examinations.

Patient Outcome	Process

PREFACE: This specific clinical information is written to facilitate the nurse's understanding of the diagnostic study and patient care needed. Before giving information the nurse should first assess the patient's anxiety level and the desire for and the ability to comprehend the information. Including the patient's family (or responsible person) in the explanation of the study usually aids the patient's understanding and provides additional reassurance. In major procedures it is essential that a person familiar to the patient be included because of the critical nature of the study.

Most patients will be apprehensive as they anticipate diagnostic studies. This may be related to what will happen during the study, or the outcome of the study—a favorable or an unfavorable diagnosis. The patient should be reassured that his anxiety is normal and that his expressions of this are acceptable. If the patient is in a very anxious state he may not hear or may exaggerate what has been said.

Every patient should have a minimum amount of information about the study which he will undergo. This information should include: a brief description of the study, any sensations the patient will experience during the study, *e.g.,* hearing, seeing, feeling, smelling, tasting, the nature of any discomfort or pain, the equipment to be used if fear provoking, and the restriction or special care involved in the study. Recognize that some patients want to know more details about the study but some would be frightened by the additional information. Each patient's individual desire to be informed should be respected.

Following the study the patient may be anxious regarding the test results. The nurse should be sensitive to this and communicate the patient's concern to the physician.

The patient experiences comfortable, safe, and expedient diagnostic studies. This includes:

1. Ascertain what tests are to be done through interview with the patient, physician, and referring to order sheet for patient.
2. Determine if any tests must be carried out prior to other studies to assure accuracy of results. Organize schedule appropriately. Examples:
   a. Radiopaque substance (barium) in the GI tract may prevent good visualization necessary to other studies, *i.e.,* intravenous pyelograms, arteriograms, Nuclear Medicine scans, ultrasonography.
   b. Iodine dyes will affect:
      • Thyroid study results for an extended length of time (several months)
      • The quantity and specific gravity of urine until the dye is excreted
      • Some 24-hour urine collections (oxylates and 17-hydroxyketosteroids)
3. Be aware of aspects of patient and his medical history which might require special nursing care and attention in scheduling. Notify diagnostic departments of patient's specific needs and indicate this on patient's chart. Consider:
   a. Critically ill or unstable patient will need to be accompanied by nurse from unit.
   b. If special equipment, *i.e.,* suction, oxygen, or monitor, is needed, make sure it will be available in study area.
   c. Patients with motor-sensory deficits cannot tolerate long periods of time on hard surfaces.
   d. Patients with cardiac and renal disease should have close monitoring of fluids to avoid over- or under-hydration. (Enemas, laxatives and the diuretic effect of dyes may alter fluid and electrolyte balance.)
   e. Confused or highly anxious patients need especially prompt attention in diagnostic departments and speedy return to familiar surroundings of ward.
   f. Patient requiring medication or nutrition at specific intervals (*e.g.,* patient with diabetes, hypoglycemia, seizures, cardiac problems, ulcers or receiving steroids) should not be held n.p.o. or have his medications delayed for long periods of time. Notify physician for questions regarding medications, fluid or nutrition needs.

A. *Is prepared for study*

4. Explain/answer questions and listen to concerns about prestudy preparation, procedure, and poststudy care.
   a. Determine if test has been introduced and/or explained by physician, if patient has had test before, or knows someone who has had test. Have patient explain his understanding of the study to determine accuracy.
   b. Clarify misunderstanding and give additional factual information.
   c. Determine if patient has gained reasonable understanding of the study. Provide opportunity for patient to talk or ask questions.
   d. Reassure patients as indicated, some of the following may be helpful:
      • Repeat explanation as needed.
      • Arrange for patient to talk with someone who has had similar procedure.
      • Arrange visit to study area to see equipment, meet personnel.
      • Call on resource people, *e.g.,* clinician, chaplain, technologist.
   e. Explain the need for and components of physical preparation.

Patient Outcome	Process
	5. Institute immediate preparation of patient for the study.
	a. Provide physical preparation for study per hospital routine.
	b. Check for signed consent form (when required).
	c. Remove patient's dentures, jewelry, prostheses, and other valuables as needed to provide for patient's safety, to expedite study, and to protect his belongings.
	d. Remove nail polish when nail beds will be observed during or after study.
	e. Provide comfort and safety for patient.
	• Have patient void before leaving unit.
	• Assist patient to move from bed to wheelchair or stretcher safely.
	• Check proper functioning of equipment, *i.e.,* patency of tubes, position of urinary drainage bag, intravenous infusion.
	• Provide sufficient cover to assure patient comfort and dignity.
	• Notify diagnostic department of any immediate needs for patient during study due to therapeutic regimen.
B. *Is free of or has minimal discomfort and complications following study*	6. Provide postprocedure care.
	a. Institute care related to specific and immediate needs of patient and physician's orders.
	b. Check that patient-care equipment such as intravenous (IVs) and drainage tubes are functioning properly.
	c. Provide nourishment to the patient as soon as possible.
	d. Maintain comfort for the patient. Consider: analgesics, positioning, and other methods used to increase patient's comfort.

Patient Outcome	Process
The patient experiences a comfortable, safe and expedient radionuclide angiocardiogram. This includes:	1. Explain/answer questions and listen to concerns about prestudy preparation, procedure and post study care. Tell patient that the technician or physician in attendance will explain the equipment and the study as it progresses. Information may include:
	a. ***Purpose:*** To collect information about heart function and blood flow through the injection of a small amount of radioactive material into a vein. A recording is made of the passage of the material through the heart and great vessels.
A. *Is prepared for study*	b. ***Procedure:*** The study takes place in a special unit as the Radionuclide Laboratory. There are two types of studies: a supine test and a rest-exercise test.
	For the supine study, the patient is asked to lie supine on an examining table. If there is not an existing intravenous line, a silastic catheter is inserted (into the antecubital vein in pediatric patients and usually in the external jugular vein in adults). A butterfly needle is often used in infants instead of the catheter. This line allows injection of the radioactive isotope and flushing with normal saline. The material injected is minimally radioactive and causes no pain or side effect. A large scintillation camera is positioned above the patient's precordial area. As the tracer is injected, the camera records the passage of the material through the heart chambers and into the arterial circulation.
	A rest-exercise study is a two-part study with both portions performed with the patient in an upright position. After an intravenous line has been inserted and the EKG leads have been applied, the patient is seated on a stabilized bicycle. The patient is asked to pedal until a predetermined heart rate is achieved or 10 minutes have elapsed. Immediately after exercise completion the patient's precordial area is positioned in front of the camera while he is still seated on the bicycle and the tracer material is injected. The rest portion of the study is performed with the patient in an upright position within the next few days (especially for pediatric patients) or after a 20-minute resting period.
	If the IV line had been started specifically for the test, it is discontinued after the pictures are taken.
	2. Institute immediate preparation of patient for study.
	a. Check for signed consent obtained by physician.
	b. Encourage parent to be present if patient is a child.
	c. Give fluids as ordered.
B. *Is free of or has minimal discomfort or complications following study*	3. Provide postprocedure care.
	a. Give diet and fluids as ordered.
	b. Resume activity as ordered.

Patient Outcome	Process

The patient experiences a comfortable, safe, and expedient arteriogram. This includes:
 	
A. *Is prepared for study*
	1. Explain/answer questions and listen to concerns about prestudy preparations, procedure, and poststudy care. Information may include:
	  a. ***Purpose:*** To detect lesions, abnormalities, or obstructions of the vessel(s) to be visualized.
	  b. ***Procedure:*** The patient lies on a hard table and is draped. The area is scrubbed by the doctor and injected with a local anesthetic. Some patients may be given a general anesthetic at the discretion of the physician. A needle is inserted into the vessel. The contrast dye is injected giving the patient a flushed and warm sensation. The patient will be instructed to hold still and not breathe for brief periods while radiographs are being taken. Patient will hear the loud noises of the automatic film changer below the table. Depending on the number of vessels visualized, the study will take at least one hour.
	2. Institute immediate preparation of patient for the study.
	  a. Interview patient for allergies to seafood or iodine or previous reactions to contrast media. Notify physician.
	  b. Check for signed consent obtained by physician.
	  c. Prepare puncture site as ordered by the physician. (Example—Shave area and give scrub using antimicrobial solution the night before procedure.)
	  d. Restrict diet and fluids if requested by radiologist.
	  e. Have patient void.
	  f. Give preprocedure medication if ordered. This may be an antihistamine, aspirin, steroids, atropine, or sedative.

B. *Is free of or has minimal discomfort or complications following study*	3. Provide postprocedure care.
	  a. Check and record physiologic responses as ordered. Frequency might be q 15 minutes × 2 hours, q 30 minutes × 2 hours, etc. Check:
	    • Radial pulse rate and character of pulses distal to puncture site
	    • Vital signs
	    • Color, temperature of skin
	    • Presence of pain which might indicate thrombus, embolus
	    • Puncture site for hematoma, bleeding (Teach patient to call nurse and apply local pressure if bleeding occurs.)
	  b. Notify physician of any abnormal physiologic reaction.
	  c. Apply small ice bag to puncture site upon return to ward as ordered.
	  d. Keep patient at bed rest 12 hours with extremity having puncture site unflexed. Head may be elevated slightly (30°).
	  e. Check for urinary retention.
	  f. Check for fluid depletion. Give diet and fluids as ordered.

Patient Outcome	Process

The patient experiences a comfortable, safe, and expedient arthrogram. This includes:
 	
A. *Is prepared for study*
	1. Explain/answer questions and listen to concerns about prestudy preparation, procedure and poststudy care. Information may include:
	  a. ***Purpose:*** To visualize cartilage, bone, ligaments and synovial structures of joints which cannot be seen on the usual radiograph
	    • Joints usually studied are shoulder, hip, knee, elbow, wrist, ankle.
	  b. ***Procedure:*** Done in the radiograph department and/or in the operating room immediately prior to surgery. Radiographs without dye are taken first. The area to be injected is prepped with antiseptic solution. Using a small needle, local anesthesia is injected making a skin wheal. Then, a larger needle is inserted into the joint. Fluoroscopy (radiograph on television screen—"live") is used to see if the needle is in the correct area. Patient may experience some discomfort if the needle is repositioned. A radiopaque dye is then injected into the joint while being observed under fluoroscopy. Patient may feel a sensation of slight swelling or pressure in the joint as the dye is injected. Needle is withdrawn. Patient is asked to exercise joint to disperse dye around joint. Then several radiographs are taken. Patient may have some slight aching and swelling in joint for 24 to 48 hours. If air is also injected into the joint for double contrast, patient may experience a bubbly or grating sensation inside joint and may have a painful joint for 3 to 4 days. Dye is absorbed in 48 hours.
	2. Institute immediate preparation of patient for study.
	  a. Check if patient is allergic to iodine (dye is 15 per cent iodine) or if he has had reaction to intravenous pyelogram dye. Report to physician.
	  b. Give "on call" sedative or other medication if ordered.

B. *Is free of or has minimal discomfort or complications following study*	3. Provide postprocedure care.
	  a. Maintain comfort for the patient. This may include:
	    • Elevation of affected extremity
	    • Application of ice bag to decrease swelling
	    • Provision of analgesics, as needed
	  b. Check for warmth and redness at puncture site.
	  c. Cover puncture site with Band-Aid.

Patient Outcome	Process

The patient experiences a safe, comfortable, and expedient arthroscopy. This includes:
 	
A. *Is prepared for study*
	1. Explain/answer questions and listen to concerns about prestudy preparation, procedure, and poststudy care. Information may include:
	  a. ***Purpose:*** Internal examination of the knee performed for diagnosis of internal derangement, *i.e.,* torn meniscus. Additional indications for arthroscopy are; to perform synovial biopsy; to determine indications for synovectomy in rheumatoid arthritis, and to remove small loose bodies or small pedicle tumors.
	  b. ***Procedure:*** The patient receives either spinal or general anesthesia in the operating room for arthroscopy. Following a small incision, an instrument with light source and irrigation tubing is inserted into joint. The joint is continually manipulated and irrigated with saline to ensure good visualization. Findings are recorded with a special camera. If an abnormality is detected that requires surgical intervention, gowns and gloves are changed and a sterile fluid reestablished for the procedure to begin.
	2. Institute immediate preparation of the patient for the study.
	  a. Give surgical scrub to area evening before and morning of study.
	  b. Check for signed consent for study.
	  c. Keep n.p.o. after midnight.
	  d. Give medications as ordered.

B. *Is free of or has minimal discomfort or complications following study*	3. Provide postprocedure care.
	  a. Provide care appropriate to operative procedure if performed, *e.g.,* menisectomy.
	  b. Monitor vital signs as indicated.
	  c. Elevate extremity and apply ice pack as ordered.
	  d. Check incision site frequently and report abnormalities to physician.
	  e. Collaborate with physician about initiating quadriceps rehabilitation program.

Patient Outcome

The patient experiences a comfortable, safe, and expedient barium enema and air contrast study. This includes:

A. *Is prepared for study*

B. *Is free of or has minimal discomfort and complications following study*

Process

1. Explain/answer questions and listen to concerns about prestudy preparation, procedure and poststudy care. Information may include:
   a. ***Purpose:*** To detect/rule out lesions, abnormalities, or obstructions of large bowel. Air contrasts are specific for polyps and inflammatory bowel disease.
   b. ***Procedure:*** Patient is placed on a radiograph table. A lubricated enema tube is inserted slowly and carefully into the rectum. This may cause a small amount of discomfort. The radiologist then allows barium to flow by gravity into the large bowel and sees the filling of the bowel with the aid of fluoroscopy (a television-like screen). As the large bowel is being filled, radiograph films are taken as the patient assumes different positions. For air contrast studies, barium and air are introduced to allow for greater distention and visualization of the bowel wall. The patient may experience "gas-pain" feeling and urge to evacuate bowel. Upon completion the patient is allowed to go to the bathroom to evacuate the barium. The films are processed and checked by the radiologist before patient is allowed to leave. Average time to complete study is one hour.
   c. ***Scheduling consideration:*** Barium may prevent good visualization necessary to other studies, *e.g.,* intravenous pyelogram, arteriogram, Nuclear Medicine examinations, ultrasonography.
2. Institute immediate preparation of the patient for study.
   a. Give laxative: Recommended preparation is 120 cc of castor oil (Neoloid) at 4:00 p.m. the day prior to study.
   b. Give clear liquid meal evening prior to study.
   c. Encourage fluids to midnight as patient's condition permits.
   d. Keep n.p.o. after midnight.
   e. Give 1500 cc tap water enema the morning of study.
3. Provide postprocedure care.
   a. Encourage diet, fluids, and activity unless restricted.
   b. Give medication to prevent abdominal discomfort and barium impactions unless contraindicated.
   c. Check that patient has a satisfactory bowel evacuation.

Bone marrow aspiration

Patient Outcome	Process

The patient experiences a comfortable, safe, and expedient bone marrow aspiration. This includes:
 	
A. *Is prepared for study*
	1. Explain/answer questions and listen to concerns about prestudy preparation, procedure and poststudy care. Information may include:
	  a. ***Purpose:*** To detect abnormalities of bone marrow cells; *i.e.,* leukemia, anemias. Areas used: sternum, anterior iliac crest, posterior iliac crest
	  b. ***Procedures:*** Patient lies supine in bed if an area on the sternum or anterior iliac crest is used. If posterior iliac crest is used, patient lies on stomach with sandbag placed under iliac areas. Area is prepped with an antiseptic solution (cool sensation), injected with local anesthetic (stinging sensation), and draped as a sterile field. The patient will feel discomfort of pressure as a large lumen needle is injected into the bone. Brief pain is felt as the marrow is aspirated. Steady pressure is applied for 5 to 15 minutes after procedure to prevent bleeding. A small sterile dressing is applied and worn for 24 hours. An elastoplast dressing is used for patients with thrombocytopenia (50,000 platelets or less).
	2. No special immediate preparation of patient for study is indicated.

B. *Is free of or has minimal discomfort or complications following study*	3. Provide postprocedure care.
	  a. Check patient for swelling or pain in area aspirated.
	  b. Alert patient to notify the nurse for swelling, and/or pain in area aspirated.
	  c. If iliac crest is site of procedure, inform patient he may feel deep soreness (similar to deep intramuscular injection) when walking the day of and for several days after the procedure.
	  d. Provide analgesics as ordered.
	  e. Check for signs of infection.

Bone scan

Patient Outcome	Process

The patient experiences a comfortable, safe, and expedient bone scan. This includes:
 	
A. *Is prepared for study*
	1. Explain/answer questions and listen to concerns about prestudy preparation, procedure, and poststudy care. Information may include:
	  a. ***Purpose:*** To observe for bone abnormalities resulting from neoplasma, trauma, infection and/or primary disease
	  b. ***Procedure:*** The patient is injected with a tracer amount of radiopharmaceutical and instructed to force fluids for one hour. The patient returns to Nuclear Medicine two hours after injection. After positioning under a scintillation camera, multiple images are obtained which take from 3 to 5 minutes each. The patient must be able to hold still voluntarily for 20-minute intervals. The female patient (childbearing age) is asked by technologist to sign a statement to verify whether or not she is pregnant.
	  c. ***Contraindication:*** Pregnancy
	2. Institute immediate preparation of patient for the study.
	  a. Evaluate potential need to sedate patient and discuss with physician for order.
	  b. Have patient and chart available to Nuclear Medicine 30 minutes prior to the study.

B. *Is free of or has minimal discomfort or complications following study*	3. No special postprocedure care is indicated.

NOTE: Restrict pregnant personnel from caring for patient for 24 hours.

Brain computerized axial tomography

Patient Outcome	Process

The patient experiences a comfortable, safe, and expedient brain computerized tomography. This includes:

A. *Is prepared for study*

1. Explain/answer questions and listen to concerns about prestudy preparation, procedure and poststudy care. Information may include:
   a. **Purpose:** To identify normalities, abnormalities of structures and spaces within the cranial vault through computerized tomography
   b. **Procedure:** Frequently this study is done in two parts. The unenhanced study requires no physical preparation. The enhanced (contrast) study, however, requires that the patient be n.p.o. prior to the study because the intravenous dye is likely to create nausea. The procedure causes no pain. The patient's cooperation is essential for accurate test results. The study room contains a large radiograph machine resembling a front-loading washing machine with a padded reclining table where the patient will lie supine with legs elevated. The technician will help the patient fit his head into a rubber cap which is inside the machine and encloses the head tightly during the study. Patient may be aware of sensation of pressure around his head. The patient's face is not covered by the machine. If the contrast phase is to be done, the physician injects contrast agent into the arm vein; the patient may experience nausea and a warm, flushed sensation. The patient is alone in the room while the radiographs are being taken. The technician observes and talks to the patient from outside the room during the study.

   It is essential that the patient not move his head during the study. He will hear the sound of the radiograph machine revolving which resembles roller-skating. The technician adjusts the machine as multiple tomograms are taken. Each part of the test lasts about 30 minutes, depending on how many radiographs are taken. The information gained is processed by a computer and printed out as photographs.
   c. **Special consideration:** Patients may be fearful of study because of appearance of machine and possible pathological findings. Postcraniotomy patient may experience (increased) headache with additional pressure of headband.
2. Institute immediate preparation of the patient for study.
   a. Interview patient for allergies to shellfish or iodine. Notify physician.
   b. Keep patient n.p.o. after midnight if enhanced part of study is scheduled for next day.
      • Contact the Radiology Department for permission to give fluids if study is delayed.
   c. Evaluate potential need to sedate patient and discuss with physician.
   d. Prepare patient and family for expectation of general anesthesia and recovery care, if appropriate.
   e. Check for written consent obtained by physician if patient is to undergo anesthesia.

B. *Is free of or has minimal discomfort or complications following study*

3. Provide postprocedure care.
   a. No special postprocedure care is necessary unless patient is recovering from sedation or anesthesia.
   b. Provide diet when appropriate.
   c. Encourage fluids, 2000 to 3000 cc daily, unless contraindicated.
   d. Resume appropriate activity.
   e. Provide mild analgesic to relieve headaches.
   f. Recognize that contrast agent causes increase in urine specific gravity for 8 to 12 hours.

Patient Outcome	Process

The patient experiences a comfortable, safe, and expedient brain scan. This includes:
 	
A. *Is prepared for study*
	1. Explain/answer questions and listen to concerns about prestudy preparation, procedure and poststudy care. Information may include:
	  a. **Purpose:** To observe for signs of cerebral infarction, contusion, abscess, neoplasm, and/or cyst
	  b. **Procedure:** The patient is positioned with head under a scintillation camera and instructed to hold still for approximately five minutes. During this time, the patient receives an intravenous injection of radioactive material and the cerebral blood distribution is recorded. Ninety minutes after injection, the patient is asked to assume multiple positions for imaging of the distribution of radioisotope within the head. The patient must be able to hold still voluntarily for 20-minute intervals. The female patient (childbearing age) is asked by technologist to sign a statement to verify whether or not she is pregnant.
	  c. **Contraindication:** Pregnancy
	2. Institute immediate preparation of patient for the study.
	  a. Evaluate potential need to sedate patient and discuss with physician for order.
	  b. Have patient and chart available to Nuclear Medicine 30 minutes prior to study.

B. *Is free of or has minimal discomfort or complications following study*	3. No special postprocedure care is indicated. **NOTE:** Restrict pregnant personnel from caring for patient for 24 hours.

Bronchogram

Patient Outcome	Process

The patient experiences a comfortable, safe, and expedient bronchogram. This includes:
 	
A. *Is prepared for study*
	1. Explain/answer questions and listen to concerns about prestudy preparation, procedure, and poststudy care. Information may include:
	  a. **Purpose:** To evaluate intrabronchial masses and to determine presence of bronchiectasis.
	  b. **Procedure:** The patient in taken to the Radiology Department and preliminary films taken. Intramuscular injections of codeine and atropine are usually given to suppress coughing and mucus production. With the patient in the seated position, the mucous membranes of the throat are anesthetized by gargling a foul tasting substance—not to be swallowed—and spraying the nose and throat with lidocaine until the gag reflex is gone. The patient is reminded not to cough at any time during the procedure.
	    The radiograph table is placed in a vertical position and the patient is asked to sit on a ledge at the base of the table. Using a fluoroscope, the physician inserts a catheter through the nasal cavity into the trachea. During insertion lidocaine (Xylocaine) is sprayed at intervals to secure further anesthesia and prevent coughing. The radiograph table is then returned to a horizontal position with the patient supine. The catheter is advanced into the lung and is visualized by using fluoroscopy. The contrast agent is injected via catheter and the patient is asked to take deep breaths. The patient may feel short of breath and/or chest tightness.
	    The patient is asked to assume different positions to facilitate radiographs. The catheter is then removed and patient encouraged to cough and expectorate as much contrast material as possible. This is facilitated through percussion as the patient lies on his stomach.
	2. Institute immediate preparation of patient for study.
	  a. Keep n.p.o. after midnight.
	  b. Give oral hygiene.
	  c. Interview patient for allergies to shellfish or iodine. Report to physician.
	  d. Remove dentures, eye glasses in Radiology Department.
	  e. Check for signed consent for study.

B. *Is free of or has minimal discomfort or complications following study*	3. Provide poststudy care.
	  a. Keep n.p.o. for 4 to 6 hours until gag reflex returns.
	  b. Give ice chips and water before resuming diet.
	  c. Observe for allergic reaction, *e.g.,* respiratory distress, bronchospasm, skin rash.
	  d. Give postural drainage and percussion q 2 hours × 4 with special attention to the lung receiving contrast agent.
	  e. Obtain chest radiographs next day as ordered.

Patient Outcome	Process
The patient experiences a comfortable, safe, and expedient bronchoscopy. This includes:	1. Explain/answer questions and listen to concerns about prestudy preparation, procedure, and poststudy care. Tell the patient that the physician in attendance will explain the study as it proceeds. Information may include:

The patient experiences a comfortable, safe, and expedient bronchoscopy. This includes:

A. *Is prepared for study*

1. Explain/answer questions and listen to concerns about prestudy preparation, procedure, and poststudy care. Tell the patient that the physician in attendance will explain the study as it proceeds. Information may include:
   a. ***Purpose:*** To allow direct visualization and access to the tracheobronchial tree for the purpose of:
      - Examining normal and abnormal structures, *e.g.*, tumor, fistula, abscess, inflammation
      - Obtaining transbronchial biopsy and/or brushing and washing of lung parenchyma
      - Loosening dry mucous plugs, removing of thick, purulent secretions or foreign objects from localized areas
   b. ***Procedure:*** The patient is taken to the study room and placed on an examining table. The physician and others in attendance are gowned and masked. While the patient is sitting, the nose and throat are sprayed with an anesthetic mist. The patient is instructed to take deep breaths and to swallow to allow deeper penetration of the spray. The patient is stimulated to cough as the spray is inhaled. The patient then assumes a reclining position with the upper portion of the body slightly elevated. A pillow is placed under the shoulders and the neck is hyperextended to facilitate placement of the flexible fiberoptic bronchoscope. The patient is draped with a sterile cloth and is reminded during the procedure to keep his hands at his side. The study equipment is assembled at the bedside and the lights are dimmed to permit better visualization of the study area. As the tube is inserted through the nose and during the procedure, the patient may be stimulated to cough Once the tube has been advanced past the vocal cords, the patient may experience a feeling of air hunger. Reassure him that there is sufficient room around the tube for him to breathe even though breathing may be more difficult. Oxygen is administered by mask during the study.

   In most cases specimens are obtained either by biopsy or a bronchial brushing and washing. Although not painful, the patient may be aware of sensations which accompany either procedure: a "snip" as the biopsy is taken, a warm flow of fluid as the bronchial washing is performed.

   After the study is completed, which usually takes about 15 to 20 minutes, the bronchoscope is removed.

2. Institute immediate preparation of the patient for study.
   a. Good oral cleaning night before and morning of the study.
   b. Check for signed consent obtained by physician.
   c. Keep patient n.p.o. for at least three hours prior to study.
   d. Remove dentures, bridges prior to study; eye glasses may be worn to study where they will be removed.
   e. Give "on-call" medications as ordered. This may be tranquilizer, atropine, analgesic, and/or sedative.
   f. Document baseline pulse, respirations and presence of breath sounds prior to leaving ward.

B. *Is free of or has minimal discomfort or complications following study.*

3. Provide postprocedure care.
   a. Check pulse, respirations, and presence of breath sounds on return to ward and as indicated. Compare with baseline.
   b. Check for symptoms that may indicate pneumothorax, *e.g.*, shortness of breath, chest pain.
   c. Keep patient n.p.o. until numbed sensation passes and gag reflex returns (at least two hours).
   d. Resume diet gradually beginning with sips of clear fluids and progressing as tolerated.
   e. Give soothing lozenges as needed for throat discomfort. Reassure patient that soreness and/or hoarseness is temporary.
   f. Discourage smoking for at least 24 hours.
   g. Resume appropriate activity.

Patient Outcome	Process

The patient experiences a comfortable safe, and expedient cardiac catheterization. This includes:
 	
A. *Is prepared for study*
	1. Explain/answer questions and listen to concerns about prestudy preparation, procedure, and poststudy care. Tell the patient the physician in attendance will explain the study as it proceeds. Information may include:
	   a. ***Purpose:*** To look for abnormalities of the heart muscle, heart valves, and/or coronary arteries
	   b. ***Procedure:*** The procedure takes place in the Cardiac Catheterization Laboratory. The patient is weighed and then placed on a narrow, padded, and contoured catheterization table. Straps are placed over the chest, thighs, and lower legs. The right groin and/or right arm and/or the left arm are scrubbed and numbed with a local anesthetic. An arterial needle is usually placed in the left arm to monitor the blood pressure and arterial and venous catheters are placed in the femoral artery and vein and/or the brachial artery and vein or both. The catheters are advanced into the heart chambers. The pressures are measured in the chambers and usually in the main vessels entering and leaving the heart. The patient usually does not experience any sensation of the catheter in the vessels. When it is in the heart he may occasionally feel palpitation. A Fick cardiac output is usually done in which the patient uses a scuba design mouthpiece to breathe, exhaling room air into a bag for a period of three minutes. Injection of a contrast material visible on radiograph is made into appropriate chambers of the heart and/or coronary arteries through the catheters. When this is injected into the major vessels or heart, a flushed sensation is often experienced by the patient which lasts several seconds. Occasionally a patient experiences headache or feels nauseated. There is usually no sensation when injections are made into the coronary arteries. When either injections are made, the patient will be asked to hold a deep breath without straining until the injection is completed, usually less than ten seconds. Cineangiocardiographs are taken at this time at a rate of 60 to 120 pictures per second, with the patient lying flat or turned to one side or the other. After the pictures are completed, the catheters are removed and the puncture sites are compressed by the physician for several minutes. The procedure usually lasts about one and a half hours. The patient is returned to the ward on a stretcher and monitoring of vital signs is continued.
	2. Institute immediate preparation of the patient for study.
	   a. Interview patient for allergies to shellfish or iodine. Notify physician.
	   b Check that results of ordered blood tests are recorded in patient's chart—such as
	     • Prothrombin time
	     • PTT or clotting time
	   c. Check for signed consent obtained by physician.
	   d. Shave and prep right groin and/or area ordered by physician.
	   e. Give sedative at bedtime, p.r.n.
	   f. Keep patient at n.p.o. after midnight, as ordered.
	   g. Document vital signs and peripheral pulses before giving ''on-call'' medications.
	   h. Have patient void.
	   i. Give ''on-call'' medications as ordered.

B. *Is free of or has minimal discomfort or complications following study*	3. Provide postprocedure care.
	   a. Check and record physiologic responses as ordered. Usual frequency: q 15 minutes × 4 times, q 30 minutes × 4 times, q 1 h × 4, q 4 h × 4. Check:
	     • Vital signs
	     • Pulses, color, and temperature of skin distal to puncture sites
	     • Sites of puncture for bleeding
	   b. Call physician if any abnormal physiologic reaction.
	   c. Elevate patient's leg slightly if blood pressure drops and pulse increases.
	   d. If bleeding at catheterization or needle site, apply pressure immediately and call physician.
	   e. Position patient on back for several hours, then turn side to side, keeping catheterized leg/arm straight. Activity is usually progressed to out of bed next a.m., after status checked by physician.
	   f. Encourage diet and fluids to 2000 cc unless restricted.
	   g. Check for symptoms of nausea, pain, wheezing, welts, rashes.
	     • Provide medication as ordered.
	     • Call physician if pain is persistent.
	     • Position for comfort.

Patient Outcome	Process

PREFACE: Includes those patients from birth to 18 years. Excludes patients with Wolff-Parkinson-White syndrome who will have specific pretest preparation and a slightly different study procedure.

The patient experiences a comfortable, safe and expedient cardiac catheterization. This includes:

A. *Is prepared for study (according to age and developmental level)*

1. Explain/answer questions and listen to concerns about prestudy preparation, procedure, and poststudy care. Information may include:
   a. *Purpose:* To look for structural abnormalities and/or malfunctions of the conduction system of the heart
   b. *Procedure:* Following sedation, the child is taken by stretcher or carried by laboratory technician to the Pediatric Catheterization Laboratory. The child is placed on a moveable table and restraints are placed on the child's arms and legs. Electrodes for monitoring the EKG, using the adhesive electrode pads, are placed on the inner aspect of the forearm and lower leg. Blood pressures are checked using an electronic device. The genital area is covered with a dressing to prevent soiling of the sterile area. The right and left groins are prepped with povidone-iodine and Phisohex; in some cases the axilla is prepped also. Local anesthesia is obtained using Xylocaine. Catheters are introduced using the artery and/or vein, usually percutaneously but sometimes by cutdown. Pressures are measured and oxygen samples removed in the heart chambers and great vessels. Contrast material is injected to diagnose structural defects and the patient should be prepared to feel a rush of heat when this occurs.

   After the procedure is completed pressure is applied over the catheter sites until homeostasis is obtained. The areas are cleaned and dressed with Neosporin and sterile pressure dressings. The patient is returned to the ward and frequent monitoring of vital signs is begun. The length of the procedure will depend upon the complexity of the heart lesion, which will be discussed with the parents by the cardiologist.
   c. Include a tour of catheterization laboratory for patient and parents, if possible.
   d. Inform parents of possible effect on child of prestudy sedation.
2. Institute immediate preparation of the patient for study.
   a. Interview parents regarding patient's allergy to shell fish or iodine. Cardiology may do this. Notify physician.
   b. Check that results of ordered laboratory tests are recorded in patient's chart. Tests may include CBC, urinalysis, chest radiograph, EKG, and echocardiogram.
   c. Check for signed consent by parents and/or legal guardian obtained by physician.
   d. Keep patient n.p.o. as ordered.
   e. Hold Digoxin until tests are completed and patient returned to ward.
   f. Check and record baseline vital signs, including blood pressure.
   g. Have patient void precardiac catheterization.
   h. Give medication "on-call" as ordered. This may be: no sedation for infants. Demerol, Phenergan or Thorazine sufficient to cause drowziness but not deep sleep.

B. *Is free of or has minimal discomfort or complications following study*

1. Provide postprocedure care.
   a. Check and record physiologic responses as ordered. Usual frequency: q 15 minutes × 4 times; q 30 minutes × 4 times; q 1 hour × 4, then per routine if stable. Check vital signs and pulses distal to puncture sites, leg color and temperature and skin sites of punctures for bleeding.
   b. Notify physician of abnormal physiologic reactions.
   c. Apply pressure immediately and call physician if any bleeding noted.
   d. Position and ambulate patient as ordered.
   e. Encourage fluids and diet unless restricted.
   f. Observe closely for rashes, urticaria, and/or wheezing, nausea, pain.
      • Provide medication as ordered.
      • Call physician if pain persists.
      • Position for comfort.
   g. Check for voiding within 4 hours.

Patient Outcome	Process

The patient experiences a comfortable, safe, and expedient cerebral angiography. This includes:
 	
A. *Is prepared for study*
 	
B. *Is free of or has minimal discomfort or complication following study*
	1. Explain/answer questions and listen to concerns about prestudy preparation, procedure, and poststudy care. Information may include:
	  a. ***Purpose:*** To visualize cerebral circulation and to detect abnormalities such as aneurysms, masses, congenital anomalies, displaced vessels (shift), hematomas, and cerebral vasospasm
	  b. ***Procedure:*** Although the patient is not usually anesthetized, sedation is given to help him relax during the procedure. He lies on a hard radiograph table with head immobilized by adhesive tape. The injection site in the groin is prepped with (cool) antiseptic solution and a (stinging) local anesthetic is injected. After the area is numb, the physician will palpate the artery (patient feels pressure), and a plastic tube is inserted and threaded up the artery. The contrast agent is injected and the patient feels an increasingly hot sensation as agent circulates. The sensation subsides in about 15 seconds. Simultaneously the patient hears the noisy clacking of radiograph plates in the radiograph changer. The patient waits while radiographs are viewed; other injections of agent may be necessary. After the test is completed, the physician removes the tube from the artery and applies firm pressure for 10 minutes. The procedure usually takes about an hour or longer. In exceptional situations, the patient may have the angiogram via carotid or brachial routes.
	  c. ***Contraindications:*** Patients who have trauma or infection near the site of injections and those who have had severe allergic reactions to the contrast agent
	2. Institute immediate preparation of the patient for study.
	  a. Interview patient for allergies to shellfish and iodine. Notify physician.
	  b. Check if the patient is on anticoagulants or has clotting problems.
	  c. Check for signed consent obtained by physician.
	  d. If ordered, keep patient n.p.o. after midnight.
	  e. Have patient void prior to test.
	  f. Give prestudy medication as ordered.
	  g. Mark pedal pulses, left and right. Check popliteal pulses.
	3. Provide postprocedure care.
	  a. Check and record physiologic responses as ordered: Usual frequency is q 15 minutes × 4 times, q 30 minutes × 4 times, then per routine if stable. Check:
	    • Vital signs
	    • Neurological status
	    • Pulses, color, and temperature of skin distal to puncture site.
	    • Puncture site for bleeding
	  b. Notify physician of any abnormal physiologic reactions.
	  c. Encourage diet and increased fluid intake unless restricted.
	  d. Discourage movement of affected leg, keep flat in bed for 12 hours, and gradually ambulate as ordered.
	  e. Expect urinary output to increase temporarily. Offer bedpan or urinal before patient is uncomfortable.
	  f. If carotid site is used:
	    • Check airway patency.
	    • Have tracheostomy set available.

Cholangiogram (T-tube)

Patient Outcome	Process

The patient experiences a comfortable, safe, and expedient cholangiogram. This includes:
 	
A. *Is prepared for study*
 	
B. *Is free of or has minimal discomfort or complications following study*
	1. Explain/answer questions and listen to concerns about prestudy preparation, procedure, and poststudy care. Information may include:
	  a. **Purpose:** To ascertain patency of the bile duct and proper healing of surgical exploration of duct
	  b. **Procedure:** Patient is placed on radiograph table. Using sterile technique, a radiologist injects dye into the bile duct via the T-tube which was placed in duct during previous surgery. Films are taken as the dye progresses through the biliary tree. The patient may experience some discomfort as the dye is injected. The procedure is usually short.
	2. Institute immediate preparation of patient for study. Interview patient for allergies to shellfish or iodine. Notify physician.
	3. Provide postprocedure care.
	  a. Encourage fluids, diet, and activity unless contraindicated.
	  b. Observe for delayed systemic reaction to dye. Symptoms include skin response, decrease in blood pressure, nausea, vomiting, and less commonly, respiratory distress and anaphylactic shock.
	  c. Check T-tube for proper positioning and any changes in drainage.
	  d. Notify physician of any abnormal responses.

Colonoscopy, proctoscopy

Patient Outcome	Process

The patient experiences a comfortable, safe, and expedient colonoscopy/ proctoscopy. This includes:
 	
A. *Is prepared for study*
 	
B. *Is free of or has minimal discomfort and complications following study*
	1. Explain/answer questions and listen to concerns about prestudy preparation, procedure, and poststudy care. Information may include:
	  a. **Purpose:** To visualize, detect, and rule out abnormalities of the rectum, sigmoid colon, and large bowel. The rectum and sigmoid colon are visualized in a proctoscopy; the entire large bowel is visualized in a colonoscopy.
	  b. **Procedure:** Patient is placed on proctoscopy table in kneeling position, head and arms are supported by table and pillows. Following digital examination of the rectum, the scope is lubricated and passed through the anus into the rectum. The obturator is then withdrawn. The rest of the examination is performed under direct vision. As the scope is passed, air may be introduced into the lumen in order to enhance visualization of the bowel wall. The patient may experience a cramping sensation which can be relieved partially by slow, deep breaths and relaxation. An additional biopsy forcep or snare may be passed through the lumen of the scope to obtain a biopsy or snare a polyp. The bowel wall contains no nerve endings; therefore, the patient will not feel pain from biopsies taken.
	2. Institute immediate preparation of the patient for study.
	  a. Give clear liquids or low residue diet as ordered one day prior to study.
	  b. Give laxatives as ordered.
	  c. Give clear liquids or n.p.o. past midnight as ordered.
	  d. Check for signed consent obtained by doctor.
	  e. Give thorough cleansing enemas (nonsudsing) until bowel is clear the night before and morning of the study.
	  f. Have patient void.
	  g. Give medications "on call", if ordered.
	3. Provide postprocedure care:
	  a. Check and record vital signs per routine or as ordered.
	  b. Encourage diet, fluids, and activity unless contraindicated.
	  c. Check stools and anus for blood.

Cystometrogram

Patient Outcome	Process

The patient experiences a comfortable, safe, and expedient cystometrogram.
This includes:
A. *Is prepared for study*
	1. Explain/answer questions and listen to concerns about prestudy preparation, procedure, and poststudy care. Information may include:
	  a. ***Purpose:*** To detect abnormalities of urethra and ureters and to evaluate abnormal bladder function, *i.e.*, to measure bladder muscle tone in relation to the volume of fluid in the bladder as well as the patient's report of sensations while bladder is being filled.
	  b. ***Procedure:*** Study is done in Urology Clinic by a nurse. The patient is asked to empty bladder completely prior to study. The patient is positioned on the examination table to facilitate insertion of Foley catheter (female in lithotomy position, and male in supine). The volume of residual urine obtained is measured and recorded. A bottle of sterile water and a catheter are attached to a recording cystometer which allows the bladder pressures to be recorded while the bladder is being filled. The patient is asked to describe all bladder sensations, *e.g.*, first urge to void, first sensation of fullness, inability to tolerate further filling. At the completion of the study the bladder is emptied and the catheter is removed. The length of study varies from 10 to 30 minutes.
	  c. ***Physical preparation:*** None

B. *Is free of or has minimal discomfort or complications following procedure*	2. Provide postprocedure care.
	  a. No restrictions of food, fluid, or activity
	  b. Patient may experience minimal bleeding and burning on urination for short time following study.
	  c. Have patient report large amounts of bright red blood in urine.
	  d. Observe for signs of infection such as chills, temperature greater than 38.5°C, continued urinary burning and frequency, and suprapubic and/or flank pain.

Cystoscopy, panendoscopy

Patient Outcome	Process

The patient experiences a comfortable, safe, and expedient cystoscopy and panendoscopy. This includes:
 	
A. *Is prepared for study*
	1. Explain/answer questions and listen to concerns about prestudy preparation, procedure, and poststudy care. Information may include:
	  a. ***Purposes:***
	    • To inspect the bladder and urethral walls by direct visualization in the diagnostic evaluation of the lower urinary tract. Biopsy of bladder wall may be performed.
	    • To facilitate treatments such as removal of bladder stones, evacuation of blood clots
	    • To allow passage of a ureteral catheter to aid in diagnosis and/or to relieve obstruction
	  b. ***Procedure:*** The study is done in the Urology Clinic by a physician. The patient is put in lithotomy position on the examination table. The external genitalia are prepped with povidone-iodine solution and draped appropriately. A topical anesthetic may be instilled into the urethra to lessen the discomfort. The patient experiences sensations similar to a urinary catheter insertion. The bladder is filled with sterile water to facilitate visualization of the bladder walls.
	    If biopsy of the bladder wall is done, a biopsy forcep is passed through the lumen of the cystoscope and bladder tissue is removed. The patient may experience this as a discomfort, but not a sharp pain.
	    If a ureteral catheter is inserted, it is threaded through the cystoscope and into the ureteral orifice. If an obstruction is present, the catheter may be passed beyond the point of obstruction to facilitate drainage of the kidney. The patient may experience colicky pain, which is usually brief.
	    At the completion of the procedure, the bladder is emptied and the instrument is removed. The length of study varies from 10 to 25 minutes.
	  c. ***Physical preparation:*** None

B. *Is free of or has minimal discomfort or complications following procedure*	2. Provide postprocedure care.
	  a. No restrictions of food, fluid or activity. Force fluids unless contraindicated.
	  b. Patient may experience minimal bleeding and burning on urination for a short time following study.
	  c. Have patient report large amounts of bright red blood in urine.
	  d. If ureteral catheterization was done, patient should be aware that colicky pain may return during the next several hours. Report if pain is severe or prolonged.
	  e. Report signs of infection such as, chills, temperature greater than 38.5°C, continued urinary burning and frequency, and suprapubic and/or flank pain.

Echocardiography

Patient Outcome	Process

The patient experiences a comfortable, safe, and expedient echocardiography
This includes:
A. *Is prepared for study*
	PREFACE: This explanation is applicable to both pediatric and adult patients even though the studies may take place in different settings and involve the use of equipment which differs in appearance and some functions. Two echocardiographic studies are offered and may be ordered by physician as one or both to be done: Time-motion Echo (still); Two-dimensional Echo (moving).
	1. Explain/answer questions and listen to concerns about procedure. Information may include:
	  a. *Purpose:* A noninvasive technique used to visualize the heart and detect structural abnormalities through the use of sound waves directed in a beam. The sound is beyond the range of human hearing (''ultrasound'').
	  b. *Procedure:* The patient lies fully extended on a bed, stretcher, or examining table. The echocardiography machine is placed next to the upper portion of the body. Initially the patient is placed in a supine position but may be examined on the left or right side and in varying degrees of the upright position. Echocardiograph leads may be applied to the limbs or on the patient's chest.
	    An ultrasonic gel material is applied to the precordial area which permits easy movement of the transducer over the skin and airless contact with the chest surface. The microphonic transducer is moved slowly multiple times back and forth over the heart in a vertical or horizontal plane. The microphone emits high frequency sound waves toward the heart where they are reflected back to the microphone. The waves that are received are used to construct a picture of the moving heart, which is temporarily visible on a luminescent screen. Continuous strip chart recordings and/or pictures are taken as a means of permanently recording the study. Because the study is partially dependent on the patient's ability to lie still, it may vary in length from 10 to 45 minutes. If the patient is an infant, study is best performed during sleep or rest period following mealtime.

B. *Is free of or has minimal discomfort or complications following study*	2. Institute immediate preparation of patient for the study.
	  a. No special preparation is indicated.
	  b. Encourage presence of child's caretaker during procedure when this provides a feeling of added security.
	  c. Encourage child to bring along his ''security object'', *e.g.*, teddy bear, pacifier.
	3. No special postprocedure care indicated.

Electromyography

Patient Outcome	Process

The patient experiences a comfortable, safe, and expedient electromyography
This includes:
A. *Is prepared for study*
	1. Explain/answer questions and listen to concerns about prestudy preparation, procedure, and poststudy care. Information may include:
	  a. *Purposes:* To measure muscle activity in response to electrical stimulation in the upper and lower extremities
	  Indications:
	  • To determine presence of neuromuscular disease and localize the site.
	  • To diagnose and differentiate specific nerve lesions, *e.g.*, herniated nucleus pulposus, neuritis, neuropathy, myopathy.
	  b. *Procedure:* The study is done in an office, Physical Therapy Department, or at the bedside. It is conducted by a physician, technician, or therapist. The patient should be in a relaxed, comfortable position, lying or seated. A large rectangular portable machine with a screen (oscilloscope) and a control panel is placed near the patient. Selected skin sites are cleansed with antiseptic solution.
	    A thin sterile needle electrode is placed in the muscle of the nerve being tested. The patient's response to this varies but most patients experience the needle insertion as a pin prick. The needle is connected to the machine which allows a brief electrical impulse to pass through the electrode to the muscle. The patient usually experiences this as a mild electrical ''shock'' followed by muscular twitching. The muscular response to the impulse can be seen as a spiked pattern moving horizontally across the screen and can be heard as a high pitched ''blipping'' sound. A number of sites may be used to compare responses. The study requires 15 to 30 minutes.

B. *Is free of or has minimal discomfort or complications following study*	2. Institute immediate preparation of patient for study.
	  • Alert patient to expect mild discomfort during study.
	3. Provide poststudy care.
	  • Give medications for relief of discomfort as indicated.

Esophagoscopy, gastroscopy, panendoscopy, endoscopic retrograde cholecystopanciatogram (ERCP)

Patient Outcome	Process

The patient experiences a comfortable, safe, and expedient esophagoscopy, gastroscopy, panendoscopy or ERCP.
This includes:
 	
A. *Is prepared for study*
 	
B. *Is free of or has minimal discomfort or complications following study*
	1. Explain/answer questions and listen to concerns about prestudy preparation, procedure, and poststudy care. Information may include:
	  a. **Purpose:** To visualize, detect, and rule out abnormalities of a specific portion of the gastrointestinal tract.
	  b. **Procedure:** Immediately prior to the study the patient is given a topical anesthetic to numb his throat and a sedative intravenously. The patient is placed on his left side and instructed to expectorate all secretions. The scope is passed through the mouth into: the esophagus by the physician who visualizes the wall of the esophagus, cardiac sphincter and may biopsy and/or photograph any lesions present when an esophagoscopy is done; the stomach, pylorus, and duodenum to visualize, biopsy, and photograph any lesions when a gastroscopy is done; the esophagus, stomach, and duodenum to visualize, biopsy, and photograph any lesions when a panendoscopy is done; the duodenum where the pancreatic and common bile ducts enter when an endoscopic retrograde cholecystopanciatogram (ERCP) is done. A retrograde injection of radiopaque dye should allow visualization of the ducts by radiograph.
	2. Institute immediate preparation of the patient for study.
	  a. Keep n.p.o. after midnight.
	  b. Check for signed consent obtained by physician.
	  c. Check for allergy to iodine and shell fish prior to ERCP. Notify physician.
	  d. Have naso-tracheal suction available at bedside.
	3. Provide postprocedure care.
	  a. Keep n.p.o. (until gag reflex returns and patient is alert—at least 3 hours).
	  b. Check and record vital signs per order.
	  c. Check for signs and symptoms of respiratory distress from aspiration such as shortness of breath, change in color, diaphoresis, restlessness.
	  d. Check for signs and symptoms of bleeding such as spitting up blood or passing blood by rectum. Guaiac test all stools for 24 hours if ordered.
	  e. Provide analgesics as ordered and soothing lozenges or ice chips after gag reflex returns.
	  f. Resume appropriate activity.

Gallium scan

Patient Outcome	Process

The patient experiences a safe, comfortable, and expedient gallium scan.
This includes:
 	
A. *Is prepared for study.*
 	
B. *Is free of or has minimal discomfort or complications following study*
	1. Explain/answer questions and listen to concerns about prestudy preparation, procedure, and poststudy care. Information may include:
	  a. **Purpose:** Type A: to observe for septic lesions
	                  Type B: to observe for neoplasms
	  b. **Procedure:** The patient is injected with a tracer amount of ^{67}GA. Imaging occurs at post injection intervals determined by Nuclear Medicine after considering patient's clinical history. An example of image intervals is 4, 24, 48, 72, and 96 hours post-injection. The patient must be able to hold still voluntarily for 20-minute intervals. The female patient (childbearing age) is asked by technologist to sign a statement to verify whether or not she is pregnant. All patients are asked to sign informed consent form.
	  c. **Contraindication:** Pregnancy
	2. Institute immediate preparation of patient for the study.
	  a. Give laxative and enemas until clear, as ordered prior to each scan.
	  b. Evaluate potential need to sedate patient and discuss with physician for order.
	  c. Have patient and chart available to Nuclear Medicine 30 minutes prior to scheduled scan time. Stress with patient need for return visits.
	3. Provide postprocedure care. Anticipate that patient may be weak as result of gastrointestinal preps and examination.

NOTE: Restrict pregnant personnel from caring for patient for one week postinjection.

Patient Outcome

Process

The patient experiences a comfortable, safe, and expedient glucose tolerance test. This includes:

A. *Is prepared for study*

1. Explain/answer questions and listen to concerns about prestudy preparation, procedure, and poststudy care. Information may include:
   a. **Purpose:** To determine the patient's ability to respond to a standard amount of glucose. It is useful in ruling out diabetes mellitus and diagnosing hyperinsulinism.
   b. **Procedure:** The patient is n.p.o. after midnight except for small amounts of water in preparation for test. Water may be given *ad lib.* during the test to ensure voidings at scheduled intervals. An initial urine specimen is collected immediately prior to administering glucose. The glucose is given in a flavored liquid form. Blood and urine specimens are gathered at one half hour after glucose and at one hour intervals until test is completed (3 to 5 hours). Often laboratory personnel and nursing staff collaborate in the steps of this procedure.
   c. **Contraindication** Patients with known diabetes. Patients whose intravenous fluids cannot be discontinued.
2. Institute immediate preparation of the patient for study.
   a. Keep patient n.p.o. after midnight, except for small amounts of water.
   b. Check with physician regarding medications that should not be deferred.
   c. Discontinue all intravenous fluids containing glucose.
   d. Permit no smoking, chewing tobacco or gum containing sugar.

B. *Is free of or has minimal discomfort or complications during study*

3. Provide care during procedure.
   a. Minimize patient activity during test. Keep available for testing.
   b. Observe for signs and symptoms of hypoglycemia such as nausea, vomiting, sweating, shakiness, hunger, change in behavior, confusion.
   c. Notify physician of any abnormal responses.
   d. Provide water *ad lib*.
   e. Observe for bleeding or hematoma as a result of blood drawing. Apply ice as necessary.
4. Provide postprocedure care.
   a. Give appropriate diet and fluids as soon as test completed.
   b. Resume appropriate activity.

Intravenous cholangiogram

Patient Outcome	Process

The patient experiences a comfortable, safe, and expedient intravenous cholangiogram. This includes:
 	
A. *Is prepared for study*
 	
B. *Is free of or has minimal discomfort or complications following study*
	1. Explain/answer questions and listen to concerns about prestudy preparation, procedure, and poststudy care. Information may include:
	  a. ***Purpose:*** To ascertain the patency or obstruction of the common bile duct and biliary tree
	  b. ***Procedure:*** The patient will lie on a hard radiograph table. A dye is given intravenously over a 15 to 30-minute period. Films are taken every 15 minutes until they show visualization of the common duct biliary tree. The study may take one to three hours.
	2. Institute immediate preparation of the patient for study.
	  a. Interview patient for allergies to shellfish or iodine. Notify physician.
	  b. Keep n.p.o. at least three hours prior to study.
	  c. Check for signed consent obtained by physician.
	3. Provide postprocedure care.
	  a. Encourage diet, fluids, and activity unless contraindicated.
	  b. Observe for delayed systemic reaction to dye. Symptoms include skin response; decrease in blood pressure; nausea; vomiting; and less commonly, respiratory distress and anaphylactic shock.
	  c. Notify physician of any abnormal physiologic responses.

Intravenous pyelogram

Patient Outcome	Process

The patient experiences a comfortable, safe, and expedient intravenous pyelogram. This includes:
 	
A. *Is prepared for study*
 	
B. *Is free of or has minimal discomfort or complications following procedure*
	1. Explain/answer question and listen to concerns about prestudy preparation, procedure, and poststudy care. Information may include:
	  a. ***Purpose:*** To detect abnormalities of kidney, renal pelvis, ureter, and bladder.
	  b. ***Procedure:*** Patient is placed on a hard radiograph table. An intravenous bolus of dye is injected into an arm vein or an established IV line may be used for the injection. The radiographs are taken as dye is filtered through the kidneys. The contrast agent may cause a hot, flushed feeling and may be accompanied by nausea. The procedure lasts about one hour.
	2. Institute immediate preparation of the patient for study.
	  a. Interview patient for allergies to shellfish or iodine. Notify physician.
	  b. Give clear liquids evening meal prior to study.
	  c. Give 4 to 6 glasses of clear liquids between evening meal and midnight.
	  d. Give laxative as ordered in p.m.
	  e. Provide fluids as ordered after midnight. Most patients are n.p.o. after midnight with exception of those who are at risk for renal failure, *e.g.,* multiple myeloma, postoperative kidney transplant.
	  f. Give enema if ordered in a.m. Assure that any previously administered barium is evacuated.
	3. Provide postprocedure care.
	  a. Encourage diet, fluids, and activity unless contraindicated.
	  b. Observe for any physiologic responses to dye as oliguria, nausea, and vomiting.
	  c. Report any abnormal physiologic reactions to physician.
	  d. Contraindications: Urine tests for sodium, specific gravity, protein and osmolality and certain 24-hour urine collections (17-hydroxyketosteroids, catecholamines, 17-hydroxy-corticoids will be significantly affected by iodine dye for 12 to 15 hours and, therefore, tests should be avoided during this time. If any PBI is done within 3 to 6 months postintravenous pyelogram, the retained iodine may affect test results.

Patient Outcome	Process

The patient experiences a comfortable, safe, and expedient kidney biopsy. This includes:
 	
A. *Is prepared for study*
	1. Explain/answer questions and listen to concerns about prestudy preparation, procedure, and poststudy care. Information may include:
	  a. ***Purpose:*** To determine the disease process present in patients with renal function abnormalities. Results of the biopsy are used to formulate prognosis and treatment plan.
	  b. ***Procedure:*** Prior to procedure patient is premedicated causing drowsiness. Patient is placed in prone position on stretcher with rolled sheet under the stomach to elevate the kidneys. Left flank is prepped with merthiolate, which feels cold, and draped as a sterile field. Area is injected with a local anesthetic, which stings when injected. Patient may be requested to hold breath during deep penetration of needle. A probe is inserted until it is resting on kidney capsule, at which time the probe will pulsate and move with inspiration and expiration. Patient feels pressure as the probe is inserted but feels no sharp pain. Patient must hold breath as requested by physician when probe is moved. Once it is positioned normal breathing may be resumed. Probe is then removed with depth of kidney noted and measurement marked on biopsy needle. Biopsy needle guide with obturator is inserted with patient holding breath, and proper position rechecked. Obturator is then removed and cutting needle inserted into guide. The cutting needle is rapidly pressed into kidney, creating a clicking sound. Tissue is obtained and needle and obturator removed. This procedure may be repeated to obtain an additional specimen. Pressure and Band-Aid are applied over puncture site and monitoring of vital signs begun.
	    This procedure may be done under fluoroscopy in which case an intravenous infusion is started and a dye is administered intravenously. The kidney is observed while the needle guide is positioned.

	2. Institute immediate preparation of the patient for study.
	  a. Check that results of bleeding and clotting studies are within normal limits and recorded in patient's chart.
	  b. Report abnormal blood pressure to physician.
	  c. Have IVP radiographs available on ward.
	  d. Check for signed consent obtained by physician.
	  e. Keep patient n.p.o. 4 to 6 hours prior to study.
	  f. Have patient void.
	  g. Place patient on stretcher if desired.
	  h. Give a medication as ordered 45 to 60 minutes prior to study.
	  i. Have available appropriate equipment and supplies for procedure such as:
	    • Stretcher with thick pad and side rails
	    • Rolled sheet
	    • Renal biopsy tray
	    • Sterile gloves
	    • Merthiolate
	    • Lidocaine (Xylocaine), 2 per cent
	    • Alcohol wipes
	    • Band-Aid
	    • Blood pressure cuff and stethoscope
	    • Sterile specimen container with desired solution

B. *Is free of or has minimal discomfort or complications following study*	3. Provide postprocedure care:
	  a. Check and record vital signs as ordered. Usual frequency is q 15 minutes × 6 hours; q 30 minutes × 6 hours; q 1 hour × 4 hours; then q 4 hours × 24 hours.
	  b. Keep prone on stretcher if used for one and a half hours then gently roll patient into bed.
	  c. Discourage coughing, sneezing, retching. Report nausea.
	  d. Observe site for bleeding, swelling. Be alert to patient reports of retro-peritoneal pain.
	  e. Notify physician of any abnormal physiologic reaction to procedure.
	4. Force fluids and provide diet unless restricted.
	5. Save and label all voidings individually (serial urines) for 24 hours. Observe for blood. (Some hematuria may be normal and should gradually clear).
	6. Keep patient on bed rest for 24 hours, on back or on side of biopsy.
	7. Check for order and record of results of hemotocrit the evening of test and the next morning.
	8. If discharge is planned, give patient instructions such as:
	  a. Avoid straining, heavy lifting, strenuous physical activity for 2 to 3 weeks.
	  b. Report hematuria, bleeding at site, swelling, or pain to physician.

Patient Outcome	Process

The patient experiences a comfortable, safe, and expedient liver biopsy. This includes:

A. *Is prepared for study*

1. Explain/answer questions and listen to concerns about prestudy preparation, procedure, and poststudy care. Information may include:
    a. **Purpose:** To determine disease process present in patients with suspected liver disease
    b. **Precautions:** Patients on anticoagulants should have them discontinued approximately two days prior to biopsy so that prothrombin time is within normal limits. Aquamephyton may be ordered to counteract reduced coagulation. Anticoagulants should not be resumed until approximately two days postbiopsy.
    c. **Procedure:** The patient is placed flat on his back, close to the right edge of bed. The patient's right arm is placed under his head. Insertion site is determined by percussion. The site is rubbed vigorously with antiseptic solution (which feels cold) and draped as a sterile field. A local anesthetic is used which stings when injected. The patient is requested to hold his breath during deep penetration of this needle. The large biopsy needle is inserted between the ribs. While this is happening, the patient must remain absolutely still and hold his breath as requested by the physician. The sudden action which follows may startle the patient. When in position, the needle is abruptly pushed through the chest wall into the liver, and liver tissue is aspirated into a saline-filled syringe. The needle is in the liver less than a second. The quantity of tissue is checked and, if sufficient, the procedure is ended. Another sample may be needed. A Band-Aid is applied and the patient assisted to right-side lying position where he will remain for two hours. Monitoring of vital signs and observing for increased severity of pain are begun.
2. Institute immediate preparation of patient for study.
    a. Check that bleeding and clotting studies are within normal limits and recorded in patient's chart.
    b. Check for signed consent obtained by physician.
    c. Interview patient for allergies to skin preparation solution or lidocaine (Xylocaine). Notify physician.
    d. Keep patient n.p.o. an hour prior to study.
    e. Have patient void immediately before procedure.
    f. Have available appropriate equipment and supplies for procedure such as,
        • Liver biopsy tray with Klapskin needle
        • Sterile gloves
        • Povidone-iodine
        • Lidocaine (Xylocaine), 1 per cent
        • Sterile saline, without preservative (15 cc)
        • Band-Aid
        • Sterile culture tubes
        • Blood pressure cuff, stethoscope

B. *Is free of or has minimal discomfort or complications following study*

3. Provide postprocedure care.
    a. Check and record physiologic responses as ordered. Usual frequency is q 15 minutes × 4; q 30 minutes × 4; q 1 hour × 4; and q 4 hours × 4. Check:
        • Vital signs
        • Puncture site for bleeding
        • Presence of severe discomfort in right upper quadrant, shortness of breath
    b. Notify physician of any abnormal physiologic reactions to procedure.
    c. Keep patient on bedrest for 24 hours.
    d. Encourage diet and fluids unless contraindicated.

Patient Outcome	Process

The patient experiences a comfortable, safe, and expedient liver scan. This includes:
 	
A. *Is prepared for study*
 	
B. *Is free of or has minimal discomfort or complications following study.*
	1. Explain/answer questions and listen to concerns about prestudy preparation, procedure, and poststudy care. Information may include:
	  a. ***Purpose:*** To observe for liver abnormalities resulting from neoplasm, trauma, infection and/or hepatocellular disease
	  b. ***Procedure:*** The patient receives an abdominal radiograph to determine the position of the kidneys, liver, and spleen. If barium is noted in the hepatic flexure, laxatives and/or enemas may be required before the study can proceed. The patient is injected with a tracer amount of radiopharmaceutical followed by scanning in six positions. The patient must be able to hold still voluntarily for 20-minute intervals. The female patient (child bearing age) is asked by technologist to sign a statement to verify whether or not she is pregnant.
	  c. ***Contraindications:*** Pregnancy or barium examinations within 96 hours prior to liver scan.
	2. Institute immediate preparation of patient for the study.
	  a. Evaluate potential need to sedate patient and discuss with physician for order.
	  b. Have patient and chart available to Nuclear Medicine 30 minutes prior to examination.
	3. No special postprocedure care is indicated.
	
	NOTE: Restrict pregnant personnel from caring for patient for 24 hours.

Lumbar puncture

Patient Outcome	Process

The patient experiences a comfortable, safe, and expedient lumbar puncture.
 This includes:
 	
 A. *Is prepared for study*
	1. Explain/answer questions and listen to concerns about prestudy preparation, procedure, and poststudy care. Information may include:
	   a. ***Purposes:***
	     • To measure cerebrospinal fluid pressure
	     • To obtain cerebrospinal fluid (CSF) for analysis (cells, protein, glucose, cytology, other chemistries, culture, sensitivity, and electrophoresis)
	     • To inject medication intrathecally (into subarachnoid space)
	     • To reduce cerebrospinal fluid pressure
	   b. ***Procedure:*** Patient is assisted into lateral, curled fetal position with back at very edge of bed. Sterile towel or absorbent pad is placed under hip. The puncture site is prepped with antiseptic, which feels cold to patient, and sterile field is maintained. A local anesthetic may be used. Patient will experience pressure as spinal needle is inserted between vertebral spines into subarachnoid space below level of spinal cord. The CSF pressure will be measured by physician with manometer. If patient experiences leg pain, reassure him that it is transient. Opening and closing pressures and appearance of CSF will be recorded in patient's chart.
	   c. ***Contraindications:*** Patients with symptoms of mass lesions in brain or spine or an open skin wound in lumbar area.
	   d. ***Special consideration:*** Determine if patient had had prior lumbar puncture. Reinforce information that most patients tolerate procedure well and have a minimum of postprocedure discomfort.
	 2. Institute immediate preparation of patient for study.
	   a. Check that consent is obtained by physician, which may be verbal.
	   b. Have available appropriate equipment and supplies, such as lumbar puncture tray, gloves, lidocaine (Xylocaine), and antiseptic solution.

B. *Is free of or has minimal discomfort or complications following study*	3. Provide postprocedure care.
	   a. Keep flat in bed (may turn side to side, or use small pillow) for 4 to 6 hours.
	   b. Encourage fluids and diet unless contraindicated.
	   c. Resume vital signs and other orders.
	   d. Provide pain medications p.r.n.
	   e. Encourage patient to lie flat, give analgesics and force fluids if he complains of headache when upright.

Lung scan

Patient Outcome	Process

The patient experiences a comfortable, safe, and expedient lung scan.
 This includes:
 	
 A. *Is prepared for study*
	1. Explain/answer questions and listen to concerns about prestudy preparation, procedure, and poststudy care. Information may include:
	   a. ***Purpose:*** To observe for pulmonary emboli
	   b. ***Procedure:*** The patient is injected with a tracer amount of radiopharmaceutical and images are taken in six positions. The patient then breathes radioactive gas for three minutes. The patient continues to breathe through a closed system until all radioactive gas has been cleared. The patient must be able to hold still voluntarily for 30-minute intervals. The female patient (childbearing age) is asked by technologist to sign a statement to verify whether or not she is pregnant.
	   c. ***Contraindication:*** Pregnancy
	 2. Institute immediate preparation of patient for the study.
	   a. Evaluate potential need to sedate patient and discuss with physician for order.
	   b. Transport patient with chart by stretcher to Nuclear Medicine 30 minutes prior to the study.

B. *Is free of or has minimal discomfort following study*	3. No special postprocedure care is indicated. **NOTE:** Restrict pregnant personnel from caring for patient for 24 hours.

Lymphangiogram

Patient Outcome	Process

The patient experiences a comfortable, safe, and expedient lymphangiogram.
This includes:
A. Is prepared for study
	1. Explain/answer questions and listen to concerns about prestudy preparation, procedure, and poststudy care. Information may include:
	  a. ***Purpose:*** To detect abnormalities of the lymphatic system, *e.g.,* lymphoma, metastatic disease, lymphedema, lymph vessel tumors
	  b. ***Procedure:*** The patient is placed in a supine position on a stretcher or radiograph table and his feet are prepped with antimicrobial solution. A small amount of Qhiline blue dye is injected into two sites on the top of each foot. As the dye moves into the lymphatic system, it permits visualization of small lymph vessels in each foot. A single vessel in each foot is selected and, by way of a "cutdown", the radiologist threads into it a tiny needle with a catheter attached. Radiopaque dye is slowly pumped into both vessels at the same time (taking approximately 40 minutes) while the patient remains as quiet as possible. Radiograph pictures are taken as the dye progresses through the entire lymphatic system. The contrast material leaves the lungs by entering the alveoli, passing through capillaries, passing through shunts in venous system, and is broken down by enzymatic activity. The needles are removed and the skin is sutured. Films of the abdomen, pelvis, and thorax are taken immediately and again 24 hours later. Length of procedure is approximately 1½ to 2 hours. Children may need to be sedated prior to the study to help them tolerate procedure and the time frame more easily. Length of procedure for children is approximately one hour.
	  c. ***Contraindications:*** Patients with severe respiratory insufficiency, known allergic response to iodine or shellfish, or concurrent radiotherapy to lungs
	2. Institute immediate preparation of the patient for study.
	  a. Scrub feet with antimicrobial solution the evening before and day of procedure.
	  b. Give diet and fluids *ad lib.*
	  c. Check for signed consent obtained by physician.
	  d. Give "on-call" medication as ordered.

B. Is free of or has minimal discomfort or complications following study	3. Provide postprocedure care.
	  a. Keep patient on bedrest with legs elevated above hips for 12 hours.
	  b. Observe for physiologic responses to procedure such as respiratory distress, hypotensive reactions, hypertensive reactions, skin reactions, nausea and vomiting, and fever.
	  c. Inspect injection sites for swelling, hematoma, or drainage.
	  d. Notify physician immediately of any abnormal reactions to study.
	  e. Be prepared to provide supportive therapy if needed such as oxygen, steroids, and antihistamines.
	  f. Encourage diet and fluids unless contraindicated.
	  g. Reassure patient that appearance of dye in feet is normal and will slowly disappear over a period of 6 to 18 months.

Metabolic bone survey

Patient Outcome	Process

The patient experiences a comfortable, safe, and expedient metabolic bone survey. This includes:
 	
A. Is prepared for study
 	
B. Is free of or has minimal discomfort or complications following study
	1. Explain/answer questions and listen to concerns about prestudy preparation, procedure, and poststudy care. Information may include:
	  a. ***Purpose:*** To diagnose presence and extent of bone abnormalities; useful in diagnosing illness which involves a loss of calcium
	  b. ***Procedure:*** Radiographs are taken in the Radiology Department of selected bones, *e.g.,* long bones, hands, clavicles, skull, and pelvis.
	2. No special immediate physical preparation or postprocedure care is indicated.

Myelogram using oil contrast, Pantopaque

Patient Outcome	Process

The patient experiences a comfortable, safe, and expedient myelogram. This includes:

A. *Is prepared for study*

1. Explain/answer questions and listen to concerns about prestudy preparation, procedure, and poststudy care. Information may include:
   a. **Purpose:** To visualize the spinal canal for identification of abnormalities, *e.g.*, disc rupture, neoplasm, arachnitis
   b. **Procedure:** The patient is usually positioned prone on a hard radiograph table with a pillow under his abdomen. The physician preps the lower back with a cool antiseptic solution prior to inserting the lumber puncture needle between the vertebrae into the subarachnoid space (below level of spinal cord). A small amount of cerebrospinal fluid is removed and sent for analysis. Contrast material is injected and the patient is tilted on the table so that the dye will flow to the spinal region(s) to be visualized. Radiographs are taken. When the contrast agent is removed by aspiration through the spinal needle, the patient may experience radicular pain (sudden, brief, electrifying pain in either leg) as a result of traction on or irritation of nerve roots. Repeated tilting may be necessary to remove the contrast agent. Entire procedure usually lasts about one hour.
   c. **Special consideration:** Determine if patient has had prior experience with a myelogram or heard reports from others having study. Reinforce information that most patients tolerate procedure well and have a minimum of postprocedure discomforts.
2. Institute immediate preparation of the patient for study.
   a. Interview patient for allergies to seafood or iodine or previous reactions to contrast media. Notify physician.
   b. Keep n.p.o. after light breakfast if study done in afternoon.
   c. Check for signed consent obtained by physician.
   d. Have patient void prior to test.
   e. Determine baseline motor and sensory function.
   f. Give medications as ordered before study.
   g. Transport to the Radiology Department on stretcher.

B. *Is free of or has minimal discomfort or complications following study*

3. Provide postprocedure care.
   a. Keep patient flat in bed 8 to 12 hours without pillow. May lie on side and flex knees. Check with physician if patient prefers pillow.
   b. Compare motor and sensory function with baseline data: if cervical myelogram done, check upper and lower extremities function and bladder control; if lumbar myelogram done, check lower extremities function and bladder control.
   c. Notify physician of any abnormal physiologic response to study.
   d. Manage postprocedure pain:
      • Reassure patient that increased pain level is usually temporary.
      • Evaluate effectiveness of analgesics. May require additional analgesic order from physician
      • Consider other measures for pain relief.
   e. Provide increased fluid intake of 2 to 3 liters daily and diet as tolerated.
   f. Facilitate voiding before patient becomes distended. Obtain premission from physician for patient to sit or stand for voiding.
   g. Anticipate that patients who have total blockage will require closer neurological observation and/or transfer to special-care area.

Patient Outcome

Process

The patient experiences a comfortable, safe, and expedient oral chole-cystogram.
This includes:
A. *Is prepared for study*

1. Explain/answer questions and listen to concerns about prestudy preparation, procedure, and poststudy care. Information may include:
   a. **Purpose:** To detect stones, obstructions, or other abnormalities of gallbladder or common duct
   b. **Procedure:** This is a very short and painless procedure. Radiographs are taken of the gallbladder in a standing and lying position. Visualization of the gallbladder is made possible by the radiopaque medications taken the evening before the study. If inadequate visualization occurs, the patient will receive additional radiopaque medications and the study will be repeated in the same manner the next day. Repeating studies the next day does not mean the gallbladder is abnormal.
2. Institute immediate preparation of the patient for study.
   a. Interview patient for allergies to shellfish or iodine.
   b. Give radiopaque medication, as ordered, prior to 9:00 p.m.
   c. Keep patient n.p.o. after midnight.

B. *Is free of or has minimal discomfort or complications following study*

3. Provide postprocedure care. Encourage food, fluids, and activity unless contraindicated.

Pneumoencephalogram, ventriculogram, cervical air myelogram

Patient Outcome	Process

The patient experiences a comfortable, safe, and expedient pneumoencephalogram, ventriculogram, and cervical air myelogram.
This includes:

A. *Is prepared for study*

1. Explain/answer questions and listen to concerns about prestudy preparation, procedure, and poststudy care. Information may include:
   a. ***Purpose:*** A pneumoencephalogram or a ventriculogram is done to visualize the size and patency of the ventricular system and identify abnormalities. A cervical air myelogram is done to visualize the high cervical and posterior fossa regions. Radiographs taken during these procedures may be used in the Operating Room to facilitate surgical approach and procedure.
   b. ***Procedure:*** Most patients have local standby anesthesia; children and confused patients may require general anesthesia. Throughout these studies there is constant monitoring of the patient's neurological and systemic status. In rare instances, unexpected lesions may be identified which will require immediate surgical intervention.
      - Pneumoencephalogram: The initial procedure followed is the same as that for a lumbar puncture except the patient may be in a seated position instead of lateral. After some cerebrospinal fluid is removed, a small amount of air is injected and skull radiographs taken to assure that it is safe to proceed with the study. More air is injected and various radiograph views are taken which require the patient to move to upright, prone, and supine positions. The physician may move the patient's head back and forth in order to distribute the air and patient may hear the air moving within his ventricles. The radiograph equipment is large and may convey the feeling that the head is "closed in". After the air is injected, the patient may experience any of the following: severe pressure headache, nausea, vomiting, diaphoresis, head "heaviness", dizziness, syncope and chills. The study usually takes one hour.
      - Ventriculogram: Air is injected directly into the ventricles in the following manner: a small area of hair in the frontal region is shaved, the skin is prepped, and local anesthetic injected. A small scalp incision is made, a hole is drilled in the skull and a spinal needle is inserted into a ventricle. The patient will feel some pressure and hear the sounds of the drill. Air is injected and the study proceeds in the same way as in a pneumoencephalogram When the study is completed, the scalp incision is sutured and a collodion dressing applied.
      - Cervical air myelogram: The procedure is the same as for pneumoencephalography except that the patient leans forward with the chin down until the cervical region is higher than the head. Air is slowly injected via lumbar puncture and multiple radiographs of the neck are obtained. The patient is then allowed to sit upright and the air rises into the head, filling the ventricular system, and films are obtained.
   c. ***Contraindications:*** A pneumoencephalogram is usually contraindicated in a patient with known increased intracranial pressure; a ventriculogram may be done instead.
2. Institute immediate preparation of the patient for the study.
   a. Keep patient n.p.o. after midnight.
   b. Check for signed consent for study including permission for a possible craniotomy obtained by physician.
   c. Have patient void prior to study.
   d. Have patient remove dentures or removable bridgework.
   e. Give medication prior to test as ordered.
   f. Give shampoo as ordered when patient is expected to go to Operating Room after the study.

B. *Is free of or has minimal discomfort or complications following study*

3. Provide postprocedure care.
   a. Monitor and record neurological status frequently. Usual frequency: q 15 minutes × 4; q 30 minutes × 4; q 1 hour × 16; then q 4 hours unless otherwise indicated
      - Level of consciousness
      - Pupil reaction
      - Motor response
      - Vital signs
   b. Report any abnormal physiologic response to study such as:
      - Increasingly difficult to arouse and pupillary change
      - Motor weakness
      - Irregular respiratory pattern
      - Marked changes in blood pressure, temperature, pulse, and respirations
   c. Anticipate temperature elevation and chills as a result of meningeal irritation due to air in cerebral spinal fluid.
   d. Provide comfort measures for headache and/or nausea such as:
      - Position flat and minimize head movement.
      - Provide antiemetics as ordered.
      - Apply cold, wet washcloth to forehead.

Patient Outcome	Process
	• Reassure patient that headache gradually diminishes, although some degree of headache may persist for days. • Provide dark, quiet environment if photophobia is present. e. Encourage extra fluids and diet as tolerated unless contraindicated. f. Individualize progression of activity according to headache.

Pulmonary function tests

Patient Outcome	Process
The patient experiences comfortable, safe, and expedient pulmonary function tests. *This includes:* **A.** *Is prepared for study*	1. Explain/answer questions and listen to concerns about prestudy preparation, study, and poststudy care. Information may include: a. ***Purpose:*** To evaluate respiratory function; to identify abnormalities of the airways, alveoli, and pulmonary vascular bed; to determine effectiveness of therapy, *e.g.,* after bronchodilation in patients with obstructive lung disease. b. ***Procedure:*** The patient is taken to the Pulmonary Function Laboratory and allowed to rest on the examining table. Blood gases are drawn by arterial puncture. The patient sits in chair next to the spirometer and is instructed by the technician in a clear, loud voice to perform a series of breathing tasks. The tasks include blowing out air forcefully through the mouth, panting, and inhaling completely. The nostrils are pinched off with a nose clip so only the mouth is used for breathing. The procedure is very tiring and may cause the patient to experience shortness of breath. The study can be interrupted to allow rest period. The study usually requires about 30 minutes.
B. *Is free of or has minimal discomfort or complications following study*	2. No special prestudy care indicated. 3. Provide poststudy care. a. Resume activity, diet, and fluids as indicated. b. Provide quiet environment to promote rest.

Schilling test

Patient Outcome	Process
The patient experiences a comfortable, safe, and expedient Schilling test. *This includes:* **A.** *Is prepared for study* **B.** *Is free of or has minimal discomfort or complications following study*	1. Explain/answer questions and listen to concerns about prestudy preparation, procedure, and poststudy care. Information may include: a. ***Purpose:*** To determine the GI absorption of vitamin B–12 to detect pernicious anemia b. ***Procedure:*** The patient is given a tracer amount of vitamin B–12 labeled radiopharmaceutical and 1000 micrograms of vitamin B–12 intramuscular (IM) 2. Institute immediate preparation of patient for the study. a. Keep n.p.o. after midnight on the day special study medications are given. 3. No special postprocedure care is indicated.

Small bowel follow-through study

Patient Outcome	Process

The patient experiences a comfortable, safe, and expedient small bowel follow-through study. This includes:
 	
A. *Is prepared for study*
 	
B. *Is free of or has minimal discomfort or complications following study*
	1. Explain/answer questions and listen to concerns about prestudy preparation, procedure, and poststudy care. Information may include:
	  a. ***Purpose:*** To detect/rule out small bowel lesions, obstructions, or abnormalities
	  b. ***Procedure:*** The patient will be asked to swallow a large cup of fruit-flavored barium. He lies on a hard table while the doctor is doing the examination, using a television-like screen (fluoroscope). The patient will need to change positions while the radiologist palpates the abdomen. Radiographs will be taken every 30 minutes until barium advances through small bowel (usually two hours).
	2. Institute immediate preparation of the patient for study.
	  a. Give laxatives and/or enemas as ordered if patient had a barium enema the previous day.
	  b. Keep patient n.p.o. after midnight.
	  c. Instruct "no smoking" day of test since smoking increases flow of digestive fluids.
	3. Provide postprocedure care.
	  a. Encourage diet, fluids, and activity unless contraindicated.
	  b. Give laxative order p.r.n.
	  c. Check that patient has a satisfactory bowel evacuation.

Stool studies

Patient Outcome	Process

The patient experiences comfortable, safe, and expedient stool studies. This includes:
 	
A. *Is prepared for study*
 	
B. *Is free of or has minimal discomfort or complications following study*
	1. Explain/answer questions and listen to concerns about prestudy preparation, procedure, and poststudy care. (Minimize embarrassment through assuring privacy and permitting patient to take as much responsibility for collecting specimen as possible.) Information may include:
	  a. ***Purpose:*** To determine the character and composition of the stool specimen
	    • Routine: For enteric pathogens (Salmonella, Shigella, Yersinia)
	    • Ova and parasites: For intestinal parasites and eggs
	    • Fat: For determination of the ability of the body to metabolize fats
	    • Guaiac: For occult blood not visible to naked eye
	  b. ***Procedure:***
	    • Routine: Collect fresh specimen, place in stool cup, label properly, and send to laboratory. Can be refrigerated.
	    • Ova, parasites: Keep specimen warm and send to laboratory immediately so that motion of parasites can be seen through microscope.
	    • Twelve-Hour Fecal Fat (Fat Balance): Obtain special container from laboratory. Give high fat diet ordered by physician. Be sure patient eats all the food. Record accurate food intake. Dietician will record calorie count. Emphasize to patient that capsules are simply colored markers and will produce temporary red stools. Give three carmen red capsules and note time on record. Instruct patient to notify nurse when he passes first red-colored stool. Discard this stool. Save *all* stools after this time and place in special container in specimen refrigerator. Seventy-two hours after first capsules are taken, administer three more carmen red capsules. Instruct patient to continue to save all stools until the next red-colored stool. Discard this stool. This ends the test. Send all stools in special container to laboratory.
	    • Guaiac: Collect fresh specimen, place in stool cup, label properly, and send to laboratory.
	2. No special immediate preparation of patient for study or postprocedure care is indicated.

Patient Outcome

Process

The patient experiences a safe, comfortable, and expedient thermogram. This includes:

A. *Is prepared for the study*

B. *Is free of or has minimal discomfort or complications following study*

1. Explain/answer questions and listen to concerns about prestudy preparation, procedure, and poststudy care. Information may include:
   a. ***Purpose:*** Diagnosis of fractures, sprains, contusions, bone tumors/metastases, back injuries, early osteomyelitis
   b. ***Procedure:*** The patient is taken to a special area. The body area to be examined is exposed and cooled to room temperature. Heat radiation from the affected area is measured by a scanning instrument. The variations in surface temperatures are photographically displayed and "hot" and "cool" areas can thus be identified.
2. No special preparation for the study is indicated.
3. No special poststudy care is indicated.

Thyroid uptake and/or scan

Patient Outcome	Process

The patient experiences a comfortable, safe, and expedient thyroid uptake and/or scan.
This includes:
 	
A. *Is prepared for study*
	1. Explain/answer questions and listen to concerns about prestudy preparation, procedure, and poststudy care. Information may include:
	  a. ***Purpose:*** To observe thyroid function and thereby to demonstrate thyroid abnormalities
	  b. ***Procedure:*** The patient is given a tracer amount of radioisotope by mouth in Nuclear Medicine. The patient is instructed to return to Nuclear Medicine in four hours, if necessary, and 24 hours in all cases. Upon return to Nuclear Medicine, the patient is positioned with the neck hyperextended under a scintillation counter. This position is held for eight minutes. The patient is then positioned under a scanner and a scan obtained. During the scan the patient cannot move, talk, or swallow. While in the hyperextended position and after the scan has been completed, the patient's thyroid gland is palpated and observations are indicated on the scan. The patient must be able to hold the neck in a hyperextended position for 40 minutes unassisted. The female patient (childbearing age) is asked by technologist to sign a statement to verify whether or not she is pregnant.
	  c. ***Contraindications:*** Rheumatoid arthritis, pregnancy
	    • Technologist will interview patient for any previous exposure to iodine preparation, *e.g.,* IVP, cholecystogram, nephrotomogram, myelogram, CT scan with enhancement, all angiograms and cardiac catheterizations, or in medications, diet, and environment.
	2. Institute immediate preparation of patient for the study. Have patient and chart available to Nuclear Medicine 30 minutes prior to the study.

B. *Is free of or has minimal discomfort or complications following study*	3. Provide postprocedure care. Provide supervision and assistance as necessary if patient is dizzy as result of positioning during study.

Total body Iodine-131 survey for thyroid cancer

Patient Outcome	Process

The patient experiences a comfortable, safe, and expedient total body ^{131}*Iodine survey.*
This includes:
 	
A. *Is prepared for study*
	1. Explain/answer questions and listen to concerns about prestudy preparation, procedure, and poststudy care. Information may include:
	  a. ***Purpose:*** To observe for metastasis of thyroid cancer. If scan is positive, the patient will be considered for ^{131}I therapy.
	  b. ***Procedure:*** The patient is given a tracer amount of ^{131}I by mouth in Nuclear Medicine. The patient has a total body scan two hours following SS enemas (this is always done early a.m.). The patient must be able to hold still voluntarily for a 90-minute interval.
	2. Institute immediate preparation of patient for the study
	  a. Check that all female patients between ages 12 to 60 have had a urinary chorionic gonadotropin test completed prior to radioisotope dose.
	  b. Give laxative as ordered the evening prior to study.
	  c. Give SS enemas until clear as ordered prior to scanning time.
	  d. Evaluate potential need to sedate patient (these patients are usually very apprehensive) and discuss with physician for order.
	  e. Have patient and chart available to Nuclear Medicine 30 minutes prior to giving drug and/or scanning.

B. *Is free of or has minimal discomfort or complications following study*	3. Provide postprocedure care. • Notify Nuclear Medicine technologist if any problem occurs or if patient has questions.

NOTE: Restrict pregnant personnel from caring for patient for five days.

Treadmill study

Patient Outcome	Process

The patient experiences a comfortable, safe, and expedient treadmill study. This includes:
 	
A. *Is prepared for study*
	1. Explain/answer questions and listen to concerns about prestudy preparation, procedure, and poststudy care. Information may include:
	  a. ***Purpose:*** To determine changes on the exercise cardiogram which would indicate ischemic coronary artery disease and/or to look for life-threatening arrhythmias which might be brought on by exercise
	  b. ***Procedure:*** Twelve-lead EKG electrodes are taped to patient's chest and arms. The patient walks on a moving belt, starting at a slow speed and slight incline. Every three minutes the speed and incline are increased slightly and a short strip of electrocardiogram is taken by a technician just before changing to the next stage. Often blood pressures are taken during the study. There may be as many as seven incline and speed changes. Many patients stop in the third stage because of fatigue, chest pain, or shortness of breath. The technician may stop the treadmill if the patient complains of any discomfort or the ST segment on the EKG changes or the patient complains of any discomfort changes. The patient can stop the treadmill by pushing a red button which is within easy reach. After the treadmill the patient will sit down until his pulse is near the preexercise rate. Usually two technicians (and sometimes a physician) are in attendance.

	2. Institute immediate preparation of the patient for study.
	  a. Keep patient n.p.o. five hours prior to the study.
	  b. Check for signed consent obtained by physician.
	  c. Instruct adult patient to wear nonskid slippers or shoes. Children may wear tennis shoes.
	  d. Encourage parents to accompany child to study.

B. *Is free of or has minimal discomfort or complications following study*	3. Provide postprocedure care. No special care is indicated unless patient has complications during study for which special orders will be written by physician.

Twenty-four-hour urine study

Patient Outcome	Process

The patient experiences a comfortable, safe, and expedient 24-hour urine study. This includes:
 	
A. *Is prepared for study*
	1. Explain/answer questions and listen to concerns about prestudy preparation, procedure, and poststudy care. Information may include:
	  a. ***Purpose:*** To determine composition and/or volume of urine
	  b. ***Procedure:*** Have patient empty bladder, discard urine and note time and date. Label container for 24-hour urine, patient's name, and time study started. Save all urine thereafter for 24 hours and place in this container. At completion of 24-hour period, have patient void again and place urine in container. Note time test completed on label, attach appropriate specimen slips, and send to proper laboratory. In the event that time period is altered from 24 hours, note actual length of time on label. If urine samples are missing, but amount is known, note this on label. To compute the results of the test, the exact amount of urine and time interval of collection must be known.

	c. ***Special considerations***
	    • Urine for catecholamines or for lead or arsenic must not touch metal such as urinal, bedpan, bottle cap, etc.
	    • Urines for lead or arsenic must be placed in special containers labeled by laboratory. These have been washed with nitric acid to remove any lead and arsenic particles.
	    • Certain collections may be altered by medications, degree of warmth. For example:
	      Catecholamines: Must be refrigerated; drug interferences include L-Dopa, Quinidine, Aldomet, iodine-based dye
	      17-hydroxycorticoids: Must be refrigerated; drug interferences are numerous and include many sedatives, antihypertensives. Check with physician or laboratory technician. Noninterfering drugs include aspirin, phenobarbital, and iodine-based dye
	      Vanillymandelic Acid (VMA): No drug or food or dye interference
	    • Urine collections for protein may be affected by menstruation. Provide careful perineal care before each specimen.
	    • Other urine collections should be refrigerated to control odor but leaving them at room temperature will not affect laboratory testing.
	    • Twenty-four-hour urine for oxylates: Add 25 cc of dilute hydrochloric acid or obtain already prepared container from laboratory.

B. *Is free of or has minimal discomfort or complications following study*	2. Institute immediate preparations of patient for study. Keep patient well hydrated unless fluid restricted. 3. No special postprocedure care is indicated.

Ultrasonography (abdominal, gall bladder, renal)

Patient Outcome	Process

The patient experiences a comfortable, safe, and expedient ultrasono-graphy.
A. *Is prepared for study*
	1. Explain/answer questions and listen to concerns about prestudy preparation, procedure, and poststudy care. Information may include:
	  a. ***Purpose:*** To identify normalities and abnormalities of structures and spaces within the abdomen or pelvis through transmission of sound waves
	    • Abdomen may include pancreas, liver, aorta, pelvis, surrounding lymph nodes
	    • Gallbladder
	    • Renal area and retroperitoneum
	    • Pelvic
	  b. ***Procedure:*** The patient is taken to the Radiology Department and placed on a stretcher in supine position (prone position for renal). Skin over the area to be studied is exposed and lubricated with mineral oil. The oil seals out any air between the skin and the transducer and decreases discomfort of the transducer rubbing on the skin. The physician or technician rubs the microphonic transducer slowly over the skin surface many times in a horizontal or vertical plane. This process communicates a visual image of structures within the area of study to a screen. Polaroid pictures are taken of the screen as a permanent record of the study. The patient will need to lie still and may be asked not to breathe for brief periods. Discomforts may include a ticklish sensation due to the transducer or abdominal discomfort. Patients who must drink large quantities of water to distend the bladder may find this fullness uncomfortable. The study usually takes 20 to 30 minutes.
	  c. ***Precautions:*** Barium interferes with ultrasound examination of the abdomen. Studies involving barium should be done after ultrasonography or at least 48 hours prior to ultrasound procedure and after vigorous bowel preparation.
	2. Institute immediate preparation of the patient for study.
	  a. Abdominal ultrasonography:
	    • Give low carbohydrate diet for 48 hours prior to study.
	    • Allow no carbonated beverages 48 hours prior to study.
	    • Encourage patient to drink large quantities of water (six cups). If unable, patient may receive nonmedicated intravenous fluids.
	    • Clamp catheter one-half hour prior to study if patient is on urinary drainage.
	  b. Gallbladder: Keep n.p.o. after midnight.
	  c. Renal: No special preparation
	  d. Pelvis: Patient must have full bladder; either by drinking large quantities of water (six cups) or receiving intravenous fluids (without medications). Patient with urinary catheter will have it clamped for one-half hour prior to study.
	  e. Give medication (sedative) if ordered.
	3. No special postprocedure care is indicated.

B. *Is free of or has minimal discomfort or complications following study*	

Upper-gastrointestinal series

Patient Outcome	Process

The patient experiences a comfortable, safe, and expedient upper-gastro-intestinal series. This includes:
 	
A. *Is prepared for study*
	1. Explain/answer questions and listen to concerns about prestudy preparation, procedure, and poststudy care. Information may include:
	  a. ***Purpose:*** To detect presence of or rule out lesions, abnormalities, or obstructions in the esophagus, stomach, and duodenum
	  b. ***Procedure:*** The patient will be asked to swallow a large cup of fruit-flavored barium. He lies on a hard table while the doctor is doing the examination using a television-like screen (fluoroscope). The patient will need to change positions while the radiologist palpates the abdomen. Radiographs will be taken throughout the procedure.
	  c. ***Scheduling considerations:*** Barium may prevent good visualization necessary to other studies, *e.g.*, intravenous pyelogram, arteriogram, Nuclear Medicine examinations, and ultrasonography.
	2. Institute immediate preparation of patient for study.
	  a. Keep patient n.p.o. after midnight.
	  b. Instruct "no smoking" day of test since smoking increases flow of digestive juices.
	3. Provide postprocedure care.

B. *Is free of or has minimal discomfort or complications following study*	a. Encourage diet, fluids, and activity unless contraindicated.
	  b. Give laxative order p.r.n.
	  c. Check that patient has a satisfactory bowel evacuation.

CHAPTER IV
Guidelines for the patient with a medical illness

INTRODUCTION: This section presents information about the care of patients who have specific medical illnesses. The effect of the understanding of the critical elements of care accomplished through key nursing activities on the desired patient outcomes is set forth.

Frequently diagnostic studies are required to confirm the diagnosis or evaluate the patient's progress. In these instances the reader is referred to Chapter 3 Guidelines For The Patient Undergoing Diagnostic Studies, p. 33. When pertinent to the skilled care requirements of patients with specific medical illnesses and the desired patient outcomes, reference is made to Chapter 1 Guidelines for General Care, and Chapter 2 Guidelines for Basic Care when There Is Deviation From Normal.

The guidelines describing nursing intervention in the care of the oncology patient are grouped in the last segment of this section to facilitate the reader's frequent need to cross-reference the material.

The care of patients with medical illness is a multidisciplinary effort. One should not hesitate to consult and plan on behalf of the patient with the patient, members of the family and various departments in the hospital setting such as Dietary, Social Services, Respiratory Therapy, Chaplaincy, Physical Therapy and such agencies as Rehabilitation Centers, Vocational Guidance Centers, Public Health Nursing Departments, and Mental Health Clinics.

Included in the appendix is an evaluation tool specifically designed and tested for use in determining the extent to which the desired outcomes of patient teaching are achieved for the patient with diabetes mellitus. This example of an assessment tool is designed to collect data concurrently by peer review through direct patient interview and observation methods.

Patient Outcome	Process
The patient functions comfortably within limitations due to angina. This includes:	**DESCRIPTION:** Angina is a symptom of coronary artery disease. It is characterized by precordial chest pain with frequent radiation to the left arm and occurs when there is an imbalance between myocardial oxygen supply and demand. Causes may include narrowing of one or more coronary arteries, valve disease, and arterial spasm. Contributing factors to the underlying disease include hypertension, hyperlipidemia, smoking.

NURSING ASSESSMENT: In addition to the general admission assessment the following information is especially important.

1. Assess and document symptoms of pain.
   a. Location
   b. Character, *e.g.,* burning, pressing, tightness
   c. Severity
   d. Duration
   e. Frequency
   f. Precipitating events: physical and emotional
   g. Associated symptoms, *e.g.,* shortness of breath, diaphoresis, nausea, vomiting, weakness, palpitations
   h. Relief measures and effectiveness
2. Assess and document physical status.
   a. Blood pressure (BP): lying and standing pressures in both arms
   b. Apical/radial pulses
   c. Peripheral pulses
   d. Electrocardiogram
   e. Heart sounds, *e.g.,* murmurs
   f. Lung sounds, *e.g.,* râles
   g. Risk factors, *e.g.,* history of cardiovascular disease and other pathophysiological states such as diabetes, obesity
3. Assess and document patient's understanding of the disease process, implications, and treatment.
4. Assess and document patient's response to information about the disease process and treatment.
   a. Apparent anxiety level
   b. Patient's self assessment of
   • Personal strengths in coping with stress
   • Support people, *e.g.,* family

A. *Is prepared for diagnostic studies*

INTERVENTION:

1. Explain/answer questions about diagnostic studies. Refer to Chapter 3 Guidelines For The Patient Undergoing Diagnostic Studies, p. 33   Studies may include:
   a. Exercise tolerance test
   b. EKG
   c. Vectorcardiogram
   d. Echocardiogram
   e. Cardiac fluoroscopy
   f. Thallium scan
   g. Radionuclide angiogram
   h. Cardiac catheterization

B. *Is achieving control of pain*

2. Provide and teach measures for pain control according to physician's orders. Refer to Chapter 2 Pain, p. 27 for specific assessment and intervention for pain.
   a. Administer nitroglycerine as ordered. The most common regimen is:
      • Preventive: One tablet sublingually 3 to 5 minutes prior to activities which have previously caused pain.
      • Therapeutic: At onset of pain one tablet sublingually, if no relief in 3 to 5 minutes, notify nurse. Do not exceed five tablets in 15 minutes.
      • Minor side effects: Headaches, flushing of face
      • Precautions:
         Report to nurse if tablet does not produce burning sensation (has lost potency).
         Store in airtight, dark container, out of sunlight. Do not mix with other medication.
            Keep no warmer than room temperature (do not carry in pocket next to body).
      • Hypotension: Take pill while sitting or lying.

Patient Outcome	Process

	b. Identify with patient pain precipitating situations, *e.g.,* physical, environmental, and emotional stresses.
	c. Discuss nonpharmacologic methods of dealing with pain.
C. *Is knowledgeable about nature of illness, self-care and continuity of care*	3. Assist patient/family to adjust to restrictions imposed by disease process.
	a. Provide opportunity for patient to express concerns, fears, and questions.
	b. Encourage patient to participate in self-care.
	c. Reinforce physician's explanation of illness and instructions regarding treatment. Include:
	• Diet modifications such as sodium and caloric restriction: consider dietician consult for assistance in teaching and counseling.
	• Drug therapy: Provide written information regarding medications.
	• Exercise program: Reinforce instructions about individualized activity programs.
	• Reduction of risk factors such as control of hypertension, smoking, stress, weight.
	d. Explore with patient needed changes in daily living pattern, *e.g.,* work schedule.
	4. Prepare patient and family as indicated for anticipated surgical intervention.
	5. Plan discharge with patient and family.
	a. Discuss community resources which may assist in continuity of care.
	b. Stress importance of follow-up care.

Patient Outcome	Process

The patient functions comfortably within limitations due to arrhythmia. This includes:

DESCRIPTION: An arrhythmia is an abnormal heart rhythm caused by disturbances in discharge or transmission of cardiac impulses. It may be due to myocardial infarction, congenital heart defects, trauma, hypoxia, electrolyte imbalance, etc.

NURSING ASSESSMENT: In addition to the general assessment, the following information is especially important.

1. Assess and document:
    a. Arrhythmia
    b. Chest pain
    c. Shortness of breath
    d. Blood pressure
    e. Mental status
    f. Presence and quality of peripheral pulses
2. Correlate known pertinent past history with symptoms. Consider:
    a. Former arrhythmias and patient response
    b. Previous response to antiarrhythmic drugs such as lidocaine, pronestyl, quinidine, Dilantin, Inderal
3. Assess and document patient's understanding of the disease process, implications, and treatment.
4. Assess and document response to information about disease process and treatment.

A. *Is achieving control of arrhythmia*

INTERVENTION:
1. Initiate immediate nursing intervention.
    a. Monitor continuously.
    b. Determine patient response to arrhythmia.
        • If patient tolerates arrhythmia (maintaining cardiac output), *i.e.,* stable blood pressure, pulses, oxygenation, mental status, no chest pain,
            Obtain 12-lead EKG
            Notify physician
            Observe closely
        • If patient does not tolerate arrhythmia (compromised cardiac output), *i.e.,* decrease in blood pressure, pulse, and oxygenation; altered mental status; chest pain:
            Refer to specific arrhythmia.

NOTE: Any arrhythmia that is compromising cardiac output is potentially life threatening.

2. Collaborate with physician and intervene to control arrhythmia.
    a. Life-threatening arrhythmias
        • Ventricular tachycardia (Fig. 4-1.)
            Administer lidocaine 50 to 100 mg IV bolus
            Defibrillate
            Initiate basic life support as needed. Refer to Chapter 9 General Guidelines for the Critical Care Patient, Life Support, p. 349
        • Ventricular fibrillation (Fig. 4-2.)
            Initiate basic life support. Refer to Chapter 9 General Guidelines for the Critical Care Patient, Life Support, p. 349,
            Defibrillate immediately
            Administer lidocaine 50 to 100 mg IV bolus.

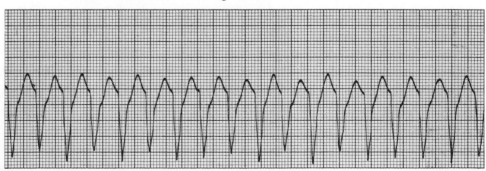

Fig. 4-1.   Ventricular tachycardia.

Patient Outcome   Process

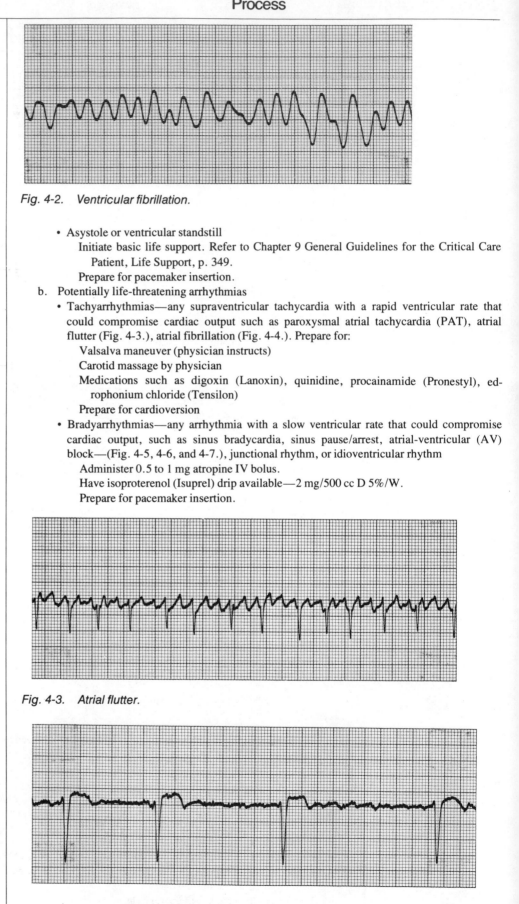

Fig. 4-2.   Ventricular fibrillation.

- Asystole or ventricular standstill
    Initiate basic life support. Refer to Chapter 9 General Guidelines for the Critical Care
        Patient, Life Support, p. 349.
    Prepare for pacemaker insertion.
b. Potentially life-threatening arrhythmias
    - Tachyarrhythmias—any supraventricular tachycardia with a rapid ventricular rate that
      could compromise cardiac output such as paroxysmal atrial tachycardia (PAT), atrial
      flutter (Fig. 4-3.), atrial fibrillation (Fig. 4-4.). Prepare for:
        Valsalva maneuver (physician instructs)
        Carotid massage by physician
        Medications such as digoxin (Lanoxin), quinidine, procainamide (Pronestyl), ed-
            rophonium chloride (Tensilon)
        Prepare for cardioversion
    - Bradyarrhythmias—any arrhythmia with a slow ventricular rate that could compromise
      cardiac output, such as sinus bradycardia, sinus pause/arrest, atrial-ventricular (AV)
      block—(Fig. 4-5, 4-6, and 4-7.), junctional rhythm, or idioventricular rhythm
        Administer 0.5 to 1 mg atropine IV bolus.
        Have isoproterenol (Isuprel) drip available—2 mg/500 cc D 5%/W.
        Prepare for pacemaker insertion.

Fig. 4-3.   Atrial flutter.

Fig. 4-4.   Atrial fibrillation.

Patient Outcome   Process

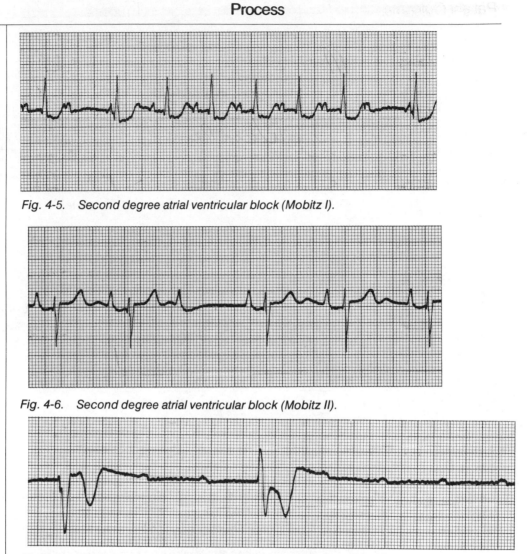

Fig. 4-5. Second degree atrial ventricular block (Mobitz I).

Fig. 4-6. Second degree atrial ventricular block (Mobitz II).

Fig. 4-7. Third degree atrial ventricular block (complete heart block).

    c. Warning arrhythmias
- Premature ventricular contractions (PVC) (Fig. 4-8.) greater than six per minute, coupling, tripling, bigeminy (Fig. 4-9.), multifocal, or R on T phenomenon administer lidocaine (IV bolus and drip per protocol) if indicated
- Premature atrial contractions (PAC) or wandering atrial pacemaker (WAP) may lead to atrial tachyarrhythmias; premature junctional contractions (PJC) may lead to junctional arrhythmias.
    No treatment indicated.
- Sinus tachycardia may be due to fever, anxiety, anemia, compromised cardiac output
    Treat underlying cause.
- First degree atrial ventricular block (AV) may lead to second degree or third degree AV block.
    No treatment indicated.

B. *Is coping with life-threatening situation*

3. Assist patient to cope with life-threatening situation.
    a. Give brief, simple and supportive explanations of equipment, procedure, and personnel.
    b. Give repetitive explanation about patient's physical status and treatment.
    c. Give reassurance of progress if appropriate.
    d. Encourage expression of feelings, concerns, and questions.
    e. Reassure patient that someone will remain with him through critical period.
    f. Demonstrate concern by providing comforting physical contact and verbal support which seems appropriate to the situation.
    g. Involve family members as appropriate.
    h. Provide general supportive care measures, *e.g.,* assistance in feeding, bathing.

Patient Outcome   Process

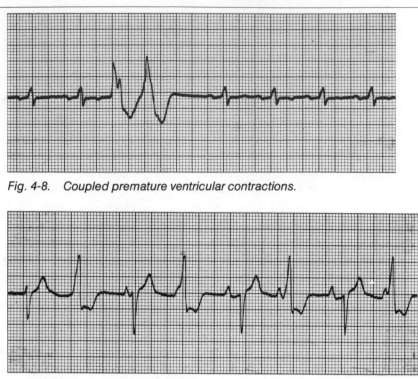

Fig. 4-8.   Coupled premature ventricular contractions.

Fig. 4-9.   Ventricular bigeminy.

C. *Is knowledgeable about nature of illness, self-care and resources for continuity of care*

4. Reinforce physician's explanations and instructions about care to include:
   a.   Medications
   b.   Activity and lifestyle
5. Teach patient to count pulse, noting rate and rhythm. Include discussion of nature of previous explained symptoms which may cause recurring arrhythmias.
6. Instruct patient to report any change in rate (plus or minus 10 beats per minute) or rhythm (regular or irregular).
7. Discuss community resources which may assist in continuity of care.
8. Initiate interagency referral as needed.

General care guidelines for the patient with cancer

Patient Outcome	Process

The patient functions comfortably within limitations due to cancer. This includes:

DESCRIPTION: Cancer is a disease characterized by development of abnormal cells which multiply and invade normal tissues and organs. Because cancer is most often thought of as totally life-threatening, it is frequently accompanied by high anxiety levels, depression, and overreactions. Careful nursing assessment, intervention, reassessment, and continual emotional support are imperative before, during, and after the diagnostic and treatment phases.

NURSING ASSESSMENT: In addition to the general admission assessment, the following information is especially important.

1. Assess and document physical status.
   a. Signs and symptoms related to cancer
      • Appearance: weight loss, malnourished, jaundice, pallor
      • Lesions, masses
      • Bruises, petechiae
      • Nausea, vomiting
      • Bowel and bladder function changes, *e.g.,* constipation
      • Bleeding and/or drainage, *e.g.,* from vagina
      • Cough, difficulty in swallowing, hoarseness
      • Pain: location, character, duration. Include effectiveness of relief methods
      • Weakness
   b. Location of primary site if known
   c. Risk factors
      • Presence of other disease states, *e.g.,* infection, liver disease, diabetes
      • Use of tobacco and alcohol
2. Assess and document patient's/family's response to information about the disease process, implications, and treatment. This includes:
   a. Apparent anxiety/fear
   b. Method of coping with past stresses, *e.g.,* illness, previous hospitalizations
   c. Inherent support systems, *e.g.,* family, friends
   d. Length of time diagnosis known
   e. Current stage of grief process
      • Shock, denial
      • Anger
      • Guilt
      • Depression
      • Bargaining
      • Acceptance
3. Assess and document patient's/family's understanding of the disease process, implications, and treatment.
4. Assess and document health habits/life-style prior to admission.
   a. Self-care ability and/or need for assistance
   b. Dietary needs/restrictions
   c. Daily activities/limitations
   d. Home health supervision/support

A. *Is prepared for diagnostic studies*

INTERVENTION:
1. Explain/answer questions about diagnostic studies. Refer to Chapter 3 Guidelines for the Patient Undergoing Diagnostic Studies, p. 33.
   a. Allow patient time and opportunity to express fears and anxieties.
   b. Be aware that specific studies depend on the type of cancer and the patient's condition. They are performed for diagnostic purposes, disease staging, and monitoring of treatment response.

B. *Understands nature of illness, chosen treatment plan, and care*

2. Reinforce physician's explanation of illness, treatment, and rehabilitation.
3. Establish general plan of care prior to initiation of treatment.
   a. Reassess patient's grief process and intervene as needed.
      • Provide continual support.
      • Consult resource persons, *e.g.,* nurse clinician, chaplain, social worker, family.
   b. Establish exercise program for optimum rehabilitation.
   c. Collaborate with physician to establish medication plan to assist in control of:
      • Pain
      • Nausea

Patient Outcome	Process
	• Constipation/diarrhea

- Constipation/diarrhea
- Anxiety/lack of sleep
- Stomatitis

   d. Provide diet based on patient's condition and preferences.
- Give frequent small feedings if necessary.
- Consult dietician.
- Modify consistency of diet as needed.
- Encourage fluids to 2 to 3 liters daily.

   e. Request aid from appropriate resource people, *e.g.,* speech therapist, physical therapist.

4. Discuss with patient the course of treatment chosen by patient and physician.
   a. Be aware of anxiety and fear of patient and family. Attempt to answer their questions.
   b. Encourage feedback.
   c. Assess the level of understanding.

C. *Is experiencing minimal discomfort or complications from chosen treatment*

5. Assist the patient undergoing surgical intervention.
   a. Discuss with patient that the aim of surgery is total removal of cancer for cure or to allow for better response to adjuvant therapy.
   b. Discuss the specific aspects of pre- and postoperative care. See Chapter 5 Preoperative Phase of Hospitalization, p. 129 and Postoperative Phase of Hospitalization, p. 130

• Surgical Intervention

   c. Provide care needed per hospital routine and physician's orders.
   d. Intervene in the critical elements of postoperative care. Refer to specific guideline appropriate to the surgical intervention, *e.g.,* mastectomy, p.187.

• Radiation therapy

6. Assist the patient undergoing radiation therapy.
   a. Be aware that radiation may be used as the primary mode of treatment, as adjunctive therapy, or palliative therapy.
   b. Discuss possible side effects of therapy. The patient may experience some or all of these depending upon treatment site. Give reassurance that all possible measures will be taken to prevent or minimize side effects.
- Discuss importance of patient's responsibilities in adhering to treatment plan.
- Instruct patient to report side effects promptly.

   c. Establish a plan of care to deal with general side effects of therapy.
- Weakness, fatigue
    Establish rest/activity program within limits of physical tolerance. Include bed exercise program.
    Request physical therapy consult as needed.
- Anorexia, nausea and vomiting
    Instruct patient to eat well-balanced meals and adhere closely to prescribed diet which may include small, frequent feedings. Consult dietician as needed. Give antiemetic as ordered.
    Monitor weight.
    If intake is inadequate, collaborate with patient and health team members.
    Establish plan for special feeding such as tube feeding.
- Skin changes in treatment area, *e.g.,* dryness, itching, sensitivity, discoloration (which may be permanent).
    Do not wash off portal marks until therapy is completed.
    Prevent further damage by avoiding washing or applying soaps, lotions, or any preparation to treatment area during therapy. Do not apply tape.
    Encourage use of soft clothing for treated area. Avoid constricting clothing.
    Keep skin folds clean and dry, especially perineal areas.
    Avoid exposure of area to sun, heating pad, ice bag, or any extreme heat or cold.
    Inspect skin daily and report to physician or nurse any skin rashes, irritations, or breaks.
- Alopecia, myelosuppression
    Refer to guidelines in the chemotherapy section, p. 81 for specific interventions.

   d. Establish a plan of care to deal with side effects related to specific treatment sites.
- Brain
    Expect hair loss, scalp itchiness, and scaling.
    Do not apply oil, soaps, rinses, or creams unless approved by physician.
    Comb hair gently; do not brush or wash.
    Suggest use of loose-fitting scarf, hat, or wig. Expose scalp to air as much as possible.

Patient Outcome	Process
	Report new or unusual central nervous system symptoms immediately.

Report new or unusual central nervous system symptoms immediately.
- Head and neck
  Expect mouth and throat soreness, difficulty in swallowing, dry mouth, hoarseness, a "lump" in throat, change in sense of taste or smell, risk of dental decay and gum disorders.
  Inspect mouth each day for irritations.
  Practice good oral hygiene; use no toothpaste or commercial mouth wash. Use a soft toothbrush and baking soda. Visit dentist regularly.
  Use electric razor for shaving.
  Avoid use of alcohol and tobacco.
- Breast
  Consult radiation therapy physician regarding use of bra or prosthesis during therapy.
  Do not wash affected axilla; use no deodorants or powders.
- Mediastinum
  Expect esophagitis, nausea, and vomiting.
  Provide small frequent meals consisting of bland diet with plenty of liquids.
- Abdomen and pelvis
  Expect nausea, vomiting, diarrhea, cramping, vaginitis, cystitis, amenorrhea.
  Provide low-residue diet with increased fluid intake.
  Avoid laxative during and for four-week period after therapy completed.
  Instruct female patient undergoing pelvic irradiation:
    Avoid vaginal creams, hygiene sprays, suppositories, douches, or tampons without specific physician orders.
    Discuss importance of sexual intercourse or "candle exercises" to maintain patent vagina following therapy.

- *Chemotherapy*

7. Assist the patient undergoing chemotherapy.
   a. Discuss with the patient that the aim of chemotherapy is to eradicate the cancer, to stop the progression of the disease and keep it under control, to facilitate remission, or to help relieve pain.
   b. Explain the type of drug(s) used, route of administration and frequency.
   c. Discuss possible side effects of therapy of which the patient may experience some or all. Give reassurance that all possible measures will be taken to prevent or minimize side effects.
      - Weakness, fatigue
      - Nausea and vomiting
      - Diarrhea and/or constipation
      - Gastrointestinal ulceration and bleeding
      - Stomatitis
      - Skin rash, hives, itching, bruises, petechiae
      - Alopecia
      - Headache
      - Myelosuppression
      - Infection
      - Peripheral neuropathy
      - Renal toxicities, hematuria
   d. Discuss the importance of patient's responsibilities in carrying out treatment plan, *e.g.*, reporting of side effects promptly. Allow patient to participate in planning care and explain/teach all procedures and routines.
      - Check for signed-consent form.
      - Stress importance of preventive measures at beginning, during, and after course of therapy.
   e. Initiate measures to control nausea and vomiting.
      - Delay food until nausea subsides.
      - Apply cold compress to forehead and neck.
      - Identify how patient has managed nausea in the past.
      - Offer ice chips and clear fluids as tolerated.
      - Give antiemetic as ordered a half hour prior to administration of chemotherapy. If nausea persists give antiemetic on a regular basis for at least 24 hours or longer if needed.
      - Collaborate with physician if nausea is uncontrolled.

Patient Outcome	Process
	• Be readily available to assist the patient who is vomiting; provide reassurance.

f. Promote optimum food and fluid intake.
  • Discuss importance of adequate nutrition to improve treatment response and to reduce side effects.
  • Consult dietician.
  • Identify patient's food preferences.
  • Have between-meal nourishment available such as milkshakes, tea, soups, eggnog, cheese, peanut butter, or crackers.
  • Encourage family to bring special foods from home.
  • Participate in dietary teaching as needed. Include family.
  • Maintain intake-output record. Initiate calorie count if necessary.
  • Weigh patient at least twice weekly.
  • Collaborate with physician, dietician, and patient if intake is inadequate. Participate in plan for special feeding such as hyperalimentation.

g. Provide and teach measures to prevent/minimize stomatitis.
  • Check patient's mouth with flashlight daily for evidence of ulcer, bleeding, and infection and notify physician if signs are present.
  • Brush teeth using toothpaste and soft toothbrush after each food intake (or q 4 hours when awake).
  • Follow brushing with warm saline gargle (1 teaspoon salt in 8 ounces of warm water). Salt-soda-borax solution may be used instead. If old blood or debris is present, use a solution of hydrogen peroxide diluted with water before the saline gargle. Diluted commercial mouth wash may then used, if desired.
  • Lubricate lips q 2 hours and p.r.n.
  • Place humidifer at bedside as needed.
  • Modify consistency of diet if necessary. May need to offer room temperature foods/ fluids.
  • Collaborate with physician for other preventive/curative measures as needed, *e.g.*, local analgesics.

h. Institute measures to maintain skin integrity.
  • Refer to Chapter 2 Skin Care Guidelines When There is Deviation From Normal p. 31   to maximize patient's ability to maintain skin integrity.
  • Apply lotion to skin several times daily.
  • Inspect skin daily, especially over bony prominences.
  • Give careful attention to skin around any stoma.
  • Give careful attention to perineal areas:
      Instruct patient in hygiene measures.
      Keep area clean and dry.
      Use sitz baths and medication as ordered.
  • Give medications as ordered to control itching.

i. Assist the patient to maintain optimum strength.
  • Refer to Chapter 2 Activity Guidelines When There is Deviation From Normal p. 21   to maximize patient's ability to maintain strength.
  • Establish with patient rest/activity program within limits of physical tolerance. Include bed exercise program.
  • Provide assistance/supervision as necessary to carry out program.
  • Request physical therapy consultation as needed.
  • Encourage family participation in activity program.

j. Institute measures to prevent complications in peripheral blood vessels.
  • Instruct patient to exercise hands by squeezing a rubber ball for 5 to 10 minutes q 4 hours while awake. This exercise should be continued after discharge.
  • Apply warm, moist packs to both arms a half hour prior to administration of therapy or venipuncture.
  • Observe drug infusion area for evidence of extravasation or infiltration and report to physician immediately.
      Reddish blue color
      Edema
      Patient complaint of moderate to severe pain in injection site
  • Give immediate care for drug extravasation/infiltration.

Patient Outcome	Process
	Have Solu-cortef available for injection.
	Apply ice packs to area for 24 hours.
	Follow with warm, moist compresses until phlebitis/cellulitis clears.

k. Intervene to prevent gastrointestinal hemorrhage.
   - Provide soft, bland diet.
   - Check stools daily for evidence of blood.
   - Document any vomitus for evidence of blood.
   - Discuss need for antacid with physician.

l. Assist the patient who has alopecia.
   - Reassure the patient that this is an expected effect and that hair growth usually resumes after completion of therapy. (Exception: Hair loss due to radiation to the head is not expected to return).
   - Suggest use of scarf, cap, or wig.

m. Promote comfort and relaxation.
   - Assess tension/apprehension state.
   - Offer back rubs at least b.i.d.
   - Discuss need for medications with physician.
   - Provide diversional activity as appropriate.

n. Monitor changes in blood component values and intervene as needed to prevent complications:
   - Decreased hematocrit and hemoglobin may necessitate blood transfusion. Refer to guidelines for Blood Transfusion, p. 407.
   - Decreased white blood count may necessitate protective isolation, antibiotics, and leukocyte transfusion. Refer to guidelines for Leukocyte Transfusion, p. 417 .
     Instruct patient to stay away from crowds and infected persons.
     Limit visitors to immediate family.
   - Decreased platelet count may necessitate platelet transfusion. Consider other measures to prevent bleeding:
     Instruct patient to use electric razor only.
     Observe stools, urine, and vomitus for evidence of blood.
     Do not allow patient to become constipated.
     Observe for vaginal bleeding; female patient may be started on oral contraceptives.

• *Immunotherapy*

8. Assist the patient undergoing immunotherapy. (With increasing evidence that deficient immune systems may play a major role in the development of cancer, increased interest is being given this mode of treatment which has fewer side effects.)
   a. Discuss with patient that the aim of immunotherapy is to stimulate production of tumor-specific antibodies by intradermal, scratch method, or intratumor injection of non-specific immune stimulator or specific vaccine made from tumor.
   b. Refer to Melanoma guideline, p. 97   for specific intervention for the patient undergoing immunotherapy.

D. *Is coping with illness*

9. Assist the patient and family to cope with life-threatening illness.
   a. Establish a trust relationship; give consistent information.
   b. Provide opportunity for expression of concerns and questions.
   c. Identify resource persons, *e.g.,* nurse clinician, chaplain, social worker.
   d. Allow family and patient as much time together as desired.
   e. Support appropriate coping strategy.
   f. Encourage participation in self-care.
   g. Facilitate interaction with other patients undergoing similar therapy, if appropriate.
   h. Assure continued support regardless of patient's decisions about therapy, *e.g.,* choosing to discontinue therapy.
   i. Give positive reinforcement and realistic hope.

10. Support patient/family in working through the grief process. Intervene appropriately.
    a. Be aware that it is essential for individual staff members to work through their own emotions before they can help the patient and family to adjust.
    b. Consider that patient and family may be in different phases of the grieving process and may fluctuate back and forth between stages.
       - ***Shock:*** Usually occurs when patient is first told of disease. Patient may not talk about disease, but may refer to it as a ''tumor'', or regard the problem as minor.
       - ***Anger:*** Hostility that this is happening; ''What did I do to deserve this?''. Patient may blame others, staff or referring physician.

Patient Outcome	Process
	• *Denial:* Patient may think there is mistaken diagnosis. Patients frequently move back and forth between anger and denial.
	• *Grief:* Patient experiences sadness, depression at having disease, at having not done certain things, may become extremely self-centered.
	• *Acceptance:* Patient can verbalize about disease to family, staff, and other patients. Able to carry out activities of daily living and may resume family role.
	c. Accept patient's responses and recognize his feelings. Allow ample time for verbalization.
	d. Demonstrate acceptance through active listening.
E. *Is knowledgeable about self-care and resources for continuity of care*	11. Plan discharge with patient and family.
	a. Reinforce physician's instructions.
	b. Reinforce teaching of knowledge/skills related to care and provide written information as needed.
	• Maintenance of adequate nutrition and fluid intake
	• Physical exercise program
	• Mouth care
	• Pain control, especially if medication is by injection
	• Other medications
	• Other care specific to type of cancer and therapy needed
	c. Instruct patient to avoid direct exposure to sunlight unless skin is covered.
	d. Assist patient to make arrangements for follow-up examinations and/or blood studies as indicated.
	e. Assist patient to obtain necessary equipment, supplies, and medications.
	f. Discuss community agencies which may assist in continuity of care, *e.g.,* American Cancer Society.
	g. Initiate interagency referral as needed.
	h. Assure patient of continued availability of physician and nurse to provide care and support. Provide telephone numbers for contact.

Patient Outcome	Process

The patient functions comfortably within limitations due to breast cancer. This includes:

DESCRIPTION: Cancer of the breast is most common in females over 40 years of age. It arises in a single focus, invades regional lymph nodes and then spreads to other areas of the body. The most likely sites for metastasis are bone, lung, liver, and the central nervous system.

Therapy is primarily surgical; radiation therapy may or may not be used. Chemotherapy and hormonal manipulation are other modes of therapy. Therapy selected depends upon staging: the universal tumor/nodal/metastatic staging is generally used.

NURSING ASSESSMENT: In addition to the general admission assessment, the following information is especially important.
1. Assess and document physical status.
    a. Signs and symptoms related to cancer
        • Breast changes, *e.g.,* masses, lesions, nipple discharge, drainage
        • Pain: location, character, duration, and successful management
        • Other masses, lesions
        • Weakness
    b. Breast skin care needs
2. Assess and document patient's/family's response to information about the disease process, implications, and treatment.
    a. Apparent anxiety level and fear
    b. Patient's self-assessment of:
        • Personal strengths in coping with stress
        • Support people, *e.g.,* family, minister
    c. Previous experience with surgery and/or diagnostic studies
    d. Length of time diagnosis known
    e. Current stage of grief process
3. Assess and document patient's/family's understanding of the disease process, implications, and treatment.
4. Assess and document health habits/life-style prior to admission.
    a. Self-care ability and/or need for assistance.
    b. Dietary needs/restrictions
    c. Daily activities/limitations
    d. Home health supervision/support

A. *Is prepared for diagnostic studies*

INTERVENTION:
1. Explain/answer questions about diagnostic studies. Refer to Chapter 3 Guidelines For The Patient Undergoing Diagnostic Studies, p. 33. Studies may include:
    a. Biopsy of lesion
    b. Chest radiograph
    c. Metastatic bone survey
    d. Bone liver, brain scans
    e. Blood studies
    f. Estrogen receptor study (biopsy of skin lesion, lymph node, bone or body fluids to determine responsiveness of tumor cells to hormonal treatment)

B. *Understands nature of illness, chosen treatment plan and care*

C. *Is experiencing minimal discomfort or complications from chosen treatment*

• *Surgical intervention*

• *Radiation therapy*

• *Chemotherapy*

2. Reinforce physician's explanation of illness and treatment.
3. Establish general plan of care prior to initiation of treatment. Refer to General Care Guidelines for the Patient With Cancer, p. 79 for specific components such as pain control.
4. Discuss with patient course of treatment chosen by patient and physician.
5. Assist the patient requiring surgical intervention.
    a. Refer to Chapter 5 Preoperative Phase of Hospitalization, p. 129 and Postoperative Phase of Hospitalization, p. 130. Provide care needed per hospital routine and physician's orders.
    b. Intervene in the critical elements of care depending upon the extent of the surgery. See Chapter 5 Mastectomy Guidelines, p. 187, for specific interventions.
6. Assist the patient receiving radiation therapy, which may be used as adjunct therapy with surgery or for palliative treatment to lungs, bone, or brain.
    • Refer to Chapter 4 General Care Guidelines for the Patient With Cancer, p. 79 for specific interventions.
7. Assist the patient undergoing chemotherapy, which may be given to patient who is estrogen/receptor negative or for recurrent disease.
    a. Refer to General Care Guidelines For the Patient With Cancer, p. 81 for specific interventions related to chemotherapy.

Patient Outcome	Process
	b. Discuss type of drug(s) used. Current drugs commonly used include: • Cyclophosphamide (Cytoxan) • Amethopterin Methotrexate (MTX) • 5-Fluorouracil (5-FU) • Doxorubicin (Adriamycin) • Vinblastine sulfate (Velban) • Vincristine sulfate (Oncovin) • Melphalan (Alkeran)

• *Hormonal therapy or manipulation*	8. Assist the patient undergoing hormonal therapy or manipulation which are used for patient who is estrogen receptor positive or over 60 years of age.
	   a. Discuss with patient that surgical manipulation is done to remove sources of estrogen:
	     • Oophorectomy in pre- or perimenopausal patient
	     • Adrenalectomy in postmenopausal patient.
	     • Hypophysectomy (ablation of pituitary gland)
	   b. Discuss expectation that patient will experience hot flashes as an effect of surgery.
	   c. Discuss hormonal replacement medications.
	     • Estrogens
	     • Antiestrogens
	     • Androgens
	     • Progestins
	   d. Discuss common side effects of hormonal medications:
	     • Vaginal bleeding or spotting, especially after drugs are discontinued
	     • Hot flashes
	     • Fluid retention
	     • Breast tenderness
	     • Nausea, vomiting
	     • Diarrhea
	     • Hyponatremia
	     • Hypercalcemia
	     • "Flare"—worsening of pain or increase in size of lesion several days after beginning hormonal agents, which soon improves
	   e. Provide measures to prevent/control side effects as indicated.
	 9. Assess patient's knowledge of response to treatment.
	   a. Clarify any misconceptions.
	   b. Reinforce information that different therapies are used at different stages of the disease depending upon response to previous therapy.
	 10. Provide and teach care of skin lesions.
	   a. Assess condition of skin lesions.
	   b. Cleanse affected area with soap and water p.r.n. unless patient is receiving radiation therapy.
	     • Use hydrogen peroxide, saline, and/or povidone-iodine solutions if area is draining or infected.
	   c. Change dressings frequently.
	   d. Control odor.
	   e. Protect surrounding skin area from infection.

D. *Is coping with illness*	11. Assist the patient and family to cope with life-threatening illness. • Refer to General Care Guidelines for the Patient With Cancer, p. 79 for specific interventions to help patient adjust to illness and therapy.

E. *Is knowledgeable about self-care and resources for continuity of care*	12. Plan discharge with patient and family.
	   a. Refer to General Care Guidelines for the Patient With Cancer, p. 84 for interventions related to discharge planning.
	   b. Observe return demonstrations of breast skin care.

Patient Outcome	Process

The patient functions comfortably within limitations due to choriocarcinoma. This includes:

DESCRIPTION: Choriocarcinoma is a trophoblastic disease that primarily occurs in women after conception. Choriocarcinoma occurs following the passage of a hydatidiform mole in 50 percent of the cases, 25 per cent after abortion, and the remainder after or along with pregnancy. A very small proportion (5 to 10 per cent) arises from trophoblast with no prior or current pregnancy. The tumor arises from the *fetal* trophoblast and not from the uterus and is thus of pregnancy origin.

NURSING ASSESSMENT: In addition to the general admission assessment, the following information is especially important.

1. Assess and document physical status.
   a. Common sites/signs/symptoms of metastasis
      • Lungs (hemoptysis, shortness of breath)
      • Brain (seizures, changes in neurological status)
      • Liver (jaundice, enzymes)
      • Vagina (profuse or irregular bleeding)
   b. Physical condition
   c. Self-care capabilities.
2. Assess and document patient's/family's response in terms of the acceptance of the disease process and treatment. Consider the following factors:
   a. Family support system
   b. Body image changes
   c. Changes in family life style
   d. Changes in maternal role
   e. Therapy/prognosis
   f. Possible loss of fertility
   g. Appropriate age-level adjustment
3. Assess and document patient's understanding of disease process, related studies, therapy, and long-term hospitalization.

A. *Is prepared for diagnostic studies and therapy*

INTERVENTION:

1. Plan with patient for diagnostic studies to obtain baseline data and to determine metastatic disease. Studies will be repeated as needed throughout hospitalization. See Chapter 3 Guidelines for the Patient Undergoing Diagnostic Studies, p. 33.
   a. IVP
   b. Ultrasound of pelvis
   c. Serum human chorionic gonadotropin (HCG)
   d. Spot urine for HCG
   e. Chest radiographs (monthly, unless known lung lesions)
   f. EKG
   g. Brain scan
   h. Liver scan
   i. Routine blood studies:
      • CBC
      • Chemistries
      • Thyroid panel
      • Serological test for syphilis
   j. Pap smear
   k. EEG
   l. Routine urinalysis
   m. Weekly 24-hour urine for HCG
   n. Computerized tomography (done in selected cases)
2. Check weekly HCG serum and urine levels, which are key studies in determining response to therapy/prognosis.
   a. Titer is determined by the BM-subunit radioimmune assay; normal titer level is less than 5.
   b. Increasing titer indicates poor response to therapy; decreasing titer indicates good response.
3. Reinforce information and answer questions regarding physician's discussion with patient regarding selected therapy. Selected therapy may be:
   a. Chemotherapy:
      • Single agent:
         Methotrexate (MTX)
         Actinomycin D (Act D)

Patient Outcome	Process
	• Triple therapy: MTX plus Actinomycin D plus Chlorambucil (or Cytoxan) given in combination. • Combinations of these drugs and others when applicable to individual cases. b. Radiation therapy: radiation given to decrease or eliminate the tumor (in brain or liver primarily) c. Surgery (refer to specific surgical procedures, *e.g.,* hysterectomy, craniotomy). See Chapter 5 p. 127 . 4. Teach prevention of pregnancy. Rationale: Assays used to test for HCG cannot distinguish between HCG, tumor, or normal pregnancy. Patients are placed on oral contraceptives for pregnancy prevention and pituitary suppression unless contraindicated.
B. *Has minimal side effects of radiation and/or chemotherapy*	5. Provide/teach care to minimize side effects of therapy. Explain to patient the reason for side effects and encourage participation in planning care. Side effects of therapy and nursing care may include: a. Nausea and vomiting: • Provide antiemetics. • Encourage fluid intake; provide for patient preference. • Record intake and output. b. Loss of hair • Reassure patient that hair will return after chemotherapy. (May or may not return after radiation therapy). Suggest wigs or scarfs as useful covers. c. Stomatitis: • Provide humidifier. • Give IV fluids. • Give antibiotics as ordered. • Provide mouth washes. d. Rashes, itching: • Give Benadryl if ordered. • Provide linen washed with a neutral soap. • Apply lotions to skin. e. Skin sensitivity: • Tell patients to avoid tight fitting clothing, shoes or prolonged pressure on skin overlying bony prominence. f. Dryness of eyes: • Give eye drops (methylcellulose). g. Loss of appetite: • Give IV fluids. • Provide selected diets and a diet consult as indicated. h. Vaginitis (usually fungal, less often bacterial, occasionally nonspecific): • Give thorough perineal care. • Give medications specific to infection. i. Myelosuppression (decreased resistance to infection; increased likelihood of bleeding from decreased white cells or platelets): • Institute protective isolation (based on WBC level) if indicated. • Watch for bruising, bleeding from any site. • Avoid IM injections. j. Increased sun sensitivity: • Tell patient to avoid sunlight. k. Hemorrhoids: • Give medications as ordered. • Provide warm sitz baths for patient. l. Neurological dysfunction: • Watch for change in speech, motor/sensory function, level of consciousness, behavior, seizure activity. m. Liver dysfunction: • Check daily liver enzyme reports.
C. *Is achieving optimal physical status*	6. Encourage independence in activities of daily living according to patient's current capabilities. Modify care plan accordingly in such areas as: a. Personal hygiene b. Physical activity regimen c. Occupational and recreational therapy

Patient Outcome	Process
	7. Provide for adequate nutritional intake.
	a. Consider patient preferences.
	b. Instruct in diet.
	c. Provide nourishment, *e.g.,* snacks.
	d. Call for diet consult as needed.
D. *Is coping with hospitalization and impact of illness*	8. Support patient's ability to cope with illness.
	a. Listen to patient and observe behaviors to determine unmet emotional needs.
	b. Hold nursing staff conference to discuss individual nursing assessments and formulate a consistent plan of care dealing with the unmet emotional needs.
	c. Make referrals to chaplain, social services, psychiatric nurse clinician, and other appropriate resource people.
	d. Encourage patient participation in diversional activities, *e.g.,* crafts, hobbies, group events (ward parties, shopping trips, movies, games). Refer to recreational therapist.
	e. Provide for school work assistance for students.
	9. Be aware that certain events will have positive or negative significance to patient/family. Be available to support patient when needed. These events may include:
	a. Weekly HCG titer reports (given to patient by physician)
	b. Other patients' favorable/unfavorable responses to therapy
	c. Campus privileges (time when patient can be away from hospital which may include home visits) may be granted unless medically contraindicated.
	d. Special personal events, *e.g.,* birthdays, anniversaries
	10. Assist patient and family in the event of impending death.
	a. Evaluate the patient's/family's response to grieving.
	b. Assist patient and family in physical and emotional comfort measures.
	c. Be aware of nurse's own feelings. Utilize support systems, *e.g.,* chaplain's service, co-workers, physician.
E. *Is knowledgeable about nature of illness, self-care, and resources for continuity of care*	11. Plan/teach care in preparation for discharge of patient such as:
	a. Reinforce physician's instructions to patient/family in regard to:
	• Medications
	• Routine blood work, *i.e.,* HCG titers as ordered
	• Skin care for itching, rashes, or dryness; mouth care
	• Gradual increase in physical activities
	• Birth control
	b. Support patient/family in relation to concerns patient may have such as:
	• Expectations of family and friends
	• Changes which may have occurred at home and among family members and friends
	• Individual fears about leaving hospital
	• Return to pretreatment appearance, *e.g.,* hair regrowth, regaining weight
	• Possible loss of fertility
	• Spouse loyalties
	c. Encourage patient to return to a normal or modified life style depending on the patient's prognosis and treatment response.
	d. Provide information about health agencies which may offer assistance in continuity of care.
	• Initiate interagency referral as needed.

Patient Outcome	Process

The patient functions comfortable within limitations due to colorectal cancer. This includes:

DESCRIPTION: Colorectal cancer is a "deep-seated" cancer that may have metastasized by the time of detection. Diagnostic staging ranges from (1) least invasive and usually requiring surgery only to (2) invasive and metastatic requiring surgery and additional treatment.

Chemotherapy is the treatment of choice; radiation therapy is rarely used. The role of immunotherapy is not yet determined.

NURSING ASSESSMENT: In addition to the general admission assessment, the following information is especially important.

1. Assess and document physical status.
   a. Signs and symptoms related to cancer:
      - Weakness
      - Weight loss
      - Change in bowel habits, *e.g.,* constipation, diarrhea, blood in stools
      - Pain: location, character, duration, method of management
   b. Risk factors
      - Presence of other disease states, *e.g.,* diabetes, arthritis
2. Assess and document patient's and family's response to information about disease process, implications and treatment.
   a. Current coping strategy
   b. Patient's self-assessment of:
      - Personal strengths in coping with stresses
      - Support persons, *e.g.,* family, minister
   c. Length of time diagnosis known
   d. Current stage of grief process
3. Assess and document health habits/life-style prior to admission.
   a. Home health supervision/support
   b. Position in family unit, *e.g.,* homemaker
   c. Dietary needs/restrictions
   d. Self-care ability and/or need for assistance
4. Assess and document understanding of the disease process, implications, and treatment.

A. *Is prepared for diagnostic studies*

INTERVENTION:
1. Explain/answer questions about diagnostic studies. See Chapter 3 Guidelines for the Patient Undergoing Diagnostic Studies, p. 33. Studies may include:
   a. Barium enema/air contrast studies
   b. Endoscopy/proctoscopy
   c. Biopsy
   d. Ultrasonography
   e. Chest radiographs
   f. Liver, spleen, bone, brain scans
   g. Blood studies

B. *Understands nature of illness, chosen treatment plan, and care*

2. Reinforce physician's explanation of illness and treatment.
3. Discuss with patient and family course of treatment chosen by patient and physician.
   a. Be aware of anxiety and fear of patient and family and attempt to answer their questions.
   b. Encourage feedback.
   c. Assess the level of understanding.
4. Establish general plan of care prior to initiation of treatment.
   - Refer to General Care Guidelines for the Patient with Cancer, p. 79 for specific components of care such as pain control.

C. *Is free of or has minimal discomfort or complications from chosen treatment*
- *Surgical intervention*

5. Assist the patient undergoing surgical intervention.
   a. Discuss the specific aspects of pre- and postoperative care. See Chapter 5 Preoperative Phase of Hospitalization, p. 129 and Postoperative Phase of Hospitalization, p. 130.
   b. Provide care needed per hospital routine and physician's orders.
   c. Intervene in the critical elements of postoperative care depending upon the nature of the surgical intervention. See Chapter 5 Colostomy, Ileostomy, Abdominoperineal Resection, p. 149 for specific aspects of care.

- *Radiation therapy*

6. Assist the patient receiving radiation therapy.
   - Refer to General Care Guidelines for the Patient With Cancer, p. 80 for specific interventions for radiation to the lower abdomen.

- *Chemotherapy*

7. Assist the patient receiving chemotherapy.

Patient Outcome	Process

	a. Refer to General Care Guidelines for the Patient With Cancer, p. 81 for interventions related to chemotherapy.
	b. Explain the type of drug(s) used. Current drugs commonly used include:
	  • 5-Fluorouracil (5-Fu)
	  • CCNU (Lomustine)
	  • Mitomycin (Mutamycin)
	  • Vincristine sulfate (Oncovin)

D. *Is coping with illness*	8. Assist the patient and family to cope with life-threatening illness and altered body image.
	  a. Refer to General Care Guidelines for the Patient With Cancer, p. 83 for specific interventions to help patient adjust to illness and therapy.
	  b. Encourage patient to participate in stoma care and application of colostomy pouch.
	  c. Exhibit therapeutically accepting attitude and behaviors toward patient and family.

E. *Is knowledgeable about self-care and resources for continuity of care*	9. Plan discharge with patient and family.
	  a. Refer to General Care Guidelines for the Patient With Cancer, p. 84 for specific intervention related to discharge planning.
	  b. Provide additional essential elements of preparation for discharge of patient with colostomy. Refer to Chapter 5 Colostomy, Ileostomy, Abdominoperineal Resection Guidelines, p. 151 for specific aspects of home care.

Patient Outcome	Process

The patient functions comfortably within limitations due to cancer of head or neck. This includes:

DESCRIPTION: Head and neck cancer progresses by local invasion with initial metastasis to regional lymph nodes. Most frequent distant metastasis sites are lung, liver, brain, and base of skull. There are eight major sites of tumor origin: nasal fossa, paranasal sinuses, oral cavity, palatine arch, larynx, hypolarynx, nasopharynx, and salivary glands. Staging of the disease is by the tumor/nodal/metastatic system.

NURSING ASSESSMENT: In addition to the general admission assessment, the following information is important.
1. Assess and document physical status.
    a. Signs and symptoms related to cancer
        • Persistent hoarseness or voice change
        • Dysphagia
        • Lesions, masses
        • Excessive salivation, lacrimation
        • Decreased hearing
        • Epistaxis
        • Nasal stuffiness, obstruction
        • Pain: location, character, duration, method of management
    b. Condition of teeth, gums, *e.g.,* bleeding, edema, pain
    c. Risk factors
        • Smoking and alcohol history
        • Presence of other disease states, *e.g.,* diabetes
    d. Ability to communicate, *e.g.,* reading and writing skills
2. Assess and document patient's/family's response to information about the disease process, implications, and treatment.
    a. Apparent anxiety level and fear
    b. Patient's self-assessment of:
        • Personal strengths in coping with stress
        • Support people, *e.g.,* family, minister
        • Self-concept and body image
    c. Previous experience with surgery and/or diagnostic studies
    d. Length of time diagnosis known
    e. Current stage of grief process
3. Assess and document patient's/family's understanding of the disease process, implications, and treatment.
4. Assess and document health habits/life-style prior to admission.
    a. Self-care ability and/or need for assistance
    b. Dietary needs/restrictions
    c. Daily activities/limitations
    d. Home health supervision/support

A. *Is prepared for diagnostic studies*

INTERVENTION:
1. Explain/answer questions about diagnostic studies. Refer to Chapter 3 Guidelines for the Patient Undergoing Diagnostic Studies, p. 33. Studies may include:
    a. Chest radiographs
    b. Special radiographs/tomograms of area(s) involved:
        • Soft tissue
        • Sinus
        • Facial
        • Mandible and/or maxilla
        • Skull
    c. Biopsy of lesion and/or nodes
    d. Bone, liver, brain scans
    e. Barium swallow
    f. Esophagoscopy
    g. Laryngoscopy
    h. Blood studies

B. *Understands nature of illness, chosen treatment plan, and care*

2. Reinforce physician's explanation of illness and treatment.
3. Establish general plan of care prior to initiation of treatment.
    a. Refer to General Care Guidelines for the Patient With Cancer, p. 79 for specific components.

Patient Outcome	Process

	b. Include additional elements of care.
	  • Consider consults to resource persons as respiratory and speech therapists and facial prosthesis department.
	  • Consider the Lost Chord Association to provide additional support.
	c. Establish with patient and family alternatives to verbal communication and method, *e.g.*, writing on pad.
	4. Discuss with patient course of treatment chosen by patient and family.

C. *Is experiencing minimal discomfort or complications from chosen treatment* • *Surgical intervention*	5. Assist the patient undergoing surgical intervention. a. Refer to Chapter 5 Preoperative Phase of Hospitalization, p. 129 and Postoperative Phase of Hospitalization, p. 130. Provide care as needed per hospital routine and physician's orders. b. Intervene in the critical elements of care depending on the extent of the surgery. See Chapter 5, Radical Neck Dissection Guidelines, p. 201 for specific intervention. c. Assess patient's specific reactions to expected change in physical appearance and body function, *e.g.*, loss of speech, taste, swallowing.
• *Radiation therapy*	6. Assist the patient receiving radiation therapy, which may be used alone or as adjunct therapy with surgery. • Refer to Chapter 4 General Care Guidelines for the Patient With Cancer, p. 80 for specific intervention.

• *Chemotherapy*	7. Assist the patient receiving chemotherapy, which may be used as adjunct therapy.
	a. Refer to General Care Guidelines for the Patient With Cancer, p. 81 for specific interventions related to chemotherapy.
	b. Discuss type of drug(s) used. Current drugs commonly used include:
	  • Vinblastine sulfate (Velban)
	  • Vincristine sulfate (Oncovin)
	  • Bleomycin sulfate (Blenoxane)
	  • Amethopterin methotrexate (MTX)
	  • 5-Fluorouracil (5-FU)
	  • Cyclophosphamide (Cytoxan)
	  • Doxorubicin (Adriamycin)
	  • BCNU (Carmustine)
	  • CCNU(Lomustine)

D. *Is coping with illness*	8. Assist the patient and family to cope with life-threatening illness and body image change. a. Refer to General Care Guidelines for the Patient With Cancer, p. 83 for specific interventions to help the patient adjust to illness and therapy. b. Demonstrate acceptance of patient and patient's appearance.
E. *Is knowledgeable about self-care and resources for continuity of care*	9. Plan discharge with patient and family. a. Refer to General Care Guidelines for the Patient With Cancer, p. 84 for interventions related to discharge planning. b. Include additional essential elements of preparation for discharge of patient with surgical intervention. See Chapter 5 Radical Neck Dissection Guideline, p. 203 for specific intervention related to self-care.

Patient Outcome	Process

The patient functions comfortably within limitations due to leukemia. This includes:

DESCRIPTION: Leukemia is a malignant disease that affects the bone marrow by the over-production of abnormal and/or immature leukocytes. This interferes with the normal production of other blood components (erythrocytes, thrombocytes). The classification, treatment, and prognosis depend upon the type of leukocyte involved. The major classifications are:

    a. Lymphocytic (acute and chronic), usually responds better to treatment.

    b. Nonlymphocytic (acute and chronic)

        Myelogenous (granulocytic)

        Monocytic

        Myelomonocytic

        Erythroleukemic

With rare exceptions, the outcome of leukemia is ultimately fatal; however, survival time has been extended. Treatment is by chemotherapy along with supportive measures as transfusion of blood components. New approaches include autologous bone marrow transplantation and immunotherapy.

NURSING ASSESSMENT: In addition to the general admission assessment, the following information is especially important.

1. Assess and document physical status.
   a. Signs and symptoms related to leukemia
   - Skin appearance, *e.g.,* bruises, petechiae, color, infection, breakdown
   - Chills and fever
   - Headache
   - Generalized weakness
   - Bleeding from any site
   - Pain, measures which effectively provide relief
   b. Previous experience with leukemia therapy
2. Assess and document patient's/family's response to information about the disease process, implications and treatment.
   a. Apparent anxiety and fear
   b. Method of coping with past stresses, *e.g.,* illness, previous hospitalizations
   c. Patient's self-assessment of support persons, *e.g.,* family, minister
   d. Length of time diagnosis known
   e. Current stage of grief process
3. Assess and document the patient's/family's understanding of the disease process, implications, and treatment.
4. Assess and document health habits/life-style prior to admission.
   a. Self-care ability and/or need for assistance
   b. Dietary needs/restrictions
   c. Daily activities/limitations
   d. Home health supervision/support

A. *Is prepared for diagnostic studies*

INTERVENTION:

1. Explain/answer questions about diagnostic studies. Refer to Chapter 3 Guidelines For The Patient Undergoing Diagnostic Studies, p. 33. Studies may include:
   a. Bone marrow aspiration and biopsy
   b. Frequent blood studies as complete blood count, platelet count, reticulocyte count
   c. Cultures of blood, urine, sputum
   d. Antibody screening
   e. Lumbar puncture

B. *Understands nature of illness, chosen treatment plan, and care*

2. Reinforce physician's explanation of illness and treatment.
3. Establish a general plan of care prior to initiation of treatment.
   a. Reassess patient's grief process and intervene as needed.
   - Provide continual support.
   - Consult resource persons, *e.g.,* nurse clinician, chaplain, social worker.
   b. Establish exercise program for optimal rehabilitation.
   c. Collaborate with physician to establish medication plan to assist in control of:
   - Nausea, vomiting
   - Constipation/diarrhea
   - Anxiety/lack of sleep
   - Stomatitis
   d. Provide diet based on patient's condition and preferences.

Patient Outcome	Process

	• Give frequent, small feedings if necessary.
	• Consult dietician.
	• Modify consistency of diet as needed.
	• Encourage fluids to 2 to 3 liters daily.

4. Discuss with patient course of treatment chosen by patient and physician.
   a. Be aware of anxiety and fear by patient and family. Attempt to answer their questions.
   b. Encourage feedback.
   c. Assess the level of understanding.

C. *Is experiencing minimal discomfort or complications from chosen treatment*
• *Chemotherapy*

5. Assist the patient undergoing chemotherapy.
   a. Discuss with patient the aim of chemotherapy is to destroy the leukemic cells by suppression of bone marrow activity so that, on recovery, the bone marrow will produce only normal cells resulting in remission of the disease process.
   b. Explain the type of drug(s) used, route of administration, and frequency. This will depend on the type of leukemia and extent of disease. Current drugs commonly used include:
      • 6-Mercaptopurine (6-mP, Purinethal)
      • Chlorambucil (Leukeran)
      • Cyclophosphamide (Cytoxan)
      • Doxorubicin (Adriamycin)
      • Daunorubicin (Daunomycin)
      • Hydroxyurea (Hydrea)
      • Methotrexate (MTX)
      • Melphalan (Alkeran)
      • Vincristine sulfate (Oncovin)
      • Prednisone
      • L-Asparaginase (Elspar)
      • 5-Azacytidine
      • Beta-deoxythioguanosine (BTG dR)
      • Busulfan (Myleran)
      • 6-Thioguaine (6-TG)
   c. Refer to General Care Guidelines for the Patient With Cancer, p. 81 for specific interventions for the patient undergoing chemotherapy.

D. *Is coping with illness*

6. Assist the patient and family to cope with life-threatening illness.
      • Refer to General Care Guidelines for the Patient With Cancer p. 83 for specific interventions to help adjust to illness and therapy.

E. *Is knowledgeable about self-care and resources for continuity of care*

7. Plan discharge with patient and family.
      • Refer to General Care Guidelines for the Patient With Cancer, p. 84 for specific interventions related to discharge planning.

Patient Outcome	Process

The patient functions comfortably within limitations due to melanoma. This includes:

DESCRIPTION: Melanoma is a cancer of the skin originating as a mole, freckle, or birthmark. Detection may occur when one of these areas undergoes changes indicating increase in size, change in color such as darkening, itching, and/or bleeding. Melanoma is more prevalent in fair skinned, light haired, sun-sensitive persons.

Choice of therapy is dictated by diagnostic categories of melanoma which range from Clark's levels I, II (least invasive and usually require surgery only) to Clark's levels III, IV, V (invasive and require surgery in addition to immunotherapy and/or chemotherapy). Many patients are hospitalized immediately after diagnosis and have little time to adjust to the gravity of the situation.

NURSING ASSESSMENT: In addition to the general admission assessment, the following information is especially important.
1. Assess and document physical status.
   a. Signs and symptoms related to melanoma (include chronology of changes)
      • Appearance of lesion, *e.g.,* pigmentation, bleeding, ulceration, progressive growth.
      • Itching
   b. Location of lesion, *e.g.,* neck, trunk
   c. Previous therapy of lesion, *e.g.,* excision
   d. Stage of disease
2. Assess and document patient's and family's response to information about the disease process, implications, and treatment.
   a. Apparent anxiety level concerning the possibility of disease control
   b. Patient's self-assessment of:
      • Personal strengths in coping with stresses
      • Support persons, *e.g.,* family, minister
   c. Current stage of grief process
3. Assess and document health habits/life-style prior to admission.
   a. Self-care ability and/or need for assistance
   b. Dietary needs/restrictions
   c. Home health supervision/support
4. Assess and document patient's understanding of the disease process, implications, and treatment.

A. *Is prepared for diagnostic studies*

INTERVENTION:
1. Explain/answer questions about diagnostic studies. See Chapter 3 Guidelines for the Patient Undergoing Diagnostic Studies, p. 33. Studies may include:
   a. Liver scan   d. Brain scan
   b. Spleen scan   e. Skin tests (to assess immunological status)
   c. Bone scan
2. Reinforce physician's explanation of illness and treatment.

B. *Understands nature of illness, chosen treatment plan, and care*

C. *Is experiencing minimal discomfort or complications from chosen treatment*

3. Discuss with the patient the course of treatment chosen by patient and physician.
   a. Be aware of anxiety and fear of patient and family and attempt to answer their questions.
   b. Encourage feedback.
   c. Assess the level of understanding.
4. Assist the patient requiring surgical excision for the melanoma.
   a. Discuss the specific aspects of pre- and postoperative care. See Chapter 5 Preoperative Phase of Hospitalization, p. 129 and Postoperative Phase of Hospitalization, p. 130. Provide care needed per hospital routine and physician's orders.
   b. Intervene in the critical elements of postoperative care depending upon the extent of excision and lymph node dissection.
      • Refer to Chapter 5 Skin Grafts and Flaps Guidelines, p. 217 for specific aspects of wound care.
      • Refer to Chapter 5 Mastectomy Guidelines, p. 187 for specific aspects of care due to extensive lymph node dissection.
      • Allow no injections, venipunctures, or blood pressures in affected limbs.
      • Use antiembolic hose as ordered.
      • Teach specific measures to avoid trauma/infection:
         File nails rather than cut with scissors.
         Avoid open-toed shoes.
         Use electric shaver on affected leg/arm.
         Do not use deodorant under arm if axillary node dissection done.

Patient Outcome	Process

• *Immunotherapy*	5. Assist the patient undergoing immunotherapy.
	   a. Discuss with patient that the aim of immunotherapy is to stimulate production of tumor specific antibodies by intradermal, scratch method, or intratumor injection of nonspecific immune stimulator or specific vaccine made from the tumor.
	   b. Follow protocol/physician's orders to continue necessary diagnostic studies which may include:
	     • Urinalysis • Skin testing to determine immunity levels
	     • Chest radiograph • Frequent blood studies
	     • Frequent liver scans, brain scans
	   c. Observe for and report to physician signs and symptoms of side effects of therapy.
	     • Anaphylactic reaction: headache, shortness of breath, dizziness, possible shock
	     • Long-range effects (1 to 2 weeks): "flu-like" syndrome, malaise, soreness and induration under injection site which may discolor and later drain
	   d. Provide and teach care for draining injection site.
	     • Clean area with soap and water. Apply sterile dressing.
	     • Dispose of soiled dressing in paper bag to prevent spread of acid fast bacilli.
	     • Apply hot or cold compresses to site to alleviate discomfort.
	   e. Reassess general condition frequently and intervene appropriately.

• *Chemotherapy*	6. Assist the patient undergoing chemotherapy.
	   a. Discuss with patient that the aim of chemotherapy is to eradicate the cancer, to stop progression of the disease and keep it under control, to facilitate remission, or to help relieve pain.
	   b. Refer to General Care Guidelines for the Patient With Cancer, p. 81 for specific interventions for the patient undergoing chemotherapy.

D. *Is coping with life-threatening illness*	7. Assist patient/family to cope with life-threatening illness.
	   a. Establish a trust relationship; give consistent information.
	   b. Provide opportunity for expression of concerns, fears, and questions.
	   c. Identify resource persons, *e.g.*, oncology nurse clinician, chaplain.
	   d. Support appropriate coping strategy.
	   e. Assure continued support regardless of patient's decisions regarding treatment.
	   f. Provide environment that is appropriate to individual needs, *e.g.*, privacy, activity, visitors, special requests.
	   g. Encourage participation in self-care.
	   h. Facilitate interactions with other patients undergoing similar therapy, if appropriate.
	   i. Give positive reinforcement and realistic hope.
	8. Support patient/family in working through grief process. Intervene appropriately.
	   a. Be aware that it is essential for individual staff members to work through their own emotions before they can help patient and family to cope with adjustment.
	   b. Consider that patient and family may be in different phases of the grief process and may move back and forth between stages.
	   c. Reassess stage of grief frequently.
	   d. Accept patient's responses and recognize his feelings.
	     • Allow ample time for verbalization.
	     • Demonstrate acceptance through active listening.

E. *Is knowledgeable about self-care and resources for continuity of care*	9. Plan discharge with patient and family.
	   a. Reinforce physician's instructions.
	   b. Reinforce teaching of knowledge/skills related to home care and provide written information as needed:
	     • Self-examination every 3 to 4 weeks for cervical, axillary, and groin nodes, subcutaneous nodules anywhere on the body.
	     • Medications: Immunotherapy patient may take previously prescribed medications with the exception of cortisone preparations. Chemotherapy patient may have cortisone preparation prescribed as part of the treatment plan.
	   c. Assist patient to make arrangements to obtain blood counts every other week as indicated by physician.
	   d. Discuss community agencies which may assist in continuity of care.
	   e. Initiate interagency referral as needed.
	   f. Give return appointment and stress importance of continued care.
	   g. Assure patient of continued availability of physician and nurse to provide care and support. Provide telephone numbers for contact.

Patient Outcome	Process

The patient functions comfortably within limitations due to cerebrovascular accident. This includes:

DESCRIPTION: Cerebrovascular accidents (stroke) occur as a result of impaired blood supply to the brain. This impairment may be due to intracerebral thrombosis, hemorrhage (ruptured blood vessel), embolism, and/or cerebral ischemia.

Strokes may be classified on the basis of the cerebral vessel(s) that is occluded or obstructed, the brain area(s) that is ischemic or infarcted, and the chronological character of the clinical episode. Therapy may be based on the following common clinical stages of stroke.

TRANSIENT ISCHEMIA ATTACK (TIA), which is characterized by transient disturbances in neurological function without residual deficit.

STROKE-IN-EVOLUTION, which is characterized by progressive and increasing neurological dysfunction over a period of hours or days with residual deficit.

COMPLETED STROKE characterized by cessation of progression of neurological dysfunction with stabilization of residual deficit. In some instances a completed stroke can become *extended* characterized by further progression of neurological dysfunction.

NURSING ASSESSMENT: In addition to the general admission assessment, the following information is especially important.
1. Assess and document physical and mental status.
   a. Level of consciousness. Describe behavioral changes and mental status.
   b. Motor/sensory function (compare right to left)
      • Weakness of facial muscles and extremities
   c. Pupillary reaction
   d. Impairments in hearing; vision, *e.g.,* diplopia; and speech, *e.g.,* dysphasia
   e. Bowel and bladder control
   f. Respiratory status, *e.g.,* color and temperature of skin, character of respiration
   g. Other important findings
      • Vertigo
      • Headache
      • Gag reflex
      • Dysphagia
2. Assess and document patient's response to information about the disease process and treatment.
   a. Apparent anxiety level, *e.g.,* life-threatening illness
   b. Patient's self-assessment of:
      • Personal strengths in coping with stress
      • Support people, *e.g.,* family, friends
3. Assess and document health habits/life-style prior to admission.
   a. Home health supervision/support
   b. Physical demands, *e.g.,* occupation
   c. Position in family unit, *e.g.,* marital status, dependent children
   d. Diet
   e. Medications
4. Assess and document patient's/family's understanding of disease process and treatment.

A. *Is prepared for diagnostic studies*

INTERVENTION:
1. Explain/answer questions about diagnostic studies. Refer to Chapter 3 Guidelines For The Patient Undergoing Diagnostic Studies, p. 33. Studies may include:
   a. CT Scan
   b. LP
   c. EEG
   d. Skull films
   e. Arteriography

B. *Is free of or has minimal complications due to immobility and/or limitation of movement*

2. Institute measures to preserve functions at optimal level and prevent further damage.
   a. Maintain respiratory function. See Chapter 2 Pulmonary Care Guideline, p. 29 for preventive and therapeutic measures.
   b. Keep patient in functional body alignment.
      • Avoid back-lying position while patient is without cough and gag reflexes.
      • Use equipment to maintain functional alignment (pillows, foot board, hand rolls, brace-booties, slings).
      • Elevate head of bed to facilitate normal feeding position when permitted.
      • Put patient's arms and legs through range of motion exercises when turned.

99

Patient Outcome	Process
	c. Assist patient to be physically active and insure joint mobility and muscle strength.
	• Collaborate with physical therapy for evaluation and treatment when patient is stabilized.
	• Encourage/teach patient to do active range of motion exercises b.i.d.
	• Schedule "out of bed" to coincide with mealtimes. Gradually lengthen time as strength and tolerance increase.
	• Use patient's maximum physical capabilities to increase participation in self-care activities.
	• Teach patient/family transfer technique using unaffected extremities.
	• Encourage ambulation using assistive devices as needed (walker, three-point cane, braces).
	• Supervise exercises and activities patient is learning in physical therapy which require practice in unit.
	d. Maintain fluid balance.
	• Keep intake and output record.
	• Weight as appropriate
	• Administer IV fluids as indicated until patient is able to tolerate oral or tube feedings.
	• Assess, daily, ability to swallow fluids.
	• Provide fluid intake of 2500 cc daily unless contraindicated.
	e. Maintain nutritional status.
	• Keep intake and output record.
	• Assess, daily, ability to swallow and chew foods.
	• Progress oral fluids to diet as tolerated, *e.g.*, edentulous diet, if able to swallow.
	• Provide nutrition via feeding tube if patient unable to swallow.
	• Evaluate caloric intake frequently.
	• Provide vitamin supplements as appropriate.
	f. Establish preventive skin care routine. See Chapter 2 Skin Care Guidelines, p. 31.
	g. Establish bladder care routine. See Chapter 2 Bladder Care Guidelines, p. 23.
	h. Establish bowel care program. See Chapter 2 Bowel Care Guidelines, p. 25.
	• Remain aware that patient may have decreased ability to communicate needs.
	• Attempt to restore regularity of bowel function.
	• Prevent constipation through use of diet and/or medications.
	• Review bowel movement record daily.
	• Institute bowel training program based on past bowel pattern:
	Suppository q.d. or q.o.d.
	Laxative or stool softener as needed
	Fluid intake of 2500 cc or more daily unless contraindicated, including prune juice
	Regularity in time of evacuation
C. *Is benefiting from therapy*	3. Administer anticoagulant therapy (heparin) as indicated by physician.
	a. Use infusion rate controller to regulate dosage per hour precisely.
	b. Prevent side effects/complications of therapy:
	• Observe for evidence of bleeding, *e.g.*, easy bruising, blood in vomitus, urine, stool.
	• Inform physician of symptoms of suspected bleeding.
	• Collaborate with physician to discontinue heparin infusion at least 6 to 12 hours prior to any invasive diagnostic study, *e.g.*, arteriogram.
	c. Keep flat in bed to promote cerebral perfusion of medication. If therapy is long term (7 to 10 days) patient may be allowed out of bed in chair.
D. *Is coping with limitations of activities of daily living*	4. Maintain verbal stimulation. Consider degree of aphasia, current evaluation of intellectual functioning, and usual manner of communicating.
	a. Encourage verbal and nonverbal attempts at communication (gestures, writing, aphasia cards).
	b. Assess need for speech therapy evaluation.
	5. Promote participation in self-care by selecting activites which the patient has the potential to accomplish.
	a. Bathing
	b. Dressing
	c. Grooming
	d. Feeding
	6. Involve family in daily care as appropriate.

Patient Outcome	Process
	7. Provide consistency in care and approach to facilitate patient response.
	a. Reorient daily to environment.
	b. Identify and use terminology used by patient to communicate needs.
	c. Provide clock and calendar.
	d. Give positive reinforcement for successful attempts in self-care activities.
E. *Is knowledgeable about the nature of illness, self-care, and resources for continuity of care*	8. Teach patient and family about illness, extent of disability, and care.
	a. Reinforce physician's explanation.
	b. Instruct in current self-care and need for assistance, stressing use of unaffected side and functional abilities.
	• Assess with patient and family the home environment in relation to limitations and care needs, *e.g.,* stairs, bathtub, chair.
	c. Support patient and family in making realistic plans for changes in life-style.
	• Counsel about realistic expectations of rehabilitation.
	• Discuss altered family role, *e.g.,* financial, vocational, social, sexual.
	d. Provide and instruct about medications and assistive devices as needed.
	• Discuss side effects of anticoagulant therapy and include reporting of any symptoms of bleeding to physician.
	• Assure that patient on anticoagulant therapy understands importance of monitoring the prothrombin time.
	• Suggest use of identification bracelet.
	e. Discuss with patient and family the feasibility of home care and alternatives.
	• Discuss available resources useful in continuity of care, *e.g.,* social worker.
	f. Initate appropriate referral to community health agencies, *e. g.,* public health nursing.

Patient Outcome	Process

The patient functions comfortably within limitations due to congestive heart failure. This includes:

DESCRIPTION: Congestive heart failure is a state of diminished cardiac function resulting in congestion of either the pulmonary or systemic circulation, or both. Congestive heart failure may be acute or chronic and is commonly described as either left-sided or right-sided although both may occur simultaneously. The condition may be due to a variety of causes such as coronary artery disease, myocardial infarction, cardiomyopathy, valvular disease, and fluid overload.

NURSING ASSESSMENT: In addition to the general admission assessment, the following information is especially important.

1. Assess and document physical status.
   a. Signs and symptoms of heart failure:
      - Shortness of breath, orthopnea
      - Râles
      - Leg and sacral edema
      - Neck vein distention
      - Abnormal heart sounds, *e.g.*, S_3, S_4
      - Tachycardia
      - Weight gain in excess of one pound per day
      - Decreased urinary output
      - Easy fatigue
      - Restlessness
      - Abdominal discomfort
   b. Current medications
   c. Associated risk factors, *e.g.*, asthma, obesity
2. Assess and document patient's response to information about the disease process, implications, and treatment.
   a. Apparent anxiety level
   b. Patient's self-assessment of:
      - Personal strengths in coping with stress
      - Support people, *e.g.*, family
3. Assess and document health habits/life style prior to admission.
   a. Home health supervision/support
   b. Position in family unit, *e.g.*, homemaker
4. Assess and document patient's understanding of the disease process, implications, and treatment.

INTERVENTION:

1. Explain/answer questions about diagnostic studies. Refer to Chapter 3, Guidelines for the Patient Undergoing Diagnostic Studies, p. 33. Studies may include:
   a. Chest radiograph
   b. Electrocardiogram
   c. Cardiac fluoroscopy
   d. Venous pressure measurement

A. *Is benefiting from therapy*

2. Institute measures to increase cardiac output.
   a. Position patient to facilitate respirations, *e.g.*, elevate head of bed.
   b. Administer oxygen
   c. Give medications as ordered, *e.g.*, diuretics, digitalis, morphine.
   d. Monitor vital signs as indicated.
   e. Restrict diet and fluid intake as ordered.
   f. Maintain intake-output record.
   g. Weigh daily.
   h. Anticipate need for indwelling urinary catheter.
   i. Apply rotating tourniquets if ordered.

B. *Is maintaining physiological function*

3. Provide supportive measures to promote other physiological functions.
   a. Establish rest/activity program with patient and physician.
      - Include active and passive range of motion exercises b.i.d.
      - Advance activity within limits of patient's physiologic tolerance.
   b. Provide pulmonary care. Refer to Chapter 2, Pulmonary Care Guidelines, p. 29.
      - Turn every two hours.
      - Encourage deep breathing and coughing.
   c. Provide bowel care. Refer to Chapter 2, Bowel Care Guidelines, p. 25.
   d. Provide skin care. Refer to Chapter 2, Skin Care Guidelines, p. 31.

Patient Outcome	Process

C. *Is coping with illness*	4. Assist patient to adjust to limitations imposed by disease process.
	    a. Provide opportunity for expression of concerns, fears, and questions.
	    b. Encourage participation in self-care within limits of patient's tolerance.
	    c. Support appropriate coping strategy.
	    d. Explore with patient necessary changes in life-style, *e.g.*, work habits.

D. *Is knowledgeable about nature of illness, self-care, and resources for continuity of care*	5. Plan discharge with patient and family.
	    a. Provide knowledge related to care:
	      • Basic anatomy and physiology of heart and circulatory system.
	      • Relationship of fluid and sodium intake to congestive heart failure.
	    b. Collaborate with physician and dietician to plan dietary modifications.
	    c. Assess with patient/family the home design in relation to prescribed activity, *e.g.*, climbing stairs.
	      • Assist in determining any needed home modifications.
	    d. Discuss stress factors and their prevention/control which may influence state of compensation, *e.g.*, infection, family conflicts.
	    e. Reinforce physician's explanations and instructions to include:
	      • Drug therapy. Emphasize consistent use of prescribed medications and signs and symptoms of toxicity.
	      • Diet and fluid modifications.
	      • Activity/rest program
	      • Reduction of risk factors such as control of hypertension.
	    f. Discuss signs and symptoms of decompensation which should be reported to physician such as:
	      • Weight gain of two pounds per day
	      • Shortness of breath
	      • Edema
	      • Easy fatigue
	      • Dry, persistent cough at night
	    g. Discuss community agencies which may assist in continuity of care, *e.g.*, vocational rehabilitation, social services.
	    h. Initiate interagency referral as needed.
	    i. Give return appointment. Emphasize importance of continued medical care.

Patient Outcome	Process

The patient functions comfortably within limitations due to diabetes mellitus. This includes:

DESCRIPTION: Diabetes mellitus is a chronic condition caused by decreased insulin production or resistance to insulin effect in peripheral tissues. Diabetes is manifested by abnormalities in carbohydrate, fat, and protein metabolism. Adults may develop diabetes with such precipitating psychophysiological factors as obesity, pregnancy, surgery, infection, and other stresses.

Diabetes may be controlled by (1) diet, (2) diet and oral hypoglycemic agent, or (3) diet and insulin. Control is dependent upon regulating activity/exercise in conjunction with dietary and pharmacologic measures.

NURSING ASSESSMENT: In addition to the general admission assessment, the following information is especially important.

1. Assess and document physical and mental status.
   a. Duration and severity of symptoms, *e.g.,* polydipsia, polyuria
   b. Current medical regimen, *e.g.,* diet, medications
   c. Nutritional status
   d. Skin condition, *e.g.,* foot or leg-ulcer, injection sites
   e. Visual acuity
   f. Circulatory status, *e.g.,* peripheral pulses, color
   g. Sensory changes, *e.g.,* numbness or pain in feet
   h. Signs of infection, *e.g.,* vaginitis
   i. Gastrointestinal, *e.g.,* bowel history
   j. Personality/behavior changes
   k. Risk factors, *e.g.,* renal impairment, hypertension
   l. Family history of diabetes
2. Assess and document patient's response to information about the disease process, implications, and treatment.
   a. Apparent anxiety level
   b. Patient's self-assessment of
      • Personal strengths in coping with stress
      • Support people, *e.g.,* family, friends
3. Assess and document health habits/life-style prior to admission.
   a. Home health supervision and support
   b. Home schedule of diabetes management including meal times, urine testing, drug administration, and activity
   c. Position in family unit, *e.g.,* meal preparation duties
4. Assess and document patient's/family's understanding of the disease process, implications, and treatment.

A. *Is prepared for diagnostic studies*

INTERVENTION:

1. Explain/answer questions about diagnostic studies. Refer to Chapter 3 Guidelines for The Patient Undergoing Diagnostic Studies, p. 33.
   a. Frequent blood chemistries
   b. Glucose tolerance test
   c. Timed urine collections
   d. Renal threshold measurement by blood drawing when urine glucose is trace to negative
   e. Additional studies if there are other problems such as infection

B. *Is achieving control of diabetes mellitus*

2. Incorporate principles of teaching to maximize effectiveness of care. Begin as early as possible in hospitalization.
   a. Reassess continuously patient's knowledge as teaching progresses.
   b. Use time periods that are realistic for the patient (do not overload patient with information at any one time).
   c. Use informal contacts to teach, reinforce information previously learned, *e.g.,* while giving medications, serving diet, helping with skin care.
   d. Encourage participation of patient and family in care as a way of reinforcing knowledge and skills.
   e. Provide positive reinforcement to increase motivation.
   f. Communicate and document positive and negative aspects of learning so plan can be modified when it is unrealistic.
   g. Provide receptive, learning environment. Control as much as possible interferences in the environment, *e.g.,* noises such as TV; talking; discomfort.
   h. Listen for cues that patient is thinking about something else or is not receptive at the time for teaching. Physiological factors such as hypo- or hyperglycemia may affect this.
   i. Make sure nursing techniques are consistent and accurate to serve as a model to patient.

Patient Outcome	Process

3. Provide and teach components of care for control of diabetes.
   a. Discuss anatomy, pathophysiology, and treatment relating to diabetes mellitus.
   b. Collaborate with patient, family, physician, and dietician to provide dietary treatment.
      - Request dietary teaching consult early in hospitalization.
      - Reinforce dietary teaching.
      - Observe for prescribed nutritional intake, *e.g.,* distribution and amounts of carbohydrate, fat, and protein.
      - Initiate calorie count if indicated.
      - Consult with physician for adjustments in diet/medications if intake is inadequate.
      - Monitor daily weight as indicated.
      - Identify need for dietary intake adjustment, *e.g.,* reduction diet for weight loss, decreased infection, change of activity postdischarge.
      - Have patient or family member responsible for meal preparation plan a day's menu based on dietary instructions.
   c. Demonstrate urine glucose/acetone testing methods and record maintenance until performed independently by patient and/or family member.
      - Teach double-voiding technique using:
         Clinitest two drop method
         Acetest
         Testape
   d. Expect patient to assume responsibility for urine testing with nurse supervision as indicated.
   e. Provide knowledge about insulin/oral agent.
      - Action, peak effect, duration
   f. Demonstrate insulin administration until performed independently by patient or family member. Include:
      - Aseptic technique
      - Injection technique, *e.g.,* subcutaneous tissue at 90° angle
      - Rotation of sites, *e. g.,* arms, thighs, abdomen, buttocks
      - Time of injection in relation to food intake
      - Single/mixed dose techniques as needed
   g. Expect patient to assume responsibility for insulin administration with nurse supervision as indicated.
   h. Observe for and teach about hypoglycemia.
      - Discuss possible contributing factors, *e.g.,* delay of meals, too much insulin, overexercise.
      - Be alert for signs and symptoms: hunger, nervousness, sweaty, headache, irritability, confusion, change in responsiveness, negative urine glucose, low blood sugar. May have rapid onset. Report to physician.
      - Treat for mild to moderate symptomatology:
         Give 10 grams of carbohydrate. Examples are 4 ounces of unsweetened orange juice or Coca-Cola, 1 tablespoon honey or 2 sugar packets.
         Repeat in 5 to 10 minutes if symptoms persist.
         Follow with 1 bread and meat exchange or 1 milk exchange if more than 1 hour to the next meal.
      - Treat for severe symptomatology, *i.e.,* decreasing level of consciousness.
         Administer 50 cc of dextrose 50 percent in water IV.
         Continue to monitor response carefully.
      - Teach the selected patient the use of glucagon.
   i. Establish with patient a consistent activity program that is compatible with life-style.
      - Discuss relationship between activity and insulin utilization.
      - Instruct patient to eat 1 extra fruit exchange (or any 10 to 15 grams carbohydrate) for every 30–60 minutes of strenuous exercise beyond usual activity, *e.g.,* tennis game, leaf raking, painting.

C. *Is free of or has minimal complications*

4. Establish with patient self-care measures to reduce risk of complications.
   a. Care of feet:
      - Bathe daily and pat dry.
      - Inspect daily for corns, bruises, trauma, rashes, ingrown toenails.
      - Apply lanolin base lotions to dry areas as needed.
      - Cut toenails straight across using appropriate instrument such as nail clippers or let someone else do it.

Patient Outcome	Process

- Wear proper-fitting shoes. Do not go barefoot.
- Avoid use of strong solutions such as antiseptics and extreme temperatures such as hot water.
- Seek physician advice for any foot problems.

b. General preventive measures
- Skin

  Bathe daily with special attention to feet, toenails, genital area, axilla, skin folds.

  Use lanolin-base lotion to prevent dryness.

  Avoid harsh soaps, detergents.

  Avoid trauma.

  Avoid constriction of extremities, *e.g.,* garters.
- Oral

  Brush teeth and use dental floss regularly.

  See dentist as indicated.
- Visual

  Discuss need for regular vision evaluation.

5. Provide therapeutic skin care as indicated.
   a. Change dry or wet dressings as needed.
   b. Observe wound condition and document changes.
   c. Prevent new trauma to wound (bulky dressings, tape).
   d. Elevate extremity.
   e. Position to avoid pressure on affected area.
   f. Allow limited activity to promote circulation and healing.

6. Teach patient/family about infection.
   a. Discuss effects of infection on management of diabetes (the effect of the increased stress usually elevates serum glucose).
   b. Teach signs and symptoms of infection. Common infections are upper respiratory, urinary tract, monilial. Report infections to physician.
   c. Instruct patient in guidelines to follow for temporary illness at home (nausea, vomiting, diarrhea, "flu-like" symptoms).
      - Take usual insulin dose.
      - Rest and keep warm.
      - Test urine for glucose and acetone at each voiding or at least four times daily.
      - Take fluids hourly.
      - Replace carbohydrates with liquids and easy-to-digest foods if unable to eat prescribed meals.
      - Call physician if the following should occur:

        Continuous urine glucose spills and presence of acetone

        Continued inability to follow meal plan after replacing four or five meals with substitute carbohydrate
      - Anticipate increased insulin requirements; a supplemental plan may be instituted based on results of urine testing.

7. Observe for and teach about hyperglycemia.
   a. Discuss possible contributing factors, *e.g.,* infection, surgery, nonadherence.
   b. Teach signs and symptoms such as polydipsia, polyuria, lethargy, weakness, skin dryness, positive urine glucose and acetone checks, high blood sugar, nausea and vomiting. Onset is slow. Report to physician.
   c. Treat for mild to moderate symptomatology:
      - Identify and treat source of hyperglycemia.
      - Always take insulin and increase dose as prescribed.
      - Increase frequency of monitoring.
   d. Treat for severe symptomatology, *e.g.,* decreased level of consciousness in addition to above.
      - Monitor blood gases and chemistries.
      - Monitor vital signs and urine volume.
      - Administer fluid and electrolyte replacement as indicated.
   e. Teach preventive measures for hyperglycemia.
      - Regular urine checks
      - Adherence to regimen, *e.g.,* rest, intake of food and fluids
      - Avoidance of undue stress, infection

Patient Outcome	Process
	• Increased monitoring of urine during illness/stress • Early reporting of symptoms/situations to physician

D. *Is willing to adapt life-style to methods of control of diabetes*	8. Assist patient/family to adapt to methods of control of diabetes.
	  a. Assess current coping strategy, *e.g.,* denial, acceptance.
	  b. Support appropriate coping strategy.
	  c. Provide opportunity for patient/family to express concerns and future plans.
	  d. Identify with patient resource persons, *e.g.,* nutritionist, social worker, family members, physician.
	  e. Encourage appropriate interactions with other persons with diabetes.
	  f. Explore with patient changes in daily living activities necessitated by incorporation of diabetes management plan, *e.g.,* work schedule, eating out, travel.
	  g. Help patient to set realistic goals, *e.g.,* weight loss, reduced insulin dose.

E. *Is knowledgeable about nature of illness, self care, and resources for continuity of care*	9. Plan discharge with patient and family.
	  a. Reinforce knowledge and skills needed to carry out management.
	  b. Provide equipment, supplies, and information about how to obtain additional supplies.
	  c. Inform about community agencies which may assist in continuity of care, *e.g.,* American Diabetes Association, employee health center.
	  d. Initiate interagency referral as needed.
	  e. Provide information about importance of wearing medical identification, *e.g.,* bracelet, wallet card.
	  f. Emphasize importance of continued medical care. Give return appointment.

Patient Outcome	Process

The patient functions comfortably within limitations due to acute viral hepatitis. This includes:

DESCRIPTION: Acute viral hepatitis is a systemic infection affecting predominantly the liver. There are two types (A and B) and the course can vary from mild to severe with destruction of liver with extensive fibrosis. Hepatitis is a reportable communicable diesease which requires investigation of contacts.

Hepatitis A or "infectious" is generally less severe than hepatitis B and the patient may not require hospitalization.

Incubation period: 15 to 45 days

Mode of transmission:

1. Oral-fecal route, contaminated water, milk, food—especially shellfish
2. Blood, serum, plasma from an infected patient; contaminated needles, syringes

Symptoms: "Flu-like": anorexia, fatigue, nausea, vomiting, diarrhea, joint pains, fever, pruritus, distaste for cigarettes, photophobia, tenderness over liver. Urine darkens due to elevated bilirubin and stools are light in color.

Pathophysiology: Inflammatory change and patchy liver cell necrosis; elevated liver enzymes. Liver generally recovers.

Treatment: Gamma globulin, symptomatic treatment, bed rest, nutritious diet

Recovery Phase: Approximately four months

Hepatitis B or "serum" is increasing in incidence. Improper handling of contaminated products has increased the incidence of the disease among hospital staff and high risk patients. Maintenance of strict precautionary measures for these enteric infections is essential. Most patients with this illness show a blood test positive for hepatitis associated antigen (HAA$^+$). The name for the antigen is HB$_s$AG. (Hepatitis B surface antigen)

Incubation period: 60 to 180 days

Mode of transmission:

1. Contaminated blood, blood products; needle punctures; open wounds; ingestion
2. Urine and stool
3. Saliva, semen and other secretions may be sources.

Virus can penetrate mucous membranes of eye, alimentary tract.

Symptoms: Same as A but usually more severe.

Pathophysiology: Patchy hepatic cell necrosis. Elevated liver enzymes: serum glutamic oxaloacetic transaminase (SGOT), serum glutamic pyruvic transaminase (SGPT), bilirubin. Liver usually recovers but patient may develop chronic progressive hepatitis resulting in hepatic failure and necrotic cirrhosis.

Treatment: Same as A, also hyperimmune gamma globulin

Recovery Phase: Depends upon severity of disease; approximately 2 to 24 weeks.

Chronic asymptomatic carriers: Remain HAA$^+$. Blood precautions should be observed for these patients.

NURSING ASSESSMENT: In addition to the general admission assessment, the following information is especially important.

1. Assess and document physical status.
   a. Signs and symptoms related to underlying disease:
      - Gastrointestinal symptoms such as anorexia, nausea and vomiting, stool changes
      - Energy level, malaise • Weight loss
      - Urine change • Jaundice
   b. Risk factors:
      - Presence of other disease states, *e.g.,* diabetes, congestive heart failure, malignancy, renal disease
2. Assess and document patient's response to information about the disease process and its treatment.
   a. Apparent anxiety level
   b. Patient's self-assessment of:
      - Personal strengths in coping with stress
      - Support people, *e.g.,* family, friends, chaplain
3. Assess and document health habits/life-style prior to admission.
   a. Home health supervision/support
   b. Physical demands, *e.g.,* occupation, recreational activities
   c. Position in family unit, *e.g.,* marital status, dependent children
   d. Potential for compliance with precautionary measures necessitated by disease
4. Assess and document patient's understanding of disease process.

Patient Outcome	Process

A. *Is prepared for diagnostic studies*	**INTERVENTION:**
	1. Explain/answer questions about diagnostic studies. These may include:
	  a. Hepatitis associated antigen and antibody. Positive antigen indicates serum hepatitis.
	  b. Prothrombin time: lowered prothrombin activity indicates severe liver damage.
	  c. Serum glutamic oxaloacetic transaminase, serum glutamic pyruvic transaminase.
	  d. Blood ammonia
	  e. Liver biopsy. See Chapter 3 Liver Biopsy, p. 57.

B. *Is protecting others from infection*	2. Establish precautionary measures according to hospital routine for isolation techniques on enteric infections. See Isolation Manual. • Explain to patient and family the reasons for the precautions used to safeguard themselves, other patients, and hospital personnel.

C. *Is achieving maximum benefit from palliative therapy*	3. Be alert to signs of liver cell damage indicated by results of blood studies such as:
	  a. Elevated SGPT and SGOT due to increased liver cell permeability and necrosis of liver cells.
	  b. Elevated bilirubin levels and bilirubin in urine
	  c. Prolonged prothrombin time; watch for signs of bleeding, prolonged clotting time.
	  d. Elevated serum ammonia levels; watch for signs of hepatic coma.
	  e. Decreased serum albumin; watch for excessive tissue edema.
	4. Deal with patient's symptoms, which may include nausea, vomiting, diarrhea, lethargy, abnormalities of taste, fever, edema, epigastric pain, itching.
	5. Restrict certain food, fluid, and drugs for patients with severe liver disease and/or renal failure. These restrictions may include:
	  a. Most drugs in the sedative, antiemetic, analgesic, and tranquilizer classes are metabolized by the liver. Drug dosage should be individualized according to patient's clinical status in order to minimize toxicity.
	    • Examples of drugs with toxic potential are:
	      Phenothiazines (Compazine, Phenergan)
	      Barbiturates
	      Paraldehyde
	      Morphine
	    • Examples of less toxic drugs are:
	      Chlordiazepoxide (Librium), Diazepam (Valium)
	      Acetominophen (Tylenol), Aspirin
	      Codeine
	      Propoxyphene (Darvon)
	  b. Some antibiotics should be avoided in patients in renal failure because this is their major route of elimination; some antibiotics are eliminated by liver metabolism and should be avoided in severe liver disease (noted by *).
	    • Examples of potentially dangerous antibiotics:
	      Tetracycline
	      Rifampin*
	      Cephalexin (Keflex)*
	      Isoniazid
	      Chloramphenicol
	    • Generally safe antibiotic:
	      Penicillin
	6. Restrict activity to bedrest with bathroom privileges or bedside commode.
	7. Provide good skin care and daily hygiene.
	8. Initiate action when signs of complications are observed such as:
	  a. Bleeding; check for further bleeding in vomitus, stool, urine, easy bruising, prolonged bleeding from puncture site.
	  b. Ascites; check abdominal girth.
	  c. Hepatic encephalopathy; monitor changes in mental status, tremors, hyperreflexia, seizures.
	  d. Hepatic coma

D. *Is coping with chronic illness and hospitalization*	9. Elicit patient's concerns about illness. Concerns may include:
	  a. Transmission of disease to family members
	  b. Return to employment, household duties, previous lifestyle
	  c. Physical discomfort
	  d. Progression of disease
	  e. Need for prolonged treatment

Patient Outcome	Process
	f. "Stigma" of disease
	g. Future physical limitations, *i.e.,* pregnancy, giving blood, fluids and diet restrictions.
E. *Is knowledgeable about nature of illness, self-care, and resources for continuity of care*	10. Teach patient and family in preparation for discharge.
	a. Reinforce patient's and family's understanding of illness.
	b. Discuss specific precautions to prevent transmission of disease at home. Specific information includes:
	• Family usually receives prophylactic gamma globulin. Check with physician.
	• Avoid sharing personal items such as washcloth, razor, toothbrush, glass.
	• Strict handwashing after using toilet, before and after meals, and brushing teeth should be practiced.
	• Launder clothes separately, if possible, in hot water with chlorine solution.
	• Handle blood-contaminated items with disposable gloves.
	• If liver enzyme levels are elevated, use disposable plates and implements. Avoid mucous membrane contact temporarily, *i.e.,* kissing, sexual contact.
	• Automatic dishwasher with hot water setting is acceptable for used utensils.
	• If separate toilet facilities unavailable, sanitize daily with chlorine solution.
	• General good cleaning of household areas, especially bathroom and kitchen is necessary.
	c. Plan with patient progressive activity as tolerated with ample rest periods.
	d. Discuss high protein diet with restrictions as prescribed. Request dietary consult.
	e. Instruct patient about prescribed medications.
	f. Alert patient that he can give no blood donations and to inform dentist or other physicians that he has hepatitis prior to care and if admitted to hospital.
	• Suggest that patient carry medical identification, *e.g.,* wallet card, arm bracelet.
	g. Encourage follow-up medical care and laboratory studies as prescribed.

Patient Outcome	Process

The patient functions comfortably within limitations due to hypertension. This includes:

DESCRIPTION: Hypertension is a condition characterized by elevation of the blood pressure beyond the level considered normal for the individual. Hypertension is a contributing factor in coronary artery disease and cerebrovascular accident. It is often hereditary and is a major health problem affecting persons of all ages.

NURSING ASSESSMENT: In addition to the general admission assessment, the following information is especially important.

1. Assess and document physical status.
   a. Blood pressure, lying and standing positions in both arms
   b. Apical/radial pulses
   c. Peripheral pulses
   d. Heart sounds, *e.g.*, S_4
   e. Lung sounds, *e.g.*, râles
   f. Associated cardiovascular risk factors, *e.g.*, obesity
2. Assess and document patient's understanding of the disease process, implications, and treatment.
3. Assess and document patient's response to information about the disease process, implications, and treatment.
   a. Apparent anxiety level
   b. Patient's self-assessment of:
      • Personal strengths in coping with stress
      • Support people, *e.g.*, family.

A. *Is prepared for diagnostic studies*

INTERVENTION:

1. Explain/answer questions about diagnostic studies. Refer to Chapter 3 Guidelines For The Patient Undergoing Diagnostic Studies, p. 33. Studies may include:
   a. EKG
   b. IVP
   c. Timed urine collections for 17-hydroxysteroids, aldosterone
   d. Renal arteriogram
   e. Renin levels

B. *Is achieving control of elevated blood pressure*

2. Provide and teach measures to prevent further elevation of blood pressure.
   a. Provide knowledge related to:
      • Chronic nature of condition
      • Effects of untreated or uncontrolled blood pressure on organ systems
      • Patient's documented acceptable range of blood pressure
   b. Administer medications as ordered. Provide verbal and written information about the use of such therapeutic drugs as diuretics, vasodilators, and sympatholytic agents.
      • Emphasize side effects which may be temporary.
      • Alert patient to potential interactions with other drugs, *e.g.*, over-the-counter drugs.
   c. Collaborate with physician, dietician, patient and family to establish dietary modifications to include weight reduction, sodium and/or fat reduction.
   d. Discuss elimination of smoking.
   e. Establish with patient a program of regular exercise, *e.g.*, walking, recretational activity.
   f. Monitor response to therapy by frequent measurements of blood pressure.
      • Teach patient/family skill of measurement of blood pressure if indicated.
   g. Counsel with patient/family to reduce physical, environmental, and emotional stresses.
      • Identify precipitating factors.
      • Determine methods of dealing with stress such as avoidance, relaxation response, biofeedback.
      • Consider referral to appropriate agencies to assist, *e.g.*, Vocational Rehabilitation.
      • Support appropriate coping strategy.
      • Explore with patient changes in life style which can reduce stress, *e.g.*, work schedule.
   h. Discuss and reinforce importance of continued medication administration even though patient begins to feel better and pressures are lowered.

D. *Is knowledgeable about nature of illness, self-care, and resources for continuity of care*

3. Plan discharge with patient/family.
   a. Reinforce knowledge needed to control blood pressure.
   b. Provide prescriptions and/or medications.
   c. Discuss community agencies which may assist in continuity of care.
   d. Initiate interagency referral as needed.
   e. Emphasize importance of continued medical care. Give return appointment.

Patient Outcome	Process

The patient functions comfortably within limitations due to lupus erythematosus. This includes:

DESCRIPTION: Systemic lupus erythematosus (SLE) is a chronic inflammatory disease of unknown etiology and characterized by periods of remissions and relapses. Single or multiple organ systems are involved including renal, cardiovascular, musculoskeletal, gastrointestinal, hematologic, integumentary and central nervous system. The disease is further characterized by autoimmune phenomena. It occurs more commonly in females with onset in the 20 to 40-year age group. The main goal of therapy is to prevent exacerbation.

NURSING ASSESSMENT: In addition to the general admission assessment, the following information is especially important.
1. Assess and document physical status.
    a. Signs and symptoms related to underlying disease:
        • Fever
        • Joint stiffness or pain
        • Anorexia
        • Weight loss
        • Fatigability
        • Extent of "butterfly" rash
    b. Risk factors:
        • Presence of other disease states
        • Extent of involvement with multiple organ systems, *e.g.*, renal
    c. Abnormal laboratory findings
2. Assess and document patient's response to information about the disease process and treatment.
    a. Apparent anxiety level
    b. Patient's self-assessment of:
        • Personal strengths in coping with stress
        • Support people, *e.g.*, family, friends
3. Assess and document health habits/life style prior to admission.
    a. Home health supervision/support
    b. Physical demands, *e.g.*, occupation
    c. Position in family unit, *e.g.*, marital status, dependent children
4. Assess and document patient's understanding of the disease process and treatment.

A. *Is free of or has minimal discomfort and complications*

INTERVENTION:
1. Give special attention to the involved body systems such as
    a. Skin
        • Provide symptomatic relief of skin irritations, *e.g.*, dryness, itching.
        • Provide skin care and general hygiene.
        • Prevent secondary infection.
    b. Musculoskeletal
        • Establish balanced rest and activity patterns.
        • Collaborate with physical therapy.
        • Give range of motion exercise to stiff joints p.r.n.
    c. Renal
        • Provide dietary and fluid modification as ordered depending on degree of renal impairment.
2. Assess response to treatment.
    a. Relief of pain
    b. Control of fever
    c. Level of fatigue
    d. Mental orientation
    e. Feeling of well-being
    f. Side effects of steroid therapy, *e.g.*, edema, weight gain, gastrointestinal irritation or bleeding, infection

B. *Is Coping with effects of chronic illness*

3. Assist patient and family to cope with illness.
    a. Provide opportunity for expression of feelings, concerns about change in life-style, limitation, and prognosis.
    b. Support realistic attempt at coping.
    c. Identify with patient ways to promote independence.
    d. Include support persons in care, *e.g.*, family, social worker.

Patient Outcome	Process

C. *Is knowledgeable about nature of illness, self-care, and resources for continuity of care*	4. Teach patient and family in preparation for discharge.
	  a. Reinforce understanding of illness and treatment.
	  b. Discuss specific measures:
	    • Avoidance of exposure to direct sunlight.
	    • Diet and fluid modifications
	    • Activity and rest modifications
	  c. Instruct about medications including prevention of side effects.
	5. Initiate interagency referral as needed. Tell patient of other agencies which may assist in continuity of care.

Myocardial infarction

Patient Outcome	Process

The patient functions comfortably within limitations due to myocardial infarction. This includes:

DESCRIPTION: Myocardial infarction is the necrosis of a portion of the myocardium due to blockage of one or more coronary arteries. Obstruction may result from a thrombus or atherosclerotic plaque.

NURSING ASSESSMENT: In addition to the general admission assessment, the following information is especially important.

1. Assess and document physical status.
   a. Pain: Location, severity, radiation, duration, quality, precipitating factors and associated symptoms as nausea, vomiting, diaphoresis, dyspnea
   b. Effectiveness of pain relief measures
   c. Blood pressure
   d. Apical/radial, peripheral pulses
   e. Presence of paradoxical pulse
   f. Presence of peripheral edema
   g. Presence of jugular vein distention
   h. Lung sounds, *e.g.,* râles
   i. Heart sounds, *e.g.,* murmur, pericardial rub
   j. History of cardiovascular disease and other pathophysiological states as obesity, diabetes
   k. Signs and symptoms of left-sided failure such as
      • Rapid pulse
      • S_3 gallop
      • Râles
      • Restlessness and/or confusion
      • Hypotension
      • Decreased urinary output
      • Cool, clammy skin
   l. Arrhythmias
   m. Signs and symptoms indicating extension of myocardial infarction
      • Recurrent chest pain
      • Significant changes in EKG
2. Assess and document patient's understanding of the disease process, implications, and treatment.
3. Assess and document response to information about the disease process, implications, and treatment.
   a. Apparent anxiety level of patient and family
   b. Patient's self-assessment of
      • Personal strengths in coping with stress
      • Support people, *e.g.,* family.

A. *Is prepared for diagnostic studies*

INTERVENTION:
1. Explain/answer questions about diagnostic studies. Refer to Chapter 3 Guidelines For The Patient Undergoing Diagnostic Studies, p. 33. Studies may include:
   a. EKG
   b. Isoenzymes
   c. Arterial blood gases
   d. Vectorcardiogram
   e. Echocardiogram
   f. Pulmonary artery pressure
   g. Myocardial scan
   h. Cardiac catheterization
2. Monitor EKG for rate, rhythm, ectopy and change in PR, QRS and QT intervals.

B. *Is benefiting from therapy*

3. Institute nursing measures to preserve injured myocardium such as
   a. Alleviate pain.
      • Administer analgesics as ordered, *e.g.,* narcotics, nitroglycerine
      • Administer O_2 as needed.
   b. Alleviate nausea.
      • Administer antiemetics as ordered.
      • Provide diet as tolerated within restrictions.
   c. Alleviate anxiety.
      • Provide reassurance and explanations about equipment, treatment, and personnel.
      • Give sedatives as ordered.

Patient Outcome	Process

d. Provide for adequate rest.
- Limit visitors.
- Coordinate scheduling of studies, treatment, and care.
- Provide periods of uninterrupted sleep.
- Administer hypnotics as ordered.

e. Control arrhythmias. Refer to Chapter 4 Arrhythmias Guidelines, p. 75.
- Monitor continuously.
- Attempt prevention of lethal ventricular arrhythmias by the prophylactic use of lidocaine. Follow physician order or protocol.
- Assess symptoms and initiate action based on physician's orders/protocol which may include:
    Administer medications, *e.g.,* lidocaine, atropine.
    Begin basic life support measures if indicated. Refer to Chapter 9 General Guideline For The Critical Care Patient, Life Support, p. 349.

4. Establish progressive activity program in relation to cardiovascular status of patient and physician's orders/protocol.
a. Explain goals to patient.
b. Give explicit instructions about activity.
c. Provide supervision as appropriate.

5. Prepare patient/family for transfer from intensive care area to intermediate care area, as appropriate.
a. Anticipate patient anxiety over transfer.
b. Assure patient of continuity of care in convalescent environment.
c. Communicate details of patient's progress to personnel in convalescent area.
d. Allow patient to take over self-care commensurate with physical status.

C. *Is knowledgeable about nature of illness, self-care, and continuity of care*

6. Assist patient/family to adjust to restrictions imposed by disease process.
a. Provide opportunity for expression of concerns, fears, and questions.
b. Encourage participation in self-care as appropriate.
c. Discuss basic knowledge of disease. This includes:
- Basic anatomy and physiology of heart and coronary arteries
- Significance of "infarcted" area
- Relationship of dietary intake to coronary artery disease
- Risk factors as they pertain to the patient

d. Reinforce physician's instructions regarding treatment. Include:
- Diet and fluid modifications: Consider dietary consult for teaching and counseling assistance.
- Drug therapy: Provide written information about medications.
- Activity/rest program
- Reduction of risk factors such as control of hypertension, stress, weight.

e. Discuss with patient features of home environment which can be conducive to convalescence.
f. Explore with patient needed changes in daily living pattern.

7. Plan discharge.
a. Discuss community resources which may assist in continuity of care.
b. Initiate interagency referral as needed.
c. Provide follow-up appointment.

Patient Outcome	Process

The patient functions comfortably within limitations due to pacemaker. This includes:

DESCRIPTION: A permanent pacemaker is an electronic device surgically implanted to assist or initiate electrical activity in the cardiac conduction system. Patients requiring pacemakers may be those with heart block, Stokes-Adams disease, sick sinus syndrome, profound bradycardia. Pacemakers function either on a fixed rate or demand rate. Depending on the type of pacemaker, the patient will require routine battery replacement at specified intervals.

NURSING ASSESSMENT: In addition to the general admission assessment, the following information is especially important.
1. Assess and document physical status.
   a. Cardiac rate and rhythm
   b. Temperature, respiration, blood pressure
   c. Peripheral pulses/edema
   d. Heart sounds
   e. Lung sounds
   f. History of syncopal episodes
   g. Medications
2. Assess and document emotional status.
   a. Current coping strategy
   b. Anxiety level
3. Assess and document patient's understanding of anticipated procedure.

A. *Is prepared for diagnostic studies and surgical procedures*

INTERVENTION:
1. Explain/answer questions about diagnostic studies. Studies may include:
   a. Routine EKG
   b. Chest radiograph
   c. Electrophysiology studies
   d. Cardiac mapping
   e. Electronic cardiac monitoring
2. Provide preoperative care according to physician's orders and hospital routine. Refer to Chapter 5 Preoperative Phase of Hospitalization, p. 129. Include additional elements of care such as:
   • Emphasize specific expectations.
   • Anesthesia may be local or general.
   • Patient may be asked to follow specific instructions during procedure, *e.g.,* coughing.
   • Patient may be required to limit activity for 24 hours.
   • Patient may have discomfort: availability of medication for relief.
   • Patient may be monitored in special cardiac care area following insertion of pacemaker. Length of time of procedure varies.
   • Usual insertion site for pacemaker is shoulder or abdomen.

B. *Is free of or has minimal discomfort or complications*

3. Provide postoperative care. See Chapter 5 Postoperative Phase of Hospitalization, p. 130.
4. Intervene in the critical elements of care following pacemaker insertion.
   a. Maintain pacemaker function.
      • Monitor continuously.
      • Observe for failure to sense, failure to capture, (Fig. 4-10.) generator failure, oversensing, competition, and runaway pacemaker.
      • Initiate action for malfunction based on assessment and physician's orders/protocol.
      • Obtain EKG with magnet placed on pacemaker site per physician's orders.

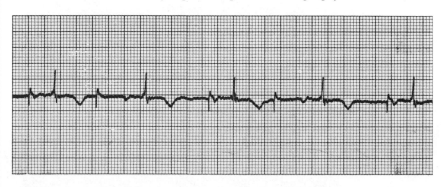

Fig. 4-10. Pacemaker—Failure to sense; failure to capture.

Patient Outcome

Process

b. Provide wound care.
- Observe sites for bleeding, infection
- Change dressing as ordered.

C. *Is knowledgeable about care and function of pacemaker, self-care, and resources for continuity of care*

5. Explain and demonstrate self-care measures to patient/family.
   a. Provide knowledge about pacemaker function. Give brochure with pacemaker and review information. Emphasize that proper, continuous functioning of pacemaker is necessary.
   b. Teach patient to count pulse for full minute and record in morning upon awakening.
   c. Determine with physician and provide explanation about:
   - Fixed rate limits (or)
   - Demand rate: 5 below lower limit as prescribed; upper limit depends upon normal physiologic response.
   d. Instruct patient to inform physician of any abnormal findings such as persistent tachycardia.
6. Provide information regarding:
   a. Projected date of battery change
   b. Avoidance of close proximity to hazards such as transmitting towers, car engines
7. Plan discharge with patient and family.
   a. Reinforce physician's explanations and instructions.
   b. Provide prescriptions and/or medications such as procainamide (Pronestyl), propranolol (Inderal), quinidine.
   c. Inform patient of availability and use of pacemaker function telephone follow-up.
   d. Instruct patient to notify physician of:
   - Trauma or infection in site of battery insertion
   - Shortness of breath, edema, angina, syncope
   e. Discuss community agencies which may assist in continuity of care.
   f. Initiate interagency referral as needed.
   g. Emphasize importance of continued medical care. Give return appointment.

Patient Outcome

Process

The patient functions comfortably within limitations due to pulmonary embolus. This includes:

DESCRIPTION: A pulmonary embolus is a foreign body such as a blood clot or other nonthrombotic material which may be fat or air dislodged from the venous system and lodged in the pulmonary vascular bed. Cardiopulmonary function is compromised and life may be threatened. Etiology of pulmonary embolism is associated with many risk factors such as thrombophlebitis, cardiovascular disease, trauma, major surgical procedures, and prolonged immobilization.

NURSING ASSESSMENT: In addition to the general admission assessment, the following information is especially important.
1. Assess and document physical and emotional status.
  a. Signs and symptoms of pulmonary embolus
    • Character of respirations, *e.g.,* rapid and shallow or deep and gasping
    • Chest and shoulder pain
    • Change in skin color, *e.g.,* dusky
    • Cough with bloody sputum
    • Change in vital signs, *e.g.,* tachycardia, hypotension, dyspnea
    • Fever
    • Positive Homan's sign
    • Blood gases (decreased PO_2 decreased PCO_2)
  b. Risk factors
    • Previous history of thrombophlebitis, calf tenderness, chest pain, etc.
    • Obesity
    • Smoking history
    • Other disease states, *e.g.,* recent abdominal surgery, polycythemia vera
  c. Apparent anxiety level

A. *Is maintaining life support*

INTERVENTION:
1. Provide life-supporting measures as indicated.
  a. Maintain patient airway and adequate oxygenation.
  b. Maintain intravenous therapy.
  c. Prepare for possible cardiopulmonary arrest. See Chapter 9 General Guidelines For the Critical Care Patient, Life Support, p. 349.
2. Collaborate with physician concerning patient who has extreme chest pain and difficulty breathing.
  a. Weigh benefits of analgesics versus the respiratory depressant effects.
  b. Position patient to facilitate breathing and yet maintain blood pressure, *e.g.,* slight elevation of head of bed and foot of bed (25° angle).

B. *Is free of or has minimal discomfort or complications*

3. Institute preparation of patient for diagnostic studies. See Chapter 3 Guidelines For the Patient Undergoing Diagnostic Studies, p. 33. Possible studies include:
  a. Lung scan
  b. Arteriogram
4. Initiate measures to decrease possibility of embolus extension or formation of new clots.
  a. For bedridden patients:
    • Turn q 1 to 2 hours.
    • Elevate foot of bed.
    • Apply antiembolic hose.
    • Check for calf tenderness.
    • Give range of motion to extremities, including extension, flexion and rotation of each foot at least q 2 hours, unless contraindicated.
  b. For ambulatory patient:
    • Encourage proper positioning such as No crossing of legs, elevate legs when sitting, keep legs elevated slightly above heart when reclining.
    • Check for calf tenderness daily.
  c. Establish bowel program.
    • Give stool softeners.
    • Avoid straining with stools.
  d. Provide supportive measures to maximize patient's ability to maintain normal physiological functions such as
    • Assess signs of decreased renal function:
        Call physician for urine output below 30 cc hourly.
        Monitor serum potassium, urea nitrogen, and creatinine levels.
    • Provide preventive skin care. See Chapter 1 Guidelines for General Care, p. 31.

Patient Outcome	Process

5. Provide for special needs of patients receiving anticoagulant therapy (heparin).
   a. Observe for evidence of bleeding from:
      • Gastrointestinal tract
      • Gums
      • Nose
      • Urinary tract
      • Intracranial area
      • Skin
   b. Test stools daily for guaiac.
   c. Apply pressure to any puncture site for 5 minutes.
   d. Monitor results of coagulation studies, *e.g.,* partial thromboplastin time (PTT).
      • For initial therapy, monitor daily.
      • For maintenance therapy, monitor weekly.
   e. For patients receiving subcutaneous heparin injections:
      • Verify correct dosage and strength.
      • Select large sites as in abdomen, leg, arm.
      • Rotate sites and note on chart at bedside.
      • Apply steady pressure to site; do not rub.
   f. For patients receiving intravenous heparin infusion:
      • Verify and give initial loading dose as ordered.
      • Use microdrip infusion chamber with controller.
      • Label medication.
      • Monitor IV intake carefully.

C. *Is coping with acute illness*

6. Provide emotional support for patient and family.
   a. Remain aware that the patient may be extremely anxious or frightened and in need of close personal contact.
   b. Provide reassurance and close attention to needs.
   c. Provide careful explanations of patient's care and response to therapy.
   d. Listen to concerns.

D. *Is knowledgeable about nature of illness, self-care, and resources for continuity of care*

7. Teach patient and family about illness and care.
   a. Reinforce physician's explanations and instruction.
   b. Discuss risk factors, *e.g.,* varicose veins, pregnancy, prolonged standing and/or sitting, medications that might interfere with normal clotting such as oral contraceptives.
   c. Discuss preventive care:
      • Keep legs elevated whenever possible.
      • Wear support hose.
      • Do not cross legs.
   d. Instruct to seek medical assistance for symptoms of calf tenderness, shortness of breath or chest pain, cyanosis of nailbeds or lips.
   e. Inform patient of special needs due to anticoagulant therapy such as:
      • Wear medical identification.
      • Return as scheduled for clotting tests.
      • Caution dentist and others caring for patient about possibility of excessive bleeding.
      • Avoid common causes of injury such as contact sports, walking barefoot, sharp razors, power machinery.
      • Report symptoms of bleeding such as:
         Fainting
         ''Weak'' feeling
         Bloody urine or stool
         Bruising
         Abdominal or back pain
      • Encourage females of child-bearing age to seek special counseling concerning birth control methods since oral contraception and intrauterine devices (IUDs) are contraindicated when receiving anticoagulants.
      • Provide patient with special medications and supplies, prescriptions, and return appointments as needed for continuity of care.

Patient Outcome	Process

The patient functions comfortably within limitations due to rheumatoid arthritis. This includes:

DESCRIPTION: Rheumatoid arthritis is a chronic, progressive, systemic disease characterized by a fluctuating inflammation of the joints. The primary symptoms are red, swollen, warm, painful joints, often first affecting the finger joints bilaterally. Women are three times more likely to have the disease than men and its onset is usually within the 20 to 40 year age range. It is thought to be caused by an autoimmune reaction because of the presence of an immunoglobulin (rheumatoid factor) in the serum and lymphocytes and plasma cells in the joint synovium. Among other rheumatic diseases are: osteoarthritis (degenerative joint disease), connective tissue diseases, gout, and suppurative arthritis.

NURSING ASSESSMENT: In addition to general admission assessment, the following information is important.
1. Assess and document physical status:
   a. Signs and symptoms related to underlying disease process
      - Pain: location, character, duration, effectiveness of relief measures
      - Joint stiffness
      - Joint deformities.
   b. Risk factors, *e.g.,* obesity
   c. Activity level
2. Assess and document patient's response to information about disease process and its treatment.
   a. Apparent anxiety level
   b. Depressive reaction
   c. Patient's self-assessment of:
      - Personal strengths in coping with stress
      - Body concept
      - Support people, *e.g.,* family, friends
3. Assess and document health habits/life-style prior to admission.
   a. Home health supervision/support
   b. Physical demands, *e.g.,* occupation, recreational activities
   c. Position in family unit, *e.g.,* marital status, dependent children
4. Assess and document patient's understanding of disease process and its treatment.

A. *Is prepared for diagnostic studies*

INTERVENTION:
1. Explain/answer questions about diagnostic studies.
   a. Sedimentation rate
   b. CBC
   c. Serum analysis for rheumatoid factor
   d. Salicylate level
   e. Joint aspiration for leukocytes, protein
   f. Radiographs for narrowing of joint space, soft tissue swelling
   g. Urinalysis

B. *Is free of or has minimal discomfort and complications*

2. Provide therapeutic measures to minimize pain, reduce inflammation, and prevent further joint damge.
   a. Give prescribed medications. Dosages are dependent upon tolerance and blood level. Analgesic should be timed to act when pain is at its peak.
      - Aspirin
      - Steroids
      - Motrin
      - Indocin
      - Butazolidin
      - Intra-articular steroid injection when other therapy is ineffective or when only one joint inflammed.
   b. Assess patient's pain level through verbal and nonverbal communication. See Chapter 2 Pain, p. 29 .
   c. Provide general comfort measures.
   d. Maintain balance between rest and activity. Plan may include:
      - Provision for rest:
         Full-night rest and daytime rest period
         Use of sedative at night if required
      - Use of comfort devices: bedboard; firm mattress; small head pillow; foot-board, if not ambulatory
      - Collaborative exercise program to preserve joint function, prevent atrophy of muscle, decalcification of bone and promote nourishment of cartilage.
         Includes range of motion, muscle-strengthening exercises designed for individual patient; caution against overexercise which may cause joint damage.

Patient Outcome	Process

	e. Provide and teach individualized rest/activity program to meet patient's needs and life style.
	   • Planned rest, *e.g.,* 5 to 10 minutes rest out of each hour, rest before exhaustion; ten hours sleep at night
	   • Activity simplification: assist patient to analyze each activity to see whether it can be simplified, eliminated, or done by others.
	      Plan activities to avoid overexertion.
	      Raise seats to prevent bending.
	      Sit whenever possible.
	      Slide objects rather than lift.
	      Store most used items within easy reach.
	      Choose clothing simple to put on and take off.
	   • Assistive devices, *e. g.,* wrist splints, cervical pillow, bathtub chair
	   • Modification of home/work schedule
	      Consider shortened work hours.
	      Work slowly.
	      Avoid using fingers when palm of hand or assistive device can be used, *e.g.,* spray cans, car door.
	   • Activities that are very important to patient should be planned for times when pain level is diminished and patient is feeling rested, *e.g.,* sexual activity may best be planned for times other than upon awakening in morning or late in evening.
	3. Assure dietary instruction for overweight, underweight, and/or potential anemic patient.

C. *Is coping with chronic illness and disability*	4. Assist patient to cope with disabilities.
	  a. Identify patient's responses, which may include anger, passive acceptance, realism.
	  b. Reinforce positive attitudes.
	  c. Identify behavioral responses, *e.g.* complaining, manipulative
	  d. Listen to the patient as he considers possible changes in life style and body image resulting from illness. Questions patient may be considering:
	    • How will I cope with the pain? Will it be constant or fluctuate?
	    • Will I be able to do the things that are most enjoyable/necessary to me? (including jobs, recreation) What activities must I stop? What will take their place?
	    • What will I look like? Will I become crippled and if so, when?
	    • Who will help me do the necessary things I can no longer do?
	    • What will be the impact on my family/friends if I can no longer function as I did before?
	    • What will be the end result? Will my life-span be shortened? Will I become bedridden? What complications might occur?
	    • Will I be on medications for the rest of my life? Will they help?
	    • If I get better, will the disease return?
	  e. Encourage independence in activities of daily living.
	    • Bathing • Feeding
	    • Dressing • Care of belongings and environment
	    • Grooming

D. *Is knowledgeable about the nature of illness, self-care, and resources for continuity of care*	5. Reinforce understanding of the disease process, its chronicity and long-term treatment.
	  • Help patient understand that acute phases of illness will fluctuate with nonacute phases and that this will determine physical capabilities.
	6. Counsel with patient and family and use resource persons as appropriate.
	  a. Realistic expectations of rehabilitation
	  b. Altered family roles (vocational, educational, financial)
	7. Plan discharge with patient and family:
	  a. Teach about drug therapy including
	    • Side effects and measures to minimize them
	    • Reinforcement of physician's instruction on how to alter drugs doses
	    • Importance of taking drugs as scheduled
	  b. Assess with patient and family the suitability of his home environment for continued care. Suggest modifications if indicated, *e.g.* stairs, doorways.
	    • Teach safety precautions, *e.g.,* slipping rugs.
	  c. Inform patient and family of community resources for assistance, *e.g.,* vocational guidance, rehabilitation center, Arthritis Foundation, physical and occupational therapy.
	  d. Initiate interagency referral as needed.
	  e. Provide medications, prescriptions and equipment as needed.

Patient Outcome	Process

The patient functions comfortably within limitations due to seizure disorder. This includes:

DESCRIPTION: Seizures are manifestations of sudden, paroxysmal, and often recurrent discharges of electrical energy in neurons of the brain. Some seizure disorders have unknown etiology and others are manifestations of underlying conditions such as trauma, brain tumor, infections, drug and alcohol withdrawal, and toxic disturbances.

Types of seizures are major motor, focal motor, and petit mal.

NURSING ASSESSMENT: In addition to the general admission assessment, the following information is especially important.
1. Assess and document physical and mental status.
   a. Signs and symptoms of seizure activity
      - Aura
      - Type
      - Frequency
      - Pattern, *e.g.,* duration, incontinence
      - Postseizure state.
   b. Anticonvulsant medications including adherence to therapy
   c. Underlying conditions, *e.g.,* infection
   d. Physical condition, *e.g.,* condition of gums and teeth, injuries due to past seizure activities
   e. Drug level in blood
2. Assess and document patient's response to information about the disorder, its implications and treatment.
   a. Apparent anxiety level
   b. Patient's self-assessment of
      - Personal strengths in coping with stress
      - Support people, *e.g.,* family
3. Assess and document health habits/life-style prior to admission.
   a. Home health supervision and support
   b. Position in family unit, *e.g.,* provider for family
4. Assess and document patient's understanding of the disorder, its implications, and treatment.

A. *Is prepared for diagnostic studies*

INTERVENTION:
1. Explain/answer questions about diagnostic studies. Refer to Chapter 3, Guidelines For the Patient Undergoing Diagnostic Studies, p. 33. Studies may include:
   a. Electroencephalogram
   b. Lumbar puncture
   c. Skull films
   d. Computerized axial tomography
   e. Brain scan
   f. Pneumoencephalogram
   g. Arteriogram
   h. Blood chemistries
   i. Psychological testing

B. *Is benefiting from therapy and safe environment*

2. Institute seizure precautions. These include:
   a. Discuss precautions with patient/family.
   b. Request patient to alert nurse if aura appears.
   c. Give medications as scheduled without fail unless otherwise ordered by physician.
   d. Restrict activity to ward unless accompanied.
   e. Tape padded tongue blade to head of bed.
   f. Pad bed as necessary.
   g. Keep bed in low position with side rails up as indicated.
   h. Take rectal temperature unless otherwise indicated.
   i. Provide darkened, quiet environment with minimal stimulation.
   j. Provide constant surveillance if status epilepticus occurs.
3. Provide care during seizure activity.
   a. Be alert to signs of impending seizure: facial expression, stare, unusual sensations or motor activity.
   b. Maintain patent airway without using extreme force.
      - Insert tongue blade or suitable alternative between teeth.
      - Insert mouth gag.
      - Position on side when possible.
      - Loosen tight clothing.

Patient Outcome	Process

c. Protect from injury.

d. Observe and document seizure activity.
  - Time of onset, duration, method of termination
  - Characteristics of involuntary contractions:
    - Site of onset, progression, unilateral or bilateral
    - Head movement, eye movement, pupillary changes
    - Type of muscle response (clonic, tonic)
  - Changes in respiratory status
  - Urinary and/or bowel incontinence
  - Loss of consciousness
  - Ability to make voluntary movements
  - Time lapse until patient regains normal alertness

e. Direct movements of patient. Do not restrain.

f. Reassure patient as appropriate.

g. Provide privacy if possible.

h. Give anticonvulsant medications as ordered.

i. Notify physician of observations and document in patient's record all observations of seizure activity pre-, during and postseizure.

4. Provide postseizure care.
  a. Reorient patient to environment.
  b. Reassure patient.
  c. Assess for injuries such as bitten tongue.
  d. Position on side.
  e. Observe for symptoms as headache, confusion.
  f. Check neurological status depending upon extent of seizures and postseizure state.
    - Level of consciousness
    - Pupillary reactions
    - Vital signs.
  g. Reassess with physician the need for changing method of administering anticonvulsant.

5. Provide knowledge about disorder and treatment to patient/family. Include:
  a. Causative factors
  b. Type of seizure activity
  c. Effects of anticonvulsant therapy in controlling seizure activity if taken regularly as prescribed by physician

6. Assist patient in identifying ways to reduce undue environmental, physical, and emotional stress.

C. *Is willing to adapt life style to methods of control of seizure disorder*

7. Assist patient/family to adapt to methods of control of seizure disorder.
  a. Assess current coping strategy.
  b. Support appropriate coping strategy.
  c. Provide opportunity for expression of concerns, questions, and future plans.
  d. Clarify any misconceptions.
  e. Identify with patient resource persons, *e.g.,* social worker, family members.
  f. Explore with patient changes in daily living activities necessitated by management goals, *e.g.,* work schedule, travel, driving, swimming.
    - Identify potentially dangerous situations.
  g. Help patient to set realistic goals.
  h. Explore with patient the importance of informing significant others of the disability.

D. *Is knowledgeable about nature of disorder, self-care, and resources for continuity of care.*

8. Plan discharge with patient and family.
  a. Reinforce knowledge needed to carry out management of disorder.
  b. Instruct to report illnesses to physician.
  c. Instruct patient/family to keep record regarding seizure activity.
  d. Stress importance of wearing medical identification, *e.g.,* bracelet, wallet card.
  e. Discuss community agencies which may assist as needed, *e.g.,* vocational rehabilitation.
  f. Initiate interagency referral as needed.
  g. Provide prescriptions and/or medications with written instructions.
  h. Emphasize importance of continued medical care. Give return appointment.

CHAPTER V
Guidelines for the patient who requires surgical intervention

INTRODUCTION: There are common features in the nursing care needed by the patient who requires surgical intervention for illness. These are considered in guidelines based on the four phases of the surgical patient's hospitalization: diagnostic, preoperative, postoperative and predischarge. Patient outcomes and related process described are applicable to a great number of patients regardless of diagnosis and therapy. Nursing interventions in the patient's diagnostic phase are described in Chapter 3 Guidelines for the Patient Undergoing Diagnostic Studies. Frequent reference is made to these guidelines for information about specific diagnostic examinations.

The critical elements of patient care due to the very nature of the specific surgical intervention (operation) are delineated in terms of desired patient outcomes and associated nursing process. There is frequent and consistent reference to the guidelines describing the four phases of hospitalization for the surgical patient.

Included in the appendix are evaluation tools specifically designed and tested for use in determining the extent to which the desired outcomes are achieved for the patient with a total hip replacement. These examples of assessment tools are designed to collect data concurrently by peer review through the methods of patient chart documentation review and direct patient interview and observation.

Patient Outcome	Process

The patient experiences an informed and comfortable preoperative phase of hospitalization. This includes:	1. Gather information about the patient's condition, planned surgical procedure, and the patient's level of understanding. Discuss the details of the surgical experiences with the patient and his family. Information may include:
	a. Purpose of procedure
	b. Physical preparation for procedure
	c. Actual procedure
	  • Location of body part
	  • Probably size of incision(s)
	  • Function of organ to be surgically altered
	  • Change in body function and appearance (if any) after surgery
	  • Probable time of surgery, visitors prior to surgery
	  • Expected length of time of surgery
	  • Preanesthesia room
	d. Postoperative expectations
	  • Immediate postoperative location (usually recovery room or special care area) and later transfer to other areas
	  • Knowledge of probable equipment, dressings, IVs, etc. to be used
	  • Provisions for relief of pain and other symptoms—when requested and limits placed on drug use and frequency
	  • Frequent observations by nursing staff
	  • Turn, cough, deep breathe routines
	  • Changes in bowel and bladder function
	  • Progressive diet changes, including IV fluids
	  • Progressive mobilization with assistance (sitting up, dangling, out of bed, ambulation)
	  • Progression of self-care

A. *Is prepared emotionally for surgery*	2. Be alert to patient's feelings and needs. a. Encourage verbalization about surgery and recognize concerns. b. Listen and observe for misconceptions and for signs of anxiety. 3. Attempt to reduce anxiety. a. Try to determine basis of anxiety with patient. b. Call chaplain for patient if indicated. c. Give medications per physician's orders. d. Provide environment that is appropriate to the needs of the individual.
B. *Is prepared physically for surgery*	4. Institute immediate preparation of patient for surgery. a. Carry out physician's written preoperative orders for medications and treatments. b. Keep n.p.o. per physician's orders. c. Give bowel preparation per physician's orders. d. Bathe patient or have patient take bath. e. Have patient empty bladder. f. Restrict activity for safety. g. Complete gown and identification bracelet. h. List allergies on preoperative record. i. Safeguard valuables and prosthesis. j. Check that signed consent form has been obtained by physician. k. Accompany patient to operating room or according to hospital policy.

Patient Outcome

Process

	IMMEDIATE Postoperative Period (1 to 24 hours)	INTERMEDIATE Postoperative Period (24 to 96 hours)

The patient experiences minor discomfort and minimal complications postoperatively. This includes:

A. *Maintains body functions*
• *Neurological*

• *Cardiovascular*

1. Observe and record level of consciousness to:
   a. Verbal stimuli
   b. Painful stimuli

2. Check and record neurological signs as indicated to include level of motor and sensory response if given spinal anesthesia.

   • Check and record neurological signs per doctors order.

3. Check and record pulse, respirations, and blood pressure q 1 hour × 4 usually, then q 4 hour if stable. Take temperature immediately and q 4 hours. Compare with previous data.

   • Check and record temperature, pulse, respirations, and blood pressure q 4 hours × 3 days depending on operative procedure, then q.i.d.

4. Intervene if symptoms of shock occur:
   a. Remain with patient.
   b. Position in modified Trendelenburg.
   c. Identify source of bleeding; apply pressure.
   d. Obtain continuous vital signs.
   e. Notify physician.
   f. Prepare for possible cardiopulmonary resuscitation.

5. Apply antiembolic hose as ordered.

6. Position with head and foot of bed elevated 30° with knees slightly flexed.

   • Remove antiembolic hose q.d. to wash legs. Provide for washing hose per hospital routine. Check for signs of thrombophlebitis such as:
   Pain in calf on dorsiflexion of toe (Homan's sign.)
   Localized warmth, swelling, tenderness, redness

7. Identify patients susceptible to cardiovascular complications such as shock, arrhythmias, hypertension, emboli. Patients may have:
   a. History of cardiac problems
   b. Prolonged anesthesia
   c. Extreme blood loss or other complication during surgery
   d. History of bleeding, clotting, or other vascular problems
   e. Obesity
   f. Cast applied

   • Remain alert to possibility of cardiovascular complications.

• *Respiratory*

8. Check and record respirations for rate, depth and clarity, skin color.

9. Encourage good pulmonary toilet which includes:
   a. Turn, cough, deep breathe q 2 hours when awake unless otherwise indicated.
   b. Incentive spirometry, intermittent positive pressure breathing (IPPB), and/or O_2 with humidity as ordered
   c. Suction p.r.n.

   • Continue pulmonary toilet.
   a. Cough and deep breathe q 4 hours when awake.
   b. IPPB usually through fourth day. Request renewal as needed.
   c. Suction for symptoms of respiratory congestion

10. Identify patients susceptible to respiratory complications. Patients may have:
    a. History of lung disease
    b. Smoking habit
    c. Thoracic surgery
    d. Chest tubes
    e. Prolonged anesthesia

    • Remain alert to possibility of respiratory complications such as pulmonary embolus, pneumonia, pneumothorax, atelectasis.

Patient Outcome   Process

	IMMEDIATE Postoperative Period (1 to 24 hours)	INTERMEDIATE Postoperative Period (24 to 96 hours)

• *Fluid balance and renal function*	11. Monitor, describe, record intake and output including tubes, drains, catheters, emesis.
	  a. Monitor IV fluid type, rate, and infusion site.
	  b. Expect patient to void 6 to 8 hours postoperatively. Check for bladder distention.
	  c. Check that hourly output is a minimum of 30 to 40 cc.
	  d. Check catheter, tubes, and drains for patency and safety.
		• Continue intake and output as needed. Give 2000 to 3000 cc per day unless contraindicated.
		  a. Continue monitoring IV fluid type, rate, infusion site every 8 hours.
		  b. Compare intake/output every 8 hours; notify physician for signs of excessive fluid retention or loss.
		
		• Maintain catheter, tubes, and drains.

• *Gastrointestinal*	12. Keep patient n.p.o. unless otherwise ordered. 13. Check for nausea, abdominal distention, and bowel sounds. 14. Alert physician for nasogastric drainage greater than 400 cc per 4 hours or signs of bleeding. Guaiac test stools and/or emesis p.r.n.	• Advance diet as tolerated after return of bowel sounds. • Check patient for possible bowel complications: impaction, constipation, diarrhea, paralytic ileus. • Plan preventive/therapeutic bowel program to facilitate patient's return to normal function. See Chapter 2 Bowel Care Guidelines, Where There is Deviation from Normal. p. 25.

• *Neuromuscular/skin*	15. Maintain good body alignment.
	  a. Reposition frequently.
	  b. Assist with active range of motion, exercises, dangling, and out of bed in chair as ordered.
	16. Identify patients susceptible to neuromuscular/skin problems.
	  a. Immobilized by physical status or equipment
	  b. Decreased sensation
	  c. Elderly, debilitated, obese
	  d. In cast, or splint
		• Continue active range of motion exercise as needed and progressive activity. Encourage independence in activities of daily living.
		• Be alert to neuromuscular/skin problems.

• *Comfort*	17. Anticipate and evaluate patient's needs for pain medication. Consider:
	  a. Wound-related pain (subjective and objective)
	  b. Pain due to required activity
	  c. Restlessness caused by pain
	Precautions:
	  a. Unstable vital signs–questionable shock
	  b. Depressed respirations
	  c. Prolonged hypotension
	  d. Patient not fully alert
	18. Evaluate need for and schedule rest periods.
	  a. Limit visitors.
	  b. Provide restful environment.
		• Continue evaluation of need for pain medication. Adjust type of medication according to patient's need and judgment of nurse and/or physician. Inform patient of decision.
		
		• Maintain a schedule for rest periods built around activities, scheduled tests, visiting hours, etc.

B. *Is emotionally able to cope with impact of surgical intervention*	19. Reorient patient to ward, equipment being used, and immediate expectations.
	20. Provide reassurance that:
	  a. Frequent observations are normal and surgery is completed.
	  b. Needs for relief of pain have been recognized. Estimate when patient can expect medication if needed.
	  c. Family can visit when immediate care needs have been met.
		• Encourage patient to verbalize about surgery, changes in physical appearance and limitations.
		
		• Discuss patient's progress with family and include them in patient's care in appropriate ways.

Patient Outcome	Process	
	IMMEDIATE Postoperative Period (1 to 24 hours)	**INTERMEDIATE** Postoperative Period (24 to 96 hours)

C. *Is healing surgical wound*	21. Provide opportunity for patient and family to ask questions. Listen to concerns.
	22. Provide wound care.
	  a. Observe dressings, casts, and wound drains. Outline current drainage on dressing, cast.
	  b. Note appearance of dressing and drainage (amount, color, consistency).
	  c. Notify physician of excessive drainage or abnormal appearance.
	  d. Reinforce or change dressings as needed.
		• Encourage patient to verbalize feelings regarding surgery and postoperative physical status.
		
		• Continue observation of wound and drainage.
		
		• Be alert to signs of wound infection such as purulent drainage, odor, fever, swelling, redness.
		• Observe wound for evidence of primary closure.
		• Change dressings as needed.

Predischarge phase of hospitalization

Patient Outcome	Process

The patient is knowledgeable about nature of illness, self care, and resources for continuity of care.	1. Discuss body image changes, limitations, and progression of activities according to patient condition and physician preference.
	2. Consult with members of other disciplines, patient, and his family in planning for patient discharge.
	3. Assist patient to gain knowledge and skills necessary for self-care after discharge. These may include:
	  a. Wound care
	  b. Stoma care
	  c. Use and care of prosthesis, other equipment
	  d. Where to buy needed equipment and supplies
	  e. Dietary modification
	  f. Teaching regarding health/illness state
	  g. Medication therapy to include symptoms of side effects
	  h. Symptoms of complications such as infection and to whom to report
	  i. Provisions for follow-up medical care
	4. Assess with patient and family suitability of home for convalescence.
	5. Suggest modifications in home situation needed to patient and family.
	6. Evaluate need for initiation of interagency referral for patients who need help in planning for and/or adjusting to an illness.
	7. Discuss community agencies available to assist patient and family as needed, for example: public health nursing services, rehabilitation center, colostomy clubs, Cancer Society.
	8. Provide patient with prescriptions, supplies and equipment, return appointment, and interagency referral as needed for continuity of care.

Patient Outcome

The patient experiences informed, comfortable, and safe preoperative, postoperative, and pre- discharge phases of hospitalization. This includes:

Process

DESCRIPTION: An aortic abdominal aneurysm consists of an enlargement of the aortic wall with a collection of plaque in the lumen. A true aneurysm involves all three layers of the artery. A false aneurysm is composed of a collection of blood and clot which forms outside the wall of the artery and is pulsatile. A dissecting aneurysm is a hemotoma which forms between the layers of the vessel. Fig. 5-1. Ninety-five per cent of abdominal aneurysms originate below the renal arteries.

The major cause of aneurysms is arteriosclerosis. Men are more often affected than women and 50 per cent have few or no symptoms. Others may be symptomatic with dull back pain or present with a ruptured aneurysm with severe pain and blood loss. The operative procedure is through a midline abdominal incision; large and small bowel are reflected and covered with saline soaked gauze while the aorta is manipulated. The aorta is clamped below the renal arteries and an incision is made down the length of the aneurysm. A woven or knitted dacron graft is sewn proximally and distally to the aneurysm and the clamp is removed to re-establish blood supply. The aneurysm sac is then closed around the graft. The bowel is replaced and the wound is closed.

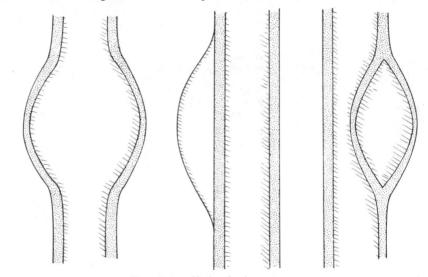

Fig. 5-1—Abdominal aneurysms.

NURSING ASSESSMENT: In addition to general admission assessment, the following information is especially important.
1. Assess and document physical status.
   a. Symptoms related to aneurysm:
      • Pain location, character, duration. Effectiveness of pain relief measures
      • Bilateral peripheral pulses (presence, absence, character)—femoral, popliteal, posterior tibial, pedal, brachial, radial, carotid
   b. Risk factors/disease states which might affect postoperative course specifically
      • Pulmonary status—note pulmonary disease, breath sounds, rate, expansion, smoking history
      • Cardiovascular status—rate and rhythm of pulse, EKG, other cardiac or vascular disease, *i.e.,* coronary artery disease
      • Renal status—voiding difficulties and infections, renal disease
      • Diabetes—method of control, type of diet.
      • Gastrointestinal status—bowel habits, girth, description of abdomen (note distention)
2. Assess and document patient's response to information about the disease process, treatment, and anticipated surgery:
   a. Apparent anxiety level
   b. Previous experience with surgery
3. Assess and document health habits prior to admission:
   a. Potential for self-care or need for supportive care
   b. Medications—especially those affecting clotting time, blood pressure, cardiac function
   c. Diet, *i.e.,* restrictions, patient's knowledge, compliance
   d. Home health supervision/support
4. Assess and document patient's understanding of disease process, treatment, and anticipated surgery.

Patient Outcome	Process

A. *Is prepared for surgery*	**INTERVENTION:**
	1. Reinforce understanding of patient and family regarding the disease process, its implications and treatment.
	2. Institute preparation of patient for diagnostic studies. See Chapter 3 Guidelines for the Patient Undergoing Diagnostic Studies p. 33.
	    a. Arteriogram c. Aortogram
	    b. Ultrasound d. Flat plate radiograph of the abdomen
	3. Summarize usual preoperative preparation and provide care per hospital procedure and physician's orders. See Chapter 5 Preoperative Phase of Hospitalization, p. 129.
	    a. Antimicrobial soap shower/bath evening before and morning of surgery
	    b. Usual skin preparation nipple to knee (early morning of surgery)
	    c. Small cleansing enema unless contraindicated. Laxative may be ordered.
	    d. Prophylactic antibiotics may be ordered.
	    e. Clear liquid diet 24 hours prior to surgery and n.p.o. after midnight
	    f. Instruction to patient regarding proper method and importance of turning, coughing, deep breathing, and leg exercises
	    g. Instruction to stop smoking before surgery
	    h. Encouragement to drink large amounts (at least 2500 cc) of fluids preoperatively unless contraindicated
	4. Summarize usual postoperative expectations.
	    a. May spend night in recovery care area for close observation
	    b. May have endotracheal tube temporarily to aid ventilation. Will not be able to speak while tube in place. Will feel discomfort in back of throat.
	    c. Mechanical ventilation for about 24 hours. Ventilator will breathe for patient.
	    d. After endotracheal tube is removed, will receive O_2 by mask. Will be instructed to turn, cough, and deep breath q 1 to 2 hours.
	    e. Peripheral pulses and abdominal girths will be checked frequently in immediate postoperative period.
	    f. Will have arm restrained for arterial line while in recovery care area
	    g. Will have urinary drainage catheter and nasogastric tube
	    h. Passive leg exercises as ordered q 1 hour until activity resumed
	    i. Bedrest for 24 hours, then gradual resumption of activity
	    j. May not be able to eat or drink for 1 to 3 days until bowel motility resumes
	    k. Smoking will not be permitted.
	    l. Pain medication available postoperatively. Patient feels free to request.

B. *Is free of or has minimal discomfort or postoperative complications*
• *Pulmonary*
 	
• *Circulatory*
	5. Provide postoperative care. See Chapter 5 Postoperative Phase of Hospitalization, p. 130.
	6. Intervene in the critical areas of patient care following surgery.
	    a. Maintain patency of airway, note signs of respiratory complications.
	     • ET tube may remain up to 24 hours or until patient's condition is stable.
	     • Frequent suctioning may be needed—note character and quantity of sputum.
	     • Pulmonary regimen is of priority due to size and location of incision and includes:
	       Turn, cough, deep breathing q 1 to 2 hours. Splint incision with pillow or folded blanket for comfort.
	       Chest physical therapy (percussion and vibration)
	       Relief of pain
	       Proper patient position
	    b. Monitor vital signs per postoperative routine.
	     • Medical management is aimed at maintaining blood pressure at safe level. Changes in blood pressure need to be reported to physician immediately. Be aware of therapeutic goals for blood pressure control especially when patient is on vasoactive drug, *e.g.*, nitroprusside (Nipride), dopamine (Intropin), hydralazine (Apresoline)
	     • Check bilateral peripheral pulses q 1 hour. Note skin color, temperature, sensation and compare with baseline. Loss of previously existing extremity pulse is an emergency; notify physician at once.
	     • Position to maintain body alignment and enhance circulation without impairing respiration.
	     • Encourage leg exercises as indicated.
	    c. Assess location and amount of any bleeding.
	     • Note drainage on abdominal dressing. Small amount of sanguineous drainage can be expected.

Patient Outcome	Process
	• Check abdominal girth (q 1 hour × 24 then with vital signs); assess abdomen for distention and bruising.
	• Note unusual bleeding at other sites, *i.e.,* arterial line site, in urine or naosgastric drainage, at injection site, or in stool.
	• Guaiac test nasogastric drainage and stool specimen
• *Renal*	d. Provide continual and careful assessment of fluid and electrolyte status.
	• Assess renal status.
	Measure and record outputs with specific gravity (q 1 hour × 24, then as appropriate).
	Diuresis may occur immediately postoperative due to diuretic which might have been given in operating room. Output usually decreases after diuretic phase of drug has passed. Call physician if output drops below 30 cc per hour.
	• Determine fluid and electrolyte status:
	Note amounts of surgical blood loss and fluid replacement.
	Notify phsycian of significant change in EKG tracing, skin turgor, central venous pressure, blood pressure, pulse, respirations, and blood chemistries.
	• Continue to monitor blood chemistries when oral diuretics and antihypertensives are administered.
• *Gastrointestinal*	e. Provide continual assessment and support of gastrointestinal function.
	• Adequate drainage is necessary through nasogastric tube to prevent abdominal distention, discomfort, and vomiting. Electrolytes are lost through nasogastric drainage and may need to be replaced.
	Measure and record drainage q 1 hour × 24, then as appropriate.
	Check position of tube initially and at least q 2 hours.
	Maintain patency by irrigation with normal saline as ordered.
	Give no ice chips since this increases sodium and potassium loss through tubes.
	• Assess for return of gastrointestinal function, *e.g.,* bowel sounds and passing flatus.
	• Nasogastric tube is usually removed when bowel sounds are present. Diet will be advanced as tolerated.
• *Neurological*	f. Assess patient for symptoms indicating neurological deficit.
	• Assess level of consciousness and mental status and compare with baseline.
	• Check for signs and symptoms of sacral nerve root ischemia such as decrease in lower extremity movement, strength, sensation.
	• Fecal or urinary incontinence.
• *Comfort*	g. Anticipate, evaluate, and provide for patient's need for pain control. See Chapter 2 Pain, p. 27.
	• Be aware that pain contributes to hypertension.
	• Administer pain medication to facilitate activity.
	• Use supportive mechanisms to reduce unnecessary incisional strain and pain:
	When assisting patient to a sitting position, raise head of bed to highest level. Have patient turn to side. Assist patient to pivot to sitting position before standing.
	To facilitate effective coughing, splint incision using pillow or folded blanket.
	An abdominal binder may be applied to support incision during ambulation.
	Patient may be more comfortable in bed with knees elevated, taking care that feet are not in a dependent position.
C. *Is knowledgeable about nature of illness, self-care, and resources for continuity of care*	7. See Chapter 5 Predischarge Phase of Hospitalization, p. 132. Include additional essential elements of preparation for discharge of patient such as
	a. Plan resumption of activities with patient and his family. These include:
	• Alternate periods of activity with rest until energy level returns to normal.
	• Avoid heavy lifting (over 10 to 15 lbs.).
	• No smoking
	• No prolonged sitting. Alternate periods of walking with sitting, *e.g.,* car trips, desk job.
	• Return to work upon advice of physician.
	b. If peripheral vascular disease is present, instruct in care of feet and legs and general precautions. See Occlusive Vascular Disease Guideline, p. 191.
	c. Instruct patient to report any of the following symptoms immediately to physician.
	• Signs of infection such as fever, incisional tenderness, drainage, or inflammation
	• Sudden or gradual development of pain, coldness, pallor in extremity(ies).
	• Development of back pain
	d. Instruct patient/family to check peripheral pulses periodically.
	e. Inform patient of community agencies which may assist in continuity of care.

Patient Outcome	Process

The patient experiences informed, comfortable, and safe preoperative, postoperative and predischarge phases of hospitalization. This includes:

DESCRIPTION: Amputations are commonly done for these reasons: advanced peripheral vascular disease, acute occlusion of a major artery, tumors (cancer), birth defects, and trauma. Depending on the type of problem, the level of amputation varies:
- Below elbow (BE)—elbow joint is preserved.
- Above elbow (AE)—shoulder joint is preserved.
- Shoulder disarticulation—arm is removed through shoulder joint.
- Forequarter amputation—arm, shoulder joint, clavicle, scapula are removed.
- Digital—fingers or toes are removed.
- Syme's—amputation is at ankle joint.
- Below Knee (BK)—knee joint is preserved.
- Knee disarticulation—removal is at the knee joint.
- Above Knee (AK)—hip joint is preserved; leg ordinarily removed at mid-thigh.
- Hip disarticulation—leg is removed at hip joint.

NURSING ASSESSMENT: In addition to general admission assessment, the following information is especially important.
1. Assess and document physical status.
    a. Symptoms related to disease process, *i.e.,* cancer, peripheral vascular disease, trauma:
       - Pain—location, character, duration, effectiveness of pain relief measures
       - Skin—temperature, color, ulceration, wounds, paresthesia
       - Movement and positioning of involved extremity
       - Swelling/edema
       - Masses
       - Peripheral pulses (presence, absence, character)
       - Presence of contractures
    b. Risk factors/disease states which might affect postoperative course specifically
       - Pulmonary status—pulmonary disease, breath sounds, rate, expansion, smoking history
       - Cardiovascular status—rate and rhythm of pulse, E.K.G., other cardiac or vascular disease, *i.e.,* coronary artery disease
       - Renal status—voiding difficulties and infections, renal disease
       - Diabetes—method of control, type of diet
       - Gastrointestinal status—bowel habits
    c. Level of activity.
       - Ambulation status, *i.e.,* use of crutches, walker, wheel chair
       - Postoperative potential of activity, *i.e.,* ability to use prosthesis, crutches, walker, or wheelchair
2. Assess and document patient's response to information about the disease process, treatment and anticipated surgery.
    a. Apparent anxiety level
    b. Previous experience with surgery
    c. Understanding of postoperative expectations
3. Assess and document patient's understanding of the disease process, treatment and anticipated surgery.
4. Assess and document health habits prior to admission:
    a. Potential for self-care or need for supportive care
       - Use of specific assistive devices such as trapeze, bed rails, alternating pressure mattress, bed cradle, sheepskins, bedside commode, and fracture pan
    b. Medications; especially those affecting clotting time, blood pressure, cardiac function and including chemotherapeutic agents
    c. Diet, *i.e.,* type, restrictions, patient's knowledge, compliance
    d. Home health supervision/support

A. *Is prepared for surgery and body image change*

INTERVENTION:
1. Reinforce understanding of patient and family regarding the disease process, implications, and treatment.
    a. Clarify misconceptions and stress preventive aspects (if appropriate).
    b. Keep informed about daily progress during long hospitalization.
    c. Explore rationale for amputation, consequences of not having amputation, and surgical procedures including level of amputation (AK, BK, etc.).

Patient Outcome	Process

2. Summarize usual preoperative preparation and provide care per hospital routine and physician's orders. See Chapter 5 Preoperative Phase of Hospitalization, p. 129. Include additional elements of preoperative care relating to amputation:
   a. Provide information about wound:
      - Form of dressing—general surgery patients may have soft, bulky dressing with or without posterior splint; orthopaedic patients may have same form of dressing, a cast, or an immediate fit prosthesis.
      - Presence of skin traction—usually used with delayed closure to prevent skin retraction.
      - Phantom sensation—some people will feel they still have the extremity present. Sensations may include: pain, burning, itching, phantom position, sense of heat or cold.
      - Use of trapeze for position changes.
      - Elevation of stump for 24 to 48 hours; be sure after this time to keep joints extended (avoid positions of contracture).
      - Presence of drains and dressings with some coloration expected.
   b. Provide additional information:
      - Infected patients may return directly from the operating room (O.R.) to the ward and will be cared for using same routines as recovery room.
      - Change of medications from preoperative such as insulin as opposed to oral agent.
   c. Encourage patient and family to express feelings, concerns, and fears:
      - Recognize patient and family may be experiencing grief response to loss of limb, *i.e.,* denial, anger, bargaining, acceptance.
      - Common fears include loss of function, social position, employment opportunities, family position, intimacy, recurrence of disease.
      - Frequent concerns involving prothesis are: appearances; financial aspects, *i.e.,* money to buy prosthesis; dealing with phantom sensation.
      - Consider use of support resources, *i.e.,* chaplain, school teacher, play therapist, recreational therapist, etc.
   d. Assess patient's postoperative ambulation goals.
      - Secure order for physical therapy consult for preoperative evaluation and instruction regarding exercises and ambulation devices.
      - Encourage patient to lie on stomach and document ability to do so.
      - Encourage patient to practice quadriceps setting and straight leg (affected leg) raising, arm chair push-ups, and hip extension exercises while lying on stomach.
      - Initiate discharge planning including home evaluation form to public health agency, if appropriate.
      - Consider referral to vocational rehabilitation.

B. *Is free of or has minimal discomfort or postoperative complications*

3. Provide postoperative care. See Chapter 5 Postoperative Phase of Hospitalization, p. 130.
4. Intervene in the critical areas of patient care following amputation.
   a. For patient who returns from O.R. without going to recovery room:
      - Spinal anesthesia
        Observe patient closely—spinal anesthesia takes a minimum of 3 to 4 hours to wear off.
        Monitor vital signs q 15 minutes until level of anesthesia is at thigh level.
        Check level of sensation q 30 minutes.
        Do not turn until level of anesthesia is below umbilicus, take vital signs V.S. when turning patient.
        Patient should remain in bed at least 6 hours.
        Patient may have difficulty voiding—observe for discomfort, distention.
      - General anesthesia
        Position patient to protect from aspirating.
        Administer O_2 as ordered; have suction available.
        Take frequent vital signs: q 15 minutes $\times$ 4 times or until awake, q 30 minutes $\times$ 4 times then q 2 hours until stable then q 4 hours.
        Call physician for decreased B.P., pulse greater than 100.
        Have medication available for reversal of narcotic, *e.g.,* naloxone (Narcan).

* *Wound healing*

   b. Observe patient closely for bleeding.
      - Check dressing and lift stump to look for bleeding; frequency as per vital signs.
      - Observe for signs of extensive bleeding/shock; low BP, increased pulse, low urine output, pallor.
      - Circle drainage on dressing, note time and date.
      - If bleeding occurs, apply pressure to wound and call physician.

Patient Outcome	Process
	c. Observe wound for healing and signs of infection.
	• If stump in cast, observe for purulent drainage, foul odor, pain, and fever 48 hours postoperative.
	• With compression dressing, physician will change first dressing; after first dressing change, clarify frequency, procedure, *i.e.,* form of dressing, and whose responsibility (physician or nurse).
	• When doing dressing change, observe and document status of incision, watching for redness, swelling, necrosis, high increase in skin temperature, drainage, and dehiscence.
	• Protect wound from contamination, *i.e.,* urine, feces.
	• Avoid constriction around stump from tight dressings. Avoid circular dressing; use spiral or figure of eight wrapping.
	• Avoid use of tape on skin of stump.
• *Musculoskeletal*	d. Prevent flexion contractures.
	• Do not allow pillows under AK or BK stump after 48 hours.
	• Patient should lie prone at least 1 hour b.i.d. and encourage patient to sleep on stomach at night if possible.
	• Collaborate with physician to have posterior plastic splint made for patient with BK (posterior splint should position knee in *full* extension).
	• Instruct patient with BK not to sit with knee bent over edge of wheelchair or bed.
	• Obtain order for physical therapy to teach range of motion and strengthening exercises.
	• Encourage patient to lie flat in bed with hip and knee (if BK) straight.
• *Safety*	e. Protect patient from accidents/trauma.
	• Patient may forget about lost limb and try to get out of bed. Remind patient limb has been removed and to call nurse for assistance. Orient patient to time, place, procedures.
	• Keep bed in low position with side rails up.
	• Keep personal items and call bell within reach, especially for patient with arm amputation.
	• Restrain patient, if necessary.
	• Consider effect of medications on mental status.
	f. Assess patient's potential and assist to maximal level of independent functioning.
	• Set goals for functioning with patient considering the following:
	Preoperative level of functioning
	Patient/family goals
	Other health factors and disease processes, age, occupation
	• Obtain order for physical therapy to begin progressive ambulation and transfers.
	• Assist patient in learning to use other hand if arm amputation.
• *Gastrointestinal*	g. Maintain normal bowel functioning.
	• Be aware that medications (iron, narcotics) and bedrest can cause constipation.
	• If patient has not returned to normal pattern:
	Encourage roughage and increased fluids in diet.
	Assess patient's choice of laxative and give to patient.
	With prolonged constipation, consider placing patient on daily regimen, *i.e.,* peri-colace, prune juice, stool softener, laxative, dietary.
• *Comfort*	h. Evaluate pain and administer pain medication considering the following:
	• Anesthesia status: Reduce analgesic to one-half dose depending upon anesthetic agent.
	• If patient returns directly from O.R., monitor B.P. closely when giving medication.
	• Phantom sensation may be extremely painful. In addition to analgestic, rubbing stump may decrease pain.
	• Consider alternatives to pain medication:
	Relaxation
	Diversion
	Touch
	Change in position
	Tender Loving Care (TLC)
• *Skin*	i. Initiate preventive skin care. See Chapter 2 Skin Care Guideline, p. 31, when there is deviation from normal skin condition.
C. *Is knowledgeable about nature of illness, self-care, and resources for continuity of care*	5. See Chapter 5 Predischarge Phase of Hospitalization. p. 132. Include additional elements of preparation for discharge of patient with amputation.
	a. Encourage patient and family to express feelings and future plans.
	b. Assess home environment considering functional status:
	• Initiate public health nurse referral if needed.

Patient Outcome	Process

	• Modify home in regard to:
	    Entry into house (may need ramp, rails, wider door)
	    Movement within house (access to bathroom, bedroom) and rearrangement of furniture
	c. Assess need for equipment at home. Collaborate with physical therapy and social service.
	    • Wheelchair—consider need for removable arms, wheelchair pad
	    • Crutches/walker
	    • Portable toilet—commode chair
	    • Bedpan/urinal
	    • Trapeze
	    • Hospital bed
	    • Ace wraps
	d. Instruct patient/family in exercises and positioning which will insure optimal mobility.
	    • Collaborate with physical therapist to establish exercise routine at home and instruct patient.
	    • Teach patient optimal positioning for home use including:
	        Lying on stomach at least two times a day for a minimum of one hour
	        Sitting/lying with knee straight (BKA's)
	        Periodically lifting self off chair if sitting for long periods of time
	        Avoid placing pillows under stump or between knees.
	e. Instruct patient/family in performing stump/wound care.
	    • Determine with physician appropriate care for stump at home.
	    • If wound is open, clarify form of dressing and solution and instruct patient/family in care of wound. Send public health referral, if appropriate.
	    • If wound is closed, usually small dry dressing will be used for protection.
	    • Daily care will involve:
	        Daily washing of stump with soap and water
	        Daily inspection of stump for injury and breakdown (ulceration)
	        Stump wrapping
	            (1) Reduce edema and mold stump for future prosthesis by wrapping
	            (2) Obtain orders from physician to begin wrapping q.i.d. Coordinate with physical therapy to stump wrap and instruct patient and family.
	            (3) Have patient/family demonstrate wrapping
	            (4) Inspect stump for healing, redness, pressure areas, breakdown.
	            (5) Provide for obtaining dressing supplies.
	f. Instruct patient/family on prevention of skin breakdown.
	    • Optimal positioning:
	        Lying on stomach at least two times a day for minimum of one hour
	        Periodically lifting self off chair if sitting for long periods of time
	        Change position q 2 hours when lying in bed.
	        Consider wheelchair cushions if wheelchair bound, sheepskin.
	    • Keep skin dry and clean.
	    • Observe skin daily using mirror, if necessary.
	    • If patient has diabetes and/or peripheral vascular disease, instruct in diabetic skin care, especially foot care.
	g. Review bowel status and suggest continuing a preventive constipation routine at home.
	h. Collaborate with physician to obtain order for appointment for amputee clinic.
	i. Establish appropriate rehabilitation goals with patient and family.

Bilateral subcutaneous mastectomy with implants or reduction mammoplasty

Patient Outcome	Process

Patient Outcome

The patient experiences informed, comfortable, and safe preoperative, postoperative, and predischarge phases of hospitalization. This includes:

Process

DESCRIPTION: Surgical procedure for fibrocystic disease: A small incision is usually made in the skin fold below the breast to facilitate removal of about 80 per cent of the patient's diseased breast tissue and insertion of a silastic envelope. For a reduction mammoplasty, excess tissue is removed.

NURSING ASSESSMENT: In addition to general admission assessment, the following information is especially important:
1. Assess and document physical status.
   a. Symptoms relating to underlying disease
   b. Presence of any other disease state
2. Assess and document patient's response to information about the disease process, treatment, and anticipated surgery.
   a. Apparent anxiety level
   b. Previous experience with surgery
   c. Patient's self-assessment of:
      • Personal strengths in coping with stresses
      • Support persons, *i.e.*, family, chaplain.
3. Assess and document patient's understanding of the disease process and anticipated surgery.

A. *Is prepared for surgery and body image change*

INTERVENTION:
1. Reinforce understanding of patient and family regarding the disease process, implications, and treatment. Information given may include discussing usual postoperative expectations with patient and family:
   • Bulky halter breast dressing
   • Skin catheters attached to bulb suction
   • Restricted movement of arms immediately following operation for several days
   • Bed rest for several days
   • Possible body image changes
2. Summarize features of preoperative phase and provide care needed per hospital routine and physician's order. See Chapter 5 Preoperative Phase of Hospitalization, p. 129.
3. Provide postoperative care, see Chapter 5 Postoperative Phase of Hospitalization, p. 130.

B. *Is free of or has minimal discomfort or postoperative complications*

4. Intervene in the critical elements of patient care following a bilateral subcutaneous mastectomy with implants or reduction mammoplasty.
   a. Provide wound care:
      • Observe and report drainage on dressing.
      • Inspect closed drainage system for proper functioning:
         Check for clots q 1 hour by milking tubing and breaking suction for first 24 hours.
         Empty drainage every 8 hours the first 24 hours: expect a total no greater than 50 to 100 cc bloody drainage. Second 24 hours: expect a total no greater than 50 cc bloody drainage.
         Usually removed by fourth postoperative day.
      • Keep on bedrest several days as ordered.
      • Restrict activity of arms.
         With arms at side, patient uses lower arm to cradle breast while nurse assists patient to make slight comfort moves.

C. *Is knowledgeable about nature of illness, self-care, and resources for continuity of care*

5. See Chapter 5 Predischarge Phase of Hospitalization, p. 132. Include additional essential elements of preparation for discharge of patient such as:
   a. Have two soft, supportive brassieres available—one same size as wearing before surgery and one next size smaller.
   b. Inform patient and family that incision will be numb temporarily; sensation to area will usually return to normal; change in activity may alter sensation.
   c. Tell patient she may resume normal activities as tolerated (exception: heavy lifting, strenuous activity involving use of arms until ordered by physician).
   d. Help patient to discuss concerns due to bilateral mastectomy or mammoplasty such as not being able to breast feed, skin care preparation, etc.

141

Patient Outcome

The patient experiences informed, comfortable, and safe preoperative, postoperative, and predischarge phases of hospitalization. This includes:

Process

DESCRIPTION: Most patients have a history of chronic neck problems sometimes causing symptoms of arm and leg numbness, pain and weakness, *e.g.*, cervical spondylosis, degenerative disc disease, and many have already used conservative methods to obtain relief such as traction and analgesics. Other patients may have had an acute cervical fracture and require a cervical fusion to stabilize the injury.

NURSING ASSESSMENT: In addition to general admission assessment, the following information is especially important.

1. Assess and document physical status.
    Symptoms related to underlying disease
    - Neurological status (upper extremities, lower extremities, strength and sensation)
    - Pain level and character
    - Previously effective means of dealing with pain
    - Use of analgesics
    - Bowel and bladder problems
    - Functional limitations due to disease process
2. Assess and document patient's response to information about the disease process, treatment, and anticipated surgery.
    a. Apparent anxiety level
    b. Previous experience with surgery
    c. Patient's self-assessment of support people (family, chaplain, etc.)
3. Assess and document health habits prior to admission.
    a. Assistive devices used
    b. Potential for self-care or need for supportive care
    c. Diet, *i.e.*, any restrictions
    d. Home health supervision/support
4. Assess and document patient's understanding of the disease process, treatment, and anticipated surgery.

INTERVENTION:

1. Reinforce understanding of patient and family regarding the disease process, implications, and treatment including the operative procedure if appropriate. Information may include:
    a. Incision site
        - *Anterior:* anterior, lateral neck (usually on left side—may be longitudinal or horizontal incision)
        - *Posterior:* posterior cervical area
        - *Graft site:* iliac crest; may have hematoma postoperatively.
    b. Drains: Penrose or closed wound drain or none
    c. Pain expectations:
        - *Anterior:* sore throat, hoarseness, discomfort on swallowing and coughing. Excessive difficulty on swallowing not expected.
        - *Posterior:* normal, incisional pain
        - *Graft site* (iliac crest): may be more painful than incision.
2. Institute preparation of patient for diagnostic studies. See Chapter 3 Guideline for the Patient Undergoing Diagnostic Studies p. 33.
    a. Myelogram
    b. Radiographs including tomograms
    c. Minnesota Multiphasic Personality Inventory
    d. Electromyography
    e. Bone Scan
3. Summarize usual features of preoperative preparation and provide care needed per hospital procedure and physician's orders. See Chapter 5 Preoperative Phase of Hospitalization, p. 129.
4. Include additional elements of preoperative care relating to cervical fusion.
    a. Respiratory routine
        - O_2 by mask
        - Diaphragmatic breathing and/or coughing are especially important to smokers and persons with chronic respiratory problems.
        - Respiratory routines especially for smokers, history of respiratory problems
        - Possible use of incentive spirometry.
    b. Cervical collar and knee length antiembolic hose per physician's orders.

A. *Is prepared for surgery*

Patient Outcome	Process
	c. Positioning and turning:

c. Positioning and turning:
- Elevate head of bed 30° to 40° to decrease edema around neck and prevent pooling of secretions.
- Position to keep neutral alignment.
- Knees can be flexed for comfort.
- Log-roll (turning head and torso as one unit-chin in line with sternum to prevent twisting).
- Motion will be restricted to log-rolling in bed until cervical collar is in place (about 36 to 48 hours). Patient then can be out of bed and ambulating with collar.

d. Leg exercises:
- Ankle "circles"
- Quadriceps setting

e. Patient will be n.p.o. then progressive diet as tolerated.

B. *Is free of or has minimal discomfort or postoperative complications.*
• Respiratory

5. Provide postoperative care. See Chapter 5 Postoperative Phase of Hospitalization, p. 130.
6. Intervene in critical elements of patient care following surgery for a cervical fusion.
   a. Institute measures to prevent respiratory problems:
   - Have tracheostomy tray ready at bedside for use.
   - Have O_2 and suction for use at bedside.
   - Be aware of patient complaints about difficult breathing or frequent swallowing of secretions. This may signal internal bleeding.
   - Check for adequate chest expansion and exhaling through nose and mouth.
   - Cough, deep breath patient q 2 hours. Reassure patient that coughing may be uncomfortable but will not disrupt sutures.
   - Avoid narcotics, barbiturates, and other drugs that depress respirations.
   - Elevate head of bed to facilitate drainage of secretions and decrease edema.
   - Use ultrasonic nebulizer to liquify secretions.
   - Encourage patient to expectorate secretions.
   - Recognize that lethargy and somnolence may indicate CO_2 buildup.

• Neurological

   b. Assess neurological status:
   - Check movement, sensation, and strength in upper and lower extremities at least q 2 hours for first 24 hours. Compare with preoperative status.
       Bilateral grips, compare right to left.
       Bilateral dorsiflexion, compare right to left.
       Probable decrease in preoperative numbness and tingling.
   - Pain levels with preoperative assessment. Expect diminished pain in affected extremity. Normal postsurgical incisional pain and graft pain are expected.
   c. Provide careful positioning and log-rolling q 2 hours. Consider patient's reluctance to turn to graft side.
   d. Progress patient's activity with cervical collar in place. Progression is:
   - Elevate head of bed,
   - Dangle,
   - Ambulate - usually begins 24 to 48 hours after surgery.
   e. Maintain position of cervical area:
   - *Anterior fusion:*
       Avoid hyperextension.
       No twisting or sudden motion
       No pulling on arms in changing positions. (Caution visitors about this.)
   - *Posterior fusion:*
       No twisting or sudden motion
       Use of sandbags by sides of head to remind patient of position
       Cervical collar as a reminder but which does not completely immobilize area
       Use of overhead trapeze to facilitate movement at discretion of physician
   f. Be alert for signs of nausea and vomiting:
   - Retching may cause sudden motion of cervical area.

C. *Is knowledgeable about nature of illness, self-care, and resources for continuity of care*

7. See Chapter 5 Predischarge Phase of Hospitalization, p. 132. Include additional elements of preparation for discharge of patient:
   a. Teach proper application of collar or brace and its care.
   - Check skin under collar or brace daily for signs of pressure. Pad with soft material and seek help if irritation continues.

Patient Outcome	Process
	• For care of cervical collar, provide stockinette material to change cover when soiled (2 feet of 4 inch tubular stockinette). b. Plan with patient and family. This may include: • Wear collar at all times—two months. • Do not twist neck—two months. • Do not drive car if peripheral vision is poor (chance of injury from sudden stop)—two months. • Do not ride in car in sitting position (may recline)—one month. • Do not lift objects weighing over 15 pounds—two months. • Resume all previous activities of daily living which don't require turning or twisting of neck. c. Instruct patient to report any of the following symptoms immediately to physician: • Infection: redness, swelling at either incision site • Difficulty swallowing • Increased pain, numbness, tingling in upper extremities • Respiratory distress • Decrease in voluntary movement or strength of extremities

Patient Outcome	Process

The patient experiences informed, comfortable, and safe preoperative, postoperative, and predischarge phases of hospitalization. This includes:

DESCRIPTION: Removal of the gall baldder may be performed for gall stones, inflammation, or cancer of the gall bladder. The common duct, pancreas, and liver may or may not be affected.

PROCEDURE: A subcostal incision is made on the right side (occasionally a midline incision is used). The cystic duct is identified and the gall bladder dissected from its bed. The duct is ligated (tied off), transected, and the gall bladder is removed. A penrose drain is brought out through a stab wound below the incision. A T-tube may be inserted to divert bile when the common duct is explored.

NURSING ASSESSMENT: In addition to general admission assessment, the following information is especially important.
1. Assess and document physical status.
    a. Symptoms related to gall bladder disease:
        • Pain: location, character, duration. Effectiveness of pain relief measures
        • Presence of jaundice
        • Bowel changes, *e.g.*, color of stools
    b. Risk factors:
        • Pulmonary status, smoking history
        • Presence of other disease states, *i.e.*, diabetes, hypertension
2. Assess and document patient's response to information about the disease process, treatment, and anticipated surgery:
    a. Apparent anxiety level
    b. Previous experience with surgery
3. Assess and document health habits prior to admission.
    a. Potential for self-care or need for supportive care
    b. Anticipated family reaction to required postoperative dietary modifications
    c. Diet, *i.e.*, restrictions, patient's knowledge and compliance
    d. Home health supervision/support
4. Assess and document patient's understanding of the disease process, treatment, and anticipated surgery.

A. *Is prepared for surgery*

INTERVENTION:
1. Reinforce understanding of patient and family regarding the disease process, implications, and treatment.
2. Summarize usual preoperative preparation and provide care per hospital procedure and physician's orders. See Chapter 5 Preoperative Phase of Hospitalization, p. 129.

B. *Is free of or has minimal discomfort or postoperative complications*
• *Gastrointestinal*

3. Provide postoperative care. See Chapter 5 Postoperative Phase of Hospitalization, p. 130.
4. Intervene in the critical areas of patient care following surgery.
    a. Monitor and record gastric drainage from nasogastric tube.
        • Consistency and color
        • Guaiac test if bleeding is suspected
    b. Monitor and record T-tube drainage.
        • Ensure patency of tube.
        • Maintain sterile collection system.
        • As patient progresses, T-tube may be clamped and bag positioned below level of incision.

• *Wound healing*

    c. Provide strict aseptic wound care. See Chapter 5 Laparotomy Guideline, p. 179.
        • Consider use of sterile collection system if penrose or other drain in wound.
        • Maintain skin integrity around site.

• *Comfort*

    d. Anticipate moderate to severe (usually) pain. Consider:
        • Effect on pulmonary function
        • Effect on early ambulation
    e. Institute measures for comfort such as:
        • Offer analgesics frequently as ordered and coordinate with pain producing activity.
        • Employ use of other measures such as backrubs, repositioning, and splinting.

C. *Is knowledgeable about nature of illness, self-care, and resources for continuity of care*

5. See Chapter 5 Predischarge Phase of Hospitalization, p. 132. Include additional essential elements of preparation for discharge of patient with a cholecystectomy:
    a. If patient is to be discharged with T-tube:
        • Consult with physician regarding schedule for clamping and/or unclamping.
    b. Teach patient how to:
        • Clamp/unclamp tube
        • Give care around tube

Patient Outcome	Process
	• Hook-up to drainage system if necessary
	• Observe for symptoms of obstruction and infection: chills, fever, jaundice, distention, feeling of tightness, change in color of urine (brownish), nausea/vomiting, clay colored stools, discharge, redness, and swelling around tube.
	c. Reinforce teaching about any dietary modifications.
	d. Discuss return appointment.
	e. Refer to public health nurse for continued monitoring of T-tube if appropriate.

Colostomy, ileostomy, abdominoperineal resection

Patient Outcome

The patient experiences informed, comfortable, and safe preoperative, postoperative, and predischarge phases of hospitalization. This includes:

Process

DESCRIPTION: Colostomy, ileostomy, and abdominoperineal resections are commonly done for treatment of tumors (cancer), trauma, perforation, diverticulitis, familial polyposis, and inflammatory bowel disease such as ulcerative colitis and Crohn's disease. A surgically created opening is made into the intestine and the stoma is brought through the abdominal wall for the purpose of diversion of intestinal contents. The diversion may be temporary or permanent depending upon the diagnosis. The most common types of procedures are:

Transverse colostomy

• *Loop colostomy (Fig. 5-2.):* A loop of colon is exteriorized and opened to provide a single large stoma with 2 openings. A plastic bridge or rod is placed under loop and remains about 8 days. Proximal opening discharges feces; distal opening secretes mucus from inactive bowel.

• *Colostomy and mucous fistula (double barrel) (Fig. 5-3.):* Colon is divided, resulting in 2 separated stomas. Proximal stoma discharges feces; distal stoma secretes mucus from inactive bowel.

Sigmoid colostomy (Fig 5-4.)

• *Colostomy and Hartman's Pouch:* The sigmoid colon is divided and the proximal end is exteriorized for fecal drainage. The distal end is sutured and left intact inside the peritoneum. Mucous drainage is through the rectum. This is usually a temporary procedure.

• *Permanent colostomy:* The sigmoid colon is divided and the proximal end is exteriorized to form a permanent stoma. The distal portion of colon is removed during the abdominoperineal resection.

Ileostomy (Fig. 5-5.): The ileum is divided and the proximal end is exteriorized for drainage of ileal contents. A total colectomy and removal of rectum usually accompanies this procedure.

Continent ileostomy (Koch's Pouch) (Fig. 5-6.): A pouch is constructed from a portion of ileum with the flush stoma formed into a nipple valve to provide continence. Ileal drainage is via bag or catheter insertion through stoma into pouch 3 to 8 times daily. A total colectomy and removal of rectum usually accompanies this procedure.

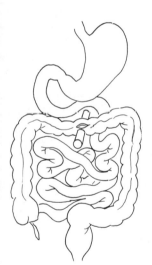
Fig. 5-2—Loop colostomy in transverse colon.

Fig. 5-3—Colostomy and mucous fistula.

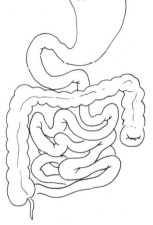
Fig. 5-4—Sigmoid colostomy with Abdominoperineal resection.

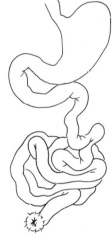
Fig. 5-5—Ileostomy with colon and rectum removed.

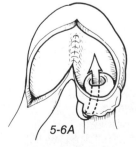
5-6A

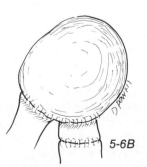
5-6B

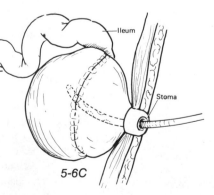
Ileum

Stoma

5-6C

Fig. 5-6—Continent ileostomy.

Patient Outcome	Process
	NURSING ASSESSMENT: In addition to the general admission assessment, the following information is especially important.

1. Assess and document physical status:
    a. Symptoms related to underlying disease
        • Pain—location, character, effectiveness of relief measures
        • Bowel habits/changes
        • Nutritional status, *e.g.*, weight loss
    b. Risk factors:
        • Presence of other disease states, *e.g.*, diabetes
        • Poor healing capacity, *e.g.*, if patient is on steroid therapy
2. Assess and document patient's response to information about the disease process, treatment, and anticipated surgery.
    a. Apparent anxiety level
    b. Previous experience with surgery
    c. Patient's self-assessment of:
        • Personal strengths in coping with stress
        • Support people, *i.e.*, family, friend
        • Concept of body image
3. Assess and document patient's understanding of disease process, treatment, and anticipated surgery.
4. Assess and document health habits/life style prior to admission:
    a. Potential for self-care and need for supportive care
    b. Position in family unit, *e.g.*, marital status
        • Sexual activity status
    c. Home health supervision/support

A. *Is prepared for surgery and body image change*

INTERVENTION:
1. Reinforce understanding of patient and his family regarding the disease process, implications and treatment.
2. Plan with patient and physician on placement of stoma.
    a. Consider skin folds, bony prominences, and waistline by observing patient in standing and sitting positions.
    b. Mark site on skin clearly.
3. Provide assistance to patient in coping with future altered body function and image. Assess need for patients with similar surgery to visit pre- and postoperatively.
4. Summarize usual preoperative preparation and provide care as needed per hospital routine and physician's orders. See Chapter 5 Preoperative phase of hospitalization, p. 129.

B. *Is free of or has minimal discomfort or postoperative complications*

• *Wound healing*

5. Provide postoperative care. See Chapter 5 Postoperative phase of hospitalization, p. 130.
6. Intervene in the critical areas of patient care following a colostomy, ileostomy, and/or abdominoperineal resection.
    a. Describe and record all output including stoma pouch, perineal drainage, and mucous fistula.
        • Expect less than 100 cc stomal bleeding; smaller amount from mucous fistula; moderate to large amount bloody/serosanguineous drainage from perineal wound. Check q 2 hours and expect to change dressing q 4 to 6 hours during first 24 hours.
        • During second 24 hour: Expect none to minimal stomal and mucous fistula drainage (stomal bleeding stops and drainage begins) if ileostomy were done. There will be no expected drainage from colostomy for 4 to 5 days. Perineal wound will drain moderate amount of serosanguineous fluid. Monitor every two hours and expect to change dressings q 6 hours.
    b. Check for adequate stomal circulation every shift and record.
        • Use clear plastic pouch for increased visibility.
        • Check pouch for proper fit allowing $\frac{1}{16}$ to ⅛-inch space to permit free circulation around stoma.
    c. Establish plan for wound care with physician and patient to promote healing.
        • Determine if abdominal wound is closed by sutures or open with packing or stay sutures.
        • Prevent wound sepsis by avoiding fecal contamination.
        • Tape dressing on wound securely to isolate from stomal area.
        • Evaluate proximity of stoma to incision and choose appliance accordingly.
        • Note advancement of drain in a partially closed wound as drainage diminishes.
            For open perineal wounds the packing is usually removed by the fourth to fifth day.

Patient Outcome	Process

	• Provide comfort:
	    Use dry heat or sitz baths if ordered.
	    Use rubber ring to minimize pressure.
	  d. Choose properly fitting appliance with Karaya seal and microporous tape or stomahesive and clear plastic drainage pouch with tape.
	    • Measure stoma with measuring card allowing $1/16$ to ⅛-inch clearance all around stoma.
	    • Order appliance as specified in precut appliance or cut appliance opening using stoma measurement.
	  e. Apply pouch properly.
	    • Start always with clean dry skin.
	    • Apply skin prep as protective film to skin when using nonporous adhesive.
	    • Center appliance over stoma and apply with firm pressure to create skin seal to prevent leakage.
	    • Secure belt tabs to skin with microporous tape if using appliance without adhesive.
	  f. Obtain physician order (unless contraindicated) for irrigation on eighth day if colostomy is located in descending or sigmoid colon.

• *Body image*
C. *Is knowledgeable about nature of illness, self-care and resources for continuity of care*
	g. Encourage participation of the patient in the care of the stoma and application of pouch.
	7. See Chapter 5 Predischarge Phase of Hospitalization, p. 132.
	8. Include additional essential elements of preparation for discharge:
	  a. Assess the acceptance by the patient and his family of the changes in body function and self-image, the stoma and its care.
	    • Discuss personal and social adjustment such as:
	      Odor control
	      Clothing
	      Sexual adjustment (confer with physician regarding possibility of impotence/interruption of innervation to perineum). Include assessment of need to provide sexual adjustment pamphlets printed by colostomy associations.
	      Colostomy association, especially for patient with permanent colostomy.
	  b. Teach/reinforce self-care activities emphasizing:
	    • Skin care around stoma
	    • Appliance application
	    • Irrigation, if appropriate
	    • Wound care
	    • Diet modifications
	    • Medications, *i.e.,* use of stool softeners; avoid any enteric-coated or long-acting drug that is not absorbed.
	  c. Refer to home health services as needed.
	  d. Provide information about location of nearest equipment and supply source and colostomy club.

Craniotomy

Patient Outcome	Process

The patient experiences informed, comfortable and safe preoperative, postoperative and predischarge phases of hospitalization. This includes:

DESCRIPTION: A craniotomy is a surgical opening into the skull to resect tumor masses, repair vascular anomalies, relieve intracranial pressure, evacuate blood clots, and approach other intracranial lesions. The patient may or may not develop permanent neurologic deficits associated with the disease process requiring craniotomy.

Most often the patient and family view brain surgery as a threat to a meaningful existence and life itself. Because of the complexity of the patient's needs, it is imperative for the nurse to include and involve the family in all phases of care.

This guideline is applicable to but not inclusive for patients with posterior fossa craniectomies and shunt procedures. The guideline includes information pertinent to both children and adults; the emphasis, however, is on the adult craniotomy patient.

NURSING ASSESSMENT: In addition to the general admission assessment, the following information is especially important:

1. Assess and document baseline neurological status.
   a. Level of consciousness (LOC). Describe behaviors and mental status.
   b. Motor function: compare right to left.
      • Present activity level
      • Focal weakness of extremities or facial muscles
   c. Sensory function
   d. Pupils: compare right to left.
      • Size
      • Reactivity to light
   e. Eye movements
   f. Seizure
      • Pattern, specify if there is aura
      • Frequency
      • Medication
   g. Communication problems: vision, speech, hearing
   h. Other important findings: symptoms of increased intracranial pressure
      • Headache
      • Nausea
      • Vomiting
      • Changes in respiratory patterns
      • Hypertension
      • Widened pulse pressure, bradycardia
   i. Loss of voluntary control of bladder and bowel
   j. Intellectual function and personality
   k. Memory; recent and long-term
   l. Coordination, gait

INTERVENTION:

A. *Experiences emotional support, concern, and caring*

1. Recognize that patient/family have certain fears about the illness, treatment, and future course.
   a. Listen for patient/family concerns and present understanding before directly questioning them about diagnostic studies/surgery.
   b. Consider the following factors that may affect patient responses:
      • Time elapsed since onset of symptoms, how and when told about problem and the need for surgery
      • Extent of symptoms and medical problem
      • Accuracy of understanding including recent information from health personnel and previous information from personal contacts, media (TV), etc.
      • Previous experience with personal crisis and patterns of coping—recent or unresolved personal crises
      • Degree of physiological stress/pain
   c. Identify and document specific fears expressed by patient/family. Examples are:
      • Death or vegetative state
      • Loss of control/independence, guilt surrounding dependent role
      • Loss of privacy, dignity
      • Change in body image, disfigurement, *e.g.,* hair loss, hemiplegia
      • Economic impact of surgery, convalescence
      • Long-term disability
         Loss of physical, intellectual, or personality function
         Changes in roles within family, previous life-styles

Patient Outcome	Process
	d. Establish plan of care directed at minimizing fears. Consider: • Be present when physician talks with patient and family. Report and document specific fears/misconceptions expressed by patient/family. Clarify misconceptions. • Note behavior and affect of patient and family that may indicate emotional response to illness. • Write nursing orders that reflect specific care needs of patient, *e.g.*, be alert to patient's aura of smelling foul odors which may precede seizure activity.
B. *Is prepared for diagnostic studies*	2. Explain scheduled diagnostic tests; provide physical preparation and postprocedure care. Refer to Chapter 3 Guidelines for the Patient Undergoing Diagnostic Studies, p. 33. a. Skull radiograph b. Brain computerized tomography c. Angiography (carotid arteriogram, brachial arteriogram) d. Pneumoencephalogram e. Electroencephalogram f. Tomograms 3. Provide information for patient regarding scheduled consults which vary according to disease process and may include the following: neurology, endocrinology, ophthalmology, otolaryngology.

C. *Is prepared for surgery and post-operative course*	4. Summarize features of preoperative preparation and provide care as needed per hospital routine and physician's orders.
	 a. Approach patient and family after considering the following:
	 • Has patient had major diagnostic procedure today?
	 • What has patient/family been told by neurosurgeon? Be present if possible during explanation.
	 • What is documented in chart and available from nursing staff about patient?
	 b. Plan patient/family teaching strategy and document individual's receptivity to teaching.
	 • Try to prearrange time when family can be present for teaching. If family cannot be there, make special effort to prepare them.
	 • Try to provide a warm, relaxed atmosphere during preoperative teaching.
	    Sit down next to patient and family.
	    Use touch, eye contact, active listening.
	 • Provide ongoing opportunities for patient/family to ask questions, express fears.
	 c. Ask patient about previous experience with surgery, any problems encountered, and what patient expects. Patient and family may have many misconceptions about brain surgery and/or surgery in general.
	 d. Give the following information to all conscious patients:
	 • Hair shaved in operating room (OR) immediately prior to surgery (will be returned to patient).
	 • Head dressing (for 7 to 10 days, then patient may wear hat, scarf, wig)
	 • Transfer from OR to Recovery Room (RR) to Intensive Care Unit (ICU)
	    Patient usually sent to RR in afternoon, may remain overnight. Family may expect to visit patient in Intensive Care Unit in early evening or in RR after 7:00 p.m. Charge nurse will assist family.
	 e. Be sensitive to anxiety level and how much information patient/family wish to know. Select from the following:
	 • Preoperative: Refer to Preoperative Phase of Hospitalization, p. 129.
	 • Immediate postoperative nursing care in RR/ICU (first 24 hours). Expectations include:
	    Frequent vital signs, neurological checks. Demonstrate neurological checks.
	    Pulmonary routine (turn, deep breath, cough, percussion). Emphasize patient participation.
	    Endotracheal tube (ET) present during surgery, usually removed before patient alert.
	    Cardiac monitor
	    If patient awakens with ET tube in place he will be unable to talk, have sore throat.
	    Prepare patient for unpleasant sounds and sensation of suctioning.
	    O_2 mask: position over mouth and nose, may feel cool moist vapor.
	    Head dressing: tight feeling
	    Headache: variable, increases during coughing. May not be able to achieve total relief of pain because only mild analgesics may be given.
	    Swelling and discoloration of eye(s): Usually begins within 24 hours.
	    IVs: minimum 24 hours

Patient Outcome	Process

                        May have arterial line.
                        Frequent IM/IV medications: usually continued for 5 days
                        Foley catheter
                        Intensive care environment is usually busy, noisy, and patients rarely have uninterrupted
                            sleep.
                        Visiting policies
                    • Progressive care expectations:
                        Anticipated stay in ICU minimum 24 hours depending upon patient condition and bed
                            availability for transfer
                        Gradual progression of diet and activity according to physician order
                        Head dressing usually on 7 to 10 days (until sutures removed). Patient may hear clicking
                            sound as bone flap heals.
               f. Support patient by giving positive aspects of surgical procedure.
                    • Surgeon(s), nursing staff, and other members of team are competent.
                    • Care is in specialized neurosurgical intensive unit.
                    • Headache may be minimal or less than patient anticipates.
                    • When patient returns from Recovery Room, family will be permitted to visit.
                    • Under certain circumstances nurse may arrange for and accompany family to RR.
                    • Medications will be given to reduce pain and to minimize swelling.
                    • Gradual progression of activity will resume within several days. If no complications,
                        patient may be ready for discharge within ten days depending on preoperative status.
               g. Consult physical therapist preoperatively for patients who need postoperative physical
                    therapy, *e.g.,* existing deficit, anticipated postoperative deficits, pulmonary problems.
               h. Provide immediate preoperative physical care:
                    • Scalp care:
                        Wash hair and scalp twice.
                        Inform physician if patient has infection of scalp or face.
                    • Measure, order, and have patient wear antiembolic hose to Operating Room.
                    • Check with physician for sedative order night before surgery for patient who does not have
                        depressed level of consciousness

D. *Is free of or has minimal postoperative complications*

• *Neurological*

5. Provide postoperative care. See Postoperative Phase of Hospitalization, p. 130.
6. Intervene in the critical areas of care following craniotomy. Refer to General Guidelines In the
   Critical Care Patient Chapter 9 Neurological, p. 359.
   a. Assess neurological status and compare with baseline data:
        • Level of consciousness
        • Pupil response
        • Motor activity
        • Vital signs
        • Speech
        • Seizure activity
        • Other abnormalities:
            Cranial nerve deficit
            Major change in headache pattern

• *Emotional support*

   b. Be particularly sensitive to patient/family needs for information and emotional support.
        • Prepare and accompany family members during initial visit to patient in postoperative
            period, *e.g.,* to explain equipment, noise, patient appearance.
        • Provide support for patient especially during frightening experiences such as suctioning,
            presence of ET tube and inability to speak.
        • If patient intubated, provide alternative means of communication, writing notes, blinks or
            finger gestures for simple "yes" or "no".

• *Wound care*

   c. Provide care of the surgical wound.
        • Keep elastic bandage over head dressing for first 4 to 6 hours to minimize subgaleal fluid
            collection. This bandage usually removed in Recovery Room.
        • If drain present, expect more drainage. Drains usually removed within 24 hours.
        • Place sterile plastic drape around bandage to prevent contamination of wet dressing.
        • Describe character of drainage and report need for dressing change to physician.
        • Prevent contamination of wound by keeping patient's fingernails clean and clipped.
            Consider use of mitts or restraints as needed.
        • If bone flap is removed (craniectomy) label dressing, "Do not turn on
            (operative) side".

Patient Outcome	Process
	• Assess fit of head dressing:
	Dressing should be intact and snug, should be able to fit two fingers under edge of dressing.
	Note swelling caused by too-tight dressing (around edge of dressing).
	Check that ears are not curled under dressing.
	• If dressing comes off, apply sterile towel and report to physician.
	• Stay with patient during dressing change.
	• Maintain dressing at least until sutures removed (7 to 14 days). Wire sutures usually remain ten days or more.
	• Observe for signs of infection and report to physician.
	Fever, especially 48 hours postoperatively
	Meningism
	Local redness, swelling, drainage
• *Intracranial bleeding*	d. Observe for rapid neurological deterioration in first 24 hours, which may be due to intracranial bleeding. (Patient may need to return to OR for evacuation of hematoma).
• *Brain swelling*	e. Observe for brain swelling, which is expected in first 24 to 72 hours postoperatively for patient with partially resected tumor or in traumatized brain. Monitor neurological status closely.
	f. Anticipate treatment modalities for increased intracranial pressure to decrease swelling. These may include:
	• Elevate head of bed 30° to facilitate venous drainage.
	• Administer steroids as ordered—May be contraindicated in recent ulcer or tuberculosis.
	Drugs may include:
	Solu-Medrol
	Cimetadine IM/IV x 5 days
	Depo-Medrol IM on fourth day
	• Monitor diabetic urines q 6 hours because of diabetogenic effect of steroids.
	• Watch for possible neurological status change after steroids discontinued.
	• Monitor GI drainage and stools for signs of bleeding.
	• Administer preventive GI regimen as ordered, *e.g.*, antacids.
	• Control ventilatory rate.
	Monitor blood gases—pCO_2 to be in low normal range.
	• Administer mannitol as ordered.
	Use administration set with filter. Dosage should be tapered.
	• Monitor urine specific gravity.
	• Maintain indwelling urinary catheter.
	• Monitor electrolytes.
	• Monitor Intake and Output. Prevent fluid overload.
	• Anticipate patient may need to return to OR to have bone flap removed (rare).
	• Anticipate use of intracranial pressure monitor.
• *Circulatory*	g. Recognize that depleted systemic blood volume compromises brain function, especially brain that has been traumatized.
	• Monitor hematocrit especially first 48 hours. Monitor for GI bleeding.
	• Monitor vital signs closely, especially when progressing patient to upright position, dangling, and out of bed.
• *Cerebral vasospasm*	h. Be aware that vasospasm of cerebral vessels may be demonstrated by decreased LOC or increased focal deficit.
	• Vasospasms are more likely to occur before and after surgery for aneurysm.
	• Patient may have one or more angiograms to determine extent of spasm.
	• IV drugs may be used to decrease spasm.
• *Seizures*	i. Anticipate that postoperative seizures are more likely in patients with preoperative seizures, subdural hematomas, meningiomas, penetrating injuries, or other lesions involving cortex.
	• Be sure anticonvulsants are resumed postoperatively. Anticonvulsants may be prescribed prophylactically in patients with no previous seizures.
	• Observe and provide care during seizure(s). Document pertinent data. Give special attention to neurological status and respiratory care during and after seizure.
	• Keep seizure record. Include onset, duration, pattern, medications given, postictal state.
	• Be aware that large loading doses of anticonvulsants may depress LOC for varying time. Usual anticonvulsants are:
	Dilantin, IV push, orally (PO) (do not give IM) Adult loading dose up to 1 gm per 24 hours. Use cardiac monitor when 1 gm loading dose is given IV push.

Patient Outcome	Process

Adults 1000 to 1500 mg per 24 hours
Child's dose calculated per kilo per 24 hours
Phenobarbital IM, IV, PO
Adults 90 to 180 mg per 24 hours
Child's dose calculated per kilo per 24 hours.

• *Pituitary dysfunction*

j. Anticipate inadequate pituitary function in patient with surgery in pituitary or parasellar region.
  • Be aware that the patient lacks adequate plasma cortisol and must receive cortisone replacement with increased doses for stress.
    Begin cortisone acetate replacement when Solu-Medrol is discontinued.
    Do not omit dose for any reason. Must give IM if oral dose not taken.
  • Monitor for diabetes insipidus:
    Report to physician excessive thirst and output of greater than 200 cc urine/hour for two consecutive hours and/or specific gravity greater than or equal to 1.005.
    Monitor electrolytes for signs of dehydration: sodium greater than 150 meq, potassium less than 3.5 meq. Collect urine and serum for osmolarity.
  • Give IV fluids of dextrose 5 percent in water to keep up with output as ordered.
    Monitor input and output very carefully.
  • Resume thyroid replacement medication if ordered preoperatively.
  • Begin patient teaching regarding the importance of cortisone replacement as soon as patient can absorb information.

• *Cerebrospinal fluid*

k. Recognize cerebrospinal fluid (CSF) leaks are more likely in patient whose dura has been torn and not repaired. Drainage may be clear or blood tinged.
  • Sites of leakage:
    Rhinorrhea—from nose (from anterior fossa)
    Otorrhea—from ear (from posterior fossa)
  • Institute nursing measures to include:
    Discourage patient from blowing nose.
    Do not suction or use IPPB unless order verified by physician.
    Confer with physician for head of bed elevation, patient position, and activity restrictions.
    Do not pack nostrils or ear.
    Collect CSF drainage in test tube for testing glucose content. Be aware that bloody CSF contains glucose.
    Change drip pad and record frequency of changes on I&O record.
    Assess degree of headache and provide analgesic and other comfort measures.
    Anticipate medical management which may include IV antibiotics and frequent lumbar punctures. Patients with severe leak may require continuous CSF drainage via lumbar drain.

• *Lobe dysfunction*

l. Be aware that lobe dysfunction may include one or more of the following depending on site and degree of damage. Deficits may be temporary or permanent. Nursing assessment should be directed toward signs related to involved lobe.
  • Frontal signs and symptoms:
    Hemiparesis/hemiplegia
    Contralateral central facial palsy (includes lack of ability to wrinkle forehead)
    Behavioral change: more likely in patients with bilateral frontal involvement *e.g.*, "frontal lobish"—flat and/or inappropriate effect
    Personality change, judgment impairment, loss of inhibitions
    Loss of voluntary bowel and bladder control
    Degree of expressive aphasia when dominant side involved (90 per cent of patients have left dominance)
    Motor seizures—usually focal facial
    Frontal release signs—emergence of primitive reflexes, *e.g.*, sucking, rooting
  • Parietal signs and symptoms:
    Difficulty with interpretation of sensory input
      Right—left confusion
      Denial of body part
      Tactile inattention
      Apraxia
      Agnosia

Patient Outcome	Process
	Sensory seizures, *e.g.*, onset of contralateral paresthesiae with or without progressive motor involvement
	Degree of receptive aphasia when dominant side involved.
	• Temporal signs and symptoms:
	Contralateral, homonymous hemianopia
	Personality change
	Loss of recent memory
	Psychomotor seizures with or without aura, *e.g.*, olfactory hallucinations
	Degree of receptive aphasia with dominant side involvement
	• Occipital signs and symptoms:
	Visual disturbances:
	Contralateral homonymous hemianopia
	Visual hallucinations
	Cortical blindness
• *Motor deficit*	m. Recognize that motor deficit is more likely in patient with frontal lobe or motor system dysfunction:
	• Deficit is contralateral to lesion, may be weakness (paresis) or paralysis (plegia).
	• Interventions to preserve and/or to restore function include:
	For all patients: Provide positioning, exercise program, use of supportive equipment, *e.g.*, footboard.
	For paresis: Provide active and passive range of motion exercise to strengthen muscles; may require cane or walker.
	For plegia: Maintain joint range of motion, possible use of sling to prevent shoulder subluxation.
	For spasticity (increased tone): Provide protective padding, passive exercise to point of joint tolerance.
• *Sensory deficit*	n. Recognize that sensory deficit is more likely with parietal lobe dysfunction:
	• Symptoms may not become obvious until patient begins activities of daily living.
	• Interventions include increasing patient's awareness of body part through visual contact, touching, verbal reminders. Consider occupational therapy consult.
• *Speech deficit*	o. Be aware that speech deficits (dysphasia) are usually seen in patients with left hemisphere (dominant) dysfunction with involvement of speech area.
	• Determine degree of dysfunction by checking verbal and written speech and patient's use of gestures. Deficit may include expressive and receptive components.
	• Interventions include:
	Recognize patient's frustration; be calm and unhurried.
	Get patient's attention; speak slowly, clearly. Use simple content and short phrases.
	Use and encourage patient's use of gestures.
	Minimize use of words; use pictures and/or alphabet board.
	Simplify environment.
	Obtain speech therapy consult. Arrange with speech therapist to schedule first evaluation when patient is rested and in quiet environment, *e.g.*, in morning, off ward.
• *Visual deficit*	p. Recognize that visual deficits may result when there is compression and/or damage to any portion of the visual pathway (optic nerve, chiasm, visual cortex).
	• Visual deficits are often unilateral.
	• Temporal hemianopia—loss of peripheral vision which may or may not be bilateral, "tunnel vision".
	Deficit occurs when lesion involves optic chiasm, *e.g*,, pituitary tumor.
	Consider safety in daily activities, especially driving—discuss restrictions with physician.
	• Homonymous hemianopia—loss of peripheral vision to one side, usually unilateral.
	Deficit is contralateral to lesion in optic tract, usually occurs in patients with lesions affecting optic tract, *i.e.*, parietal, temporal lobes.
	Approach patient in functioning field of vision.
	Teach patient to adapt by turning head to scan full visual field.
	• Diplopia—Double vision
	Usually occurs after head trauma; commonly occurs with sixth cranial nerve palsy; patient loses ability to look laterally.
	Patient tends to turn head toward the side of the sixth nerve lesion.

Patient Outcome	Process
	Suggest patching schedule.
	• Blindness—may be unilateral of bilateral.
	Often unilateral is a result of local trauma to optic nerve (second cranial nerve).
	Bilateral blindness results from damage to optic chiasm or lesions involving occipital lobe cortex.
	Check with physician to assure that this deficit has been explained to patient/family.
	Help patient's adaptation to blindness by simplifying environment and giving careful verbal cues, *e.g.*, announce arrival upon entering room, explain placement of food items in clock-like arrangement.
	Recognize appropriate behaviors of newly blind person may indicate feelings of denial, anger, or loss.
• *Common cranial nerve deficits*	q. Be aware that many cranial nerve deficits are permanent; however, some may resolve gradually over many months.
	• Anosmia—loss of smell (second cranial nerve—olfactory)
	Deficit may be consequence of head trauma, anterior fossa lesion, surgery for aneurysm.
	Check ability to smell and taste in patient likely to have this deficit.
	Check with physician if this deficit has been explained to patient/family.
	• Ptosis, opthalmoplegia—loss of ability to elevate eyelid, to rotate eyeball medially (third cranial nerve—oculomotor)
	Extent of "third nerve palsy" is determined by degree of compression on nerve.
	Opthalmoplegia—complete deficit of third nerve, includes ptosis, dilated fixed pupil and pupil deviated down and out. May occur with aneurysm of internal carotid artery, lesion of cavernosus sinus, herniation, diabetes mellitus.
	Inform patient of need for medical identification for this deficit, *e.g.*, bracelet.
	• Diplopia—double vision (sixth cranial nerve—abducens)
	Occurs with head trauma, increased intracranial pressure.
	Patch one eye and alternate eye patched at least daily.
	• Loss of corneal blink reflex (fifth cranial nerve—trigeminal)
	May occur with tumors of middle fossa, large acoustic neuromas, after open operative procedure for gasserian ganglion rhizotomy.
	Use opthalmic ointment and watch glass to prevent keratitis.
• *Pulmonary*	r. Promote adequate pulmonary function.
	• Be aware of acute need for adequate oxygenation following brain surgery. Potential complications in early postoperative period include:
	Anesthetic complications
	Apnea, laryngospasm, abnormal blood gases in postextubation period.
	Shallow respirations due to depressed LOC.
	• Identify patient who is at high risk for pulmonary complications and who also may be intubated for longer periods. Consider those with:
	Prolonged depressed LOC
	Chronic obstructive pulmonary disease
	History of heavy smoking
	Obesity
	Congestive heart failure.
	• Assess rate and depth of respirations; auscultate breath sounds bilaterally and compare. Usual frequency:
	Q 1 hour x 12 hour; then, q 4 hours until acute phase ended
	• Implement aggressive pulmonary management appropriate to patient situation to include:
	Patient who is extubated and able to participate:
	Turn, cough, and deep breathing exercises
	Humidity
	Percussion if congested
	IV/PO fluids
	Incentive spirometry
	Recognize degree of headache as related to patient participation in coughing.
	• Patient who is intubated and unable to participate: In addition to the above:
	Monitor frequent blood gases. Carry out proper care of patient with arterial line.

Patient Outcome	Process

If patient cannot maintain adequate perfusion and ventilatory rate (as evidenced by blood gases) mechanical support of ventilation may be indicated, *i.e.*, (PEEP), intermittent mandatory ventilation.

Be aware of incidence of O_2 toxicity in patients who are in high concentrations for prolonged intervals.

Daily chest radiographs as ordered
- Collaborate with physician for modifications needed in pulmonary regimen. Report changes noted in pulmonary status.
- Assess effectiveness of pulmonary regimen and change plan as needed.

- *Cardiovascular*

s. Promote adequate cardiovascular function.
- Identify patient at high risk for cardiovasuclar complications. Use cardiac monitor for at least 24 hours.

Previous cardiovascular disease, *e.g.*, congestive heart disease, myocardial infarction, phlebitis, pulmonary embolus, arteriosclerosis

Hypertension

Elderly

Obese

History of heavy smoking

Electrolyte disturbances

Patients receiving drugs affecting cardiovascular system
- Assess apical, radial pulse rate, rhythm, presence of peripheral pulses, color and skin temperature. Usual frequency:

Q 1 hour × 12 hours

Then q 4 hours until acute phase is ended.
- Call physician for change in cardiovascular status and for appropriate management.

- *Fluid/electrolyte balance*

t. Assist patient to maintain fluid and electrolyte balance.
- Monitor and record all intake and output to include IV fluids, ice chips, emesis and other drainage.
- Test specific gravity of urine q 1 hour or as ordered.
- Notify physician for any of the following:

Output less than 30cc per hour

Discrepancy between 24 per hour intake and output totals, *e.g.*, greater than 1000cc difference.

Abnormal blood chemistries, particularly sodium and potassium

Symptoms of diabetes insipidus:

Excessive output of 200cc per hour for two consecutive hours in the presence of specific gravity greater than or equal to 1.005

Extreme thirst
- Monitor IV therapy closely to include:

Volume and rate of infusion

Electrolyte content of solution and additives

Preserve and protect IV site(s)—may need to restrain or mitt patient.
- Avoid fluid overload. Be aware of these considerations:

Maximum fluid intake for first 72-hour period should be less than 2000cc per 24 hours.

Normal saline is usually contraindicated because of its relationship to brain swelling.

- *Bladder*

u. Assist patient to maintain bladder function.
- Consult physician to discontinue indwelling catheter as soon as possible.
- After catheter removal:

Monitor for volume and frequency of voiding. Compare with patient's intake and normal pattern.

Check residual urine if retention suspected.

Send specimen for analysis and culture and sensitivity if catheter in place for longer than 48 to 72 hours.
- Refer to Bladder care guideline, when there is deviation from normal bladder function p. 23 for patient who has problems voiding after catheter discontinued.

- *Nutrition*

v. Assist patient to achieve adequate nutritional status.
- Progress diet as tolerated after patient is alert.
- Identify patient likely to have poor nutrition. Examples are:

Preoperative nutritional problems, *e.g.*, alcoholic, elderly

Patient Outcome	Process
	Prolonged depressed level of consciousness Loss of gag reflex • Implement appropriate nutritional regimen: tube feedings, high protein feedings, supplemental vitamins, dietary consult.
• *Bowel*	w. Assist patient to maintain bowel function. • Identify patient who may have bowel function problems, *e.g.*, chronic constipation. • Implement appropriate bowel regimen.

F. *Achieves optimal level of activity*	7. Assist the patient to achieve optimal level of activity.
	 a. Formulate individualized daily activity plan in collaboration with patient, family, physician, and physical therapist. Consider the following components:
	 • Realistic progressive goals: sitting balance, standing, walking
	 • Timing, frequency, duration of activities
	 • Timing of analgesics with activity; intersperse rest periods
	 • Family's expectation of patient's resumption of function
	 • Deficits affecting patient's activity
	 • Environmental constraints, *e.g.*, indwelling lines, catheter.
	 b. Intervene for patient with deficit affecting patient's activity. Consider the following:
	 • Depressed level of consciousness:
	   Maximize patient's highest level of activity with timed periods of sensory stimulation. Provide reinforcement to patient/family.
	   Select sensory stimulation based on patient's interest, abilities, personality, *e.g.*, family pictures, radio, TV, conversations.
	   Consider sensory deprivation versus overload.
	   Determine if patient has disturbed sleep–wake cycle. Attempt to gradually reorient to normal cycle with lighting, information giving, pacing of activity and rest periods.
	   Provide patient with consistent reality orientation: time, date, place, person, explanation of noises, other sensations patient may be experiencing.
	 • Weakness
	   Establish extent and permanence of loss. Discuss with physician.
	   Carry out exercise program at least b.i.d.
	   Support limbs in functional position, *e.g.*, use sling for flaccid arm, use trochanter roll for rotation of leg, use foot support to prevent foot drop.
	   Assist patient to maximize capabilities, *e.g.*, place bed in room so that patient can use affected side, order finger foods to facilitate feeding self. Coordinate efforts with family and staff.
	   Arrange physical therapy consult as early as possible.
	 • Denial of body part
	   Reorient patient to body part. Talk about, have patient look at, recognize, move part.
	   Visual disturbances (field cuts, diplopia, blindness) and associated loss of balance.
	   Establish extent of deficit.
	   Field cuts:
	    Approach patient within functional field of vision.
	    Place bed in room to facilitate visual input.
	    Encourage scanning to increase field of vision as patient improves.
	   Diplopia:
	    Follow individualized plan for alternating eye patched.
	   Blindness:
	    Announce presence and identity when entering room.
	    Simplify number of items on meal tray, describe location of item using clock analogy.
	    Remove unnecessary obstacles in room.
	    Describe location of objects and do not rearrange without informing patient.
	    Encourage development of other senses (touch, hearing, smell, taste).
	    Interpret sounds, other sensations patient may be experiencing.
	   Loss of balance/impaired safety when ambulating.
	    Be aware that visual loss affects patient's balance and will make ambulation more difficult. Provide appropriate and safe assistance, *e.g.*, walker, assistance of another person.
	    Recognize fear and denial often accompanying new visual deficit.

161

Patient Outcome	Process
G. *Has knowledge and skills related to home care including resources for continuity of care*	8. Initiate and coordinate discharge planning.

8. Initiate and coordinate discharge planning.
   a. Collaborate with physician about tentative discharge date and medical plans.
   b. Determine where patient will be going after discharge, *e.g.,* home, rehabilitation unit, nursing home, local hospital; transportation needed to get there.
   c. Determine who will be consistent care giver and and responsible person (decision maker).
   d. Assess patient/family concerns about home care. Attempt to provide information about priority questions before giving general information.
   e. Plan and implement discharge program with patient/family including skills and knowledge to be learned. Check for accurate verbal feedback, and watch return demonstration of skills. Document what patient has learned and what needs further teaching. Components include:

   • *Scalp care*
   • Scalp care:
       Teach one of the following, as appropriate:
         If no head dressing or sutures: Demonstrate scalp washing; have patient/family assist.
         If no sutures, but head dressing is still needed and to be used at home:
           Give family date when dressing is to be removed. Describe how to remove it and to begin routine scalp care.
         If head dressing and sutures are in place, and dressing is not to be removed at home:
           Emphasize importance of keeping dressing dry and intact. Caution against placing fingers or foreign objects under edge of dressing.
           Reassure patient/family that some scalp itching and some fluid collection under scalp may be expected.
           Differentiate between fluid collection and swelling resulting from infection.
   • Head covering:
       Suggest form of head coverings that are attractive and provide comfort and ventilation, *e.g..* scarf, cap, wig with mesh lining.
       If large skull defect (especially in child), determine with physician if patient needs protective helmet.

   • *Activity*
   • Activity
       Assess patient/family response to perceived level of illness, then establish goals for home activity dependent upon any deficit, current level of activity, and independence and patient/family participation.
       Collaborate with physician and physical therapist to determine need for continuing physical therapy at home.
       Discuss safety in home environment, prevention of falls.
       Encourage gradual resumption of activity interspersed with rest preiods.
       Limit visitors during first two weeks of convalescence.
       No restrictions on resuming sexual activity.
       The following may not be resumed until approved by physician:
         Strenuous physical activities such as sports, housework, yardwork
         Return occupation   Driving or long trips

   • *Medication*
   • Medication:
       Assure that prescriptions have been written for all needed medications, especially anticonvulsants, antibiotics, steroids, pituitary replacements (cortisone, thyroid, androgens, estrogens), iron, previous medications for chronic health problems.
       Review medications with patient/family including purpose, dosage, frequency, side effects. Emphasize drugs that must be taken without fail.

   • *Diet*
   • Diet/alcoholic beverages:
       Encourage patient to eat well-balanced diet.
       Avoid alcoholic beverages until approved by physician.

   • *Illness*
   • Signs and symptoms to report to physician:
       Infection: drainage from suture, redness, tenderness, increased swelling.
       Severe headache   Seizures
       Nausea, vomiting   Check with physician for any others that need to be reported.

   • *Resources*
   • Appropriate home care needs/agencies.
       Determine if patient/family needs public health, social services or other referral and initiate accordingly.
       Equipment, *e.g.,* commode chair, cane, walker   Radiation therapy
       Speech therapy   Vocational counseling

   f. Write nursing discharge note to include the following:
   • Appearance of wound   • Patient outcomes met and unmet at discharge
   • Level of independent activity   • Plan for home care
   • Mode of travel when leaving ward   • Referrals made

Patient Outcome	Process

The patient experiences informed, comfortable, and safe preoperative, postoperative, and predischarge phases of hospitalization. This includes:

DESCRIPTION: Kidney donors are blood relatives of patients with end stage renal disease for whom transplantation is indicated. A donor can be a parent, sibling, or infrequently, a child (of age) and is considered to be in a normal state of health as documented by complete physical examination and diagnostic studies. There are no expected changes in status of renal function. Kidney, artery, vein and ureter are removed through a flank incision with resection of 11th or 12th rib and immediately perfused before transplanting into recipient.

NURSING ASSESSMENT: In addition to the general admission assessment, the following information is important.

1. Assess and document physical status.
    a. Blood pressure
    b. Signs and symptoms of any recent or present infection
    c. Risk factors:
        • Pulmonary status, smoking history

2. Assess and document patient's response to information about the proposed surgery.
    a. Apparent anxiety level
    b. Previous experience with surgery
    c. Expectations regarding outcome of transplantation to family member
    d. Patient's self-assessment of ability to cope with stressful experience
    e. Identify support persons, *i.e.,* spouse, chaplain.

3. Assess and document patient's understanding of anticipated surgery.

A. *Is prepared for surgery*

INTERVENTION:

1. Reinforce understanding of patient and his family regarding the surgical intervention, implications, and treatment.
Encourage patient to verbalize about surgery and acknowledge concerns. Listen and observe for misconceptions and for signs of anxiety. Call physician, chaplain, renal transplant nurse clinician as necessary.
    • Arrange discussion with another donor if possible.
    • Reinforce information given by renal transplant nurse clinician who routinely visits donor several times on days preceding surgery.
    • Help patient accept fact that some degree of threatened graft rejection is expected in recipient.

2. Summarize features of preoperative phase and provide care as needed per hospital routine and physician's orders. See Preoperative Phase of Hospitalization Chapter 5, p. 129.

3. Include additional elements of preoperative care due to nephrectomy.
    a. Prepare patient for specimen collection (blood and urine) and collect specimens as ordered:
        • Day 1 preoperative 12-hour urine specimen for routine chemical analysis
        • Day 2 preoperative urine culture and sensitivity
        • Day 3 preoperative urine 50 cc for cytology
    b. Explain need for Foley catheter and collection bag which are usually removed day after surgery, and include:
        • Immediate preoperative preparation in addition to usual care:
            Force fluids 8:00 p.m. to 12:00 midnight night prior to surgery up to 1500 to 2000 cc.
            Soap suds enema
            IV evening prior to surgery or early morning
            At 6:00 a.m. increase IV rate to run in 1500 cc within the next one to one and a half hours.

B. *Is free of or has minimal discomfort or postoperative complications*
• *Pulmonary*
• *Urinary*

4. Provide postoperative care. See Chapter 5 Postoperative Phase of Hospitalization, p. 130.

5. Intervene in the critical elements of patient care following donor nephrectomy.
    a. Maintain pulmonary status:
        • Frequent monitoring of respirations for rate, depth
        • Provide good pulmonary toilet.
    b. Maintain adequate intake and output:
        • Record intake and output.

Patient Outcome	Process
	• Regulate fluid intake as ordered. IV is removed when oral intake reaches 1500 cc per day.
	• Maintain good Foley catheter care and observe for urinary tract infection.
• *Body image*	c. Reinforce preoperative information concerning loss of kidney and ability to live a normal life.
	• Encourage patient to verbalize concerns about kidney recipient.
	• Reinforce information given by renal transplant nurse-clinician regarding recipient progress.
	• Assist patient to visit recipient when both are physically able.
C. *Is knowledgeable about self-care and resources for continuity of care*	6. See Chapter 5 Predischarge Phase of Hospitalization, p. 132. Include additional essential elements of preparation for discharge.
	a. Instruct patient to report any symptoms of wound or urinary infection to physician.
	b. Instruct patient it is normal to continue to feel some slight incisional discomfort for several weeks.
	c. Give return appointment in six weeks.

Facelift with blepharoplasty, dermabrasion

Patient Outcome	Process

The patient experiences informed, comfortable, and safe preoperative, postoperative, and predischarge phases of hospitalization. This includes:

DESCRIPTION: Surgical facelift is the excision and removal of excess skin and superficial subcutaneous tissue in the forehead, cheek, and neck. Incisions are made in the scalp near the hair line and anterior and posterior to the ear. Blepharoplasty is the removal of excess skin and fat pockets in the upper and lower eyelids. Dermabrasion is a technique of sanding superficial skin to smooth surface irregularities.

NURSING ASSESSMENT: In addition to the general admission assessment, the following information is especially important.

1. Assess and document patient's response to information about the anticipated surgery.
   a. Apparent anxiety level
   b. Previous experience with surgery
   c. Patient's self-assessment of:
      • Expectation of final results when weighed in light of immediate postoperative appearance
      • Support people, *i.e.,* spouse, friend. Often patient comes alone or only one person knows of hospitalization at patient's request.
2. Assess and document patient's understanding of anticipated surgery.

A. *Is prepared for surgery*

INTERVENTION:

1. Reinforce understanding of patient and family regarding the treatment and implications of face lifts.
2. Summarize usual postoperative expectations with patient and family. These include:
   a. Local or general anesthesia; immediate return to ward from operating room
   b. Bulky head dressings for 5 to 7 days
   c. Eye patches for several hours
   d. Bruises and swelling about eyes and face
   e. Drainage system may be used in posterior neck involvement.
3. Summarize features of preoperative care. See Chapter 5 Preoperative Phase of Hospitalization, p. 129.
4. Provide postoperative care. See Chapter 5 Postoperative Phase of Hospitalization, p. 130.

B. *Is free of or has minimal discomfort or postoperative complications*

• *Safety*

• *Wound healing*

5. Intervene in the critical elements of patient care following a face lift with blepharoplasty or dermabrasion.
   a. Provide total nursing care until patient has eye patches removed and vision is adequate for patient to safely resume own care.
   b. Place items for patient's safe use such as: bell cord, side rails, personal items, drinking cup.
   c. Observe for and respond to signs and symptoms of extreme swelling and bruising.
      • Check that dressing is loose enough to permit a finger under edge.
      • Explain to patient that tightness is due to stretching of skin over tissue which is now swollen.
      • Give iced saline compresses for comfort after eye patches are removed.
      • Obtain order for protective eye drops for patients unable to blink eye due to swelling.
   d. Apply wound dryer for 15 minutes, q 4 hours, first day; then p.r.n. until dry when dressing removed from dermabrasion.

• *Comfort*

   e. Plan comfort measures with patient such as:
      • Diet soft enough for patient to eat without difficulty in chewing
      • Obtain permission from physician for shampoo after head dressing removed.
   f. Help patient cope with immediate appearance. Reinforce fact that swelling and bruising will decrease very gradually.

C. *Is knowledgeable about self-care and resources for continuity of care*

6. See Chapter 5 Predischarge Phase of Hospitalization, p. 132. Include additional essential elements of preparation for discharge such as:
   Clarify with patient and family any special details due to surgical procedure such as:
      • No restrictions in activity
      • Sutures to be removed gradually within a month after surgery
      • May give usual hair and skin care except check with physician about skin preparations, *e.g.,* sun screen, cosmetics, moisturizer.

Patient Outcome	Process
The patient functions comfortably within limitations due to gastrointestinal hemorrhage. This includes:	**DESCRIPTION:** Acute, massive gastrointestinal hemorrhage commonly occurs from one or more upper or lower tract sites. Massive hemorrhage may occur in:

DESCRIPTION: Acute, massive gastrointestinal hemorrhage commonly occurs from one or more upper or lower tract sites. Massive hemorrhage may occur in:
(1) Esophageal varices (due to portal hypertension secondary to liver disease)
(2) Gastric ulcer (due to loss of tissue in an area that is in contact with hydrochloric acid—most often in the duodenum, esophagus, and stomach. The lack of resistance to the acid may be related to physical and/or emotional stress, fatigue, drugs such as steroids.)
(3) Gastritis
(4) Advanced carcinoma
(5) Diverticulitis
(6) Ulcerative colitis
(7) Hemorrhoids

NURSING ASSESSMENT: In addition to the general admission assessment, the following information is especially important.
1. Assess and document signs and symptoms of shock throughout acute bleeding phase.
   a. Rapid, thready pulse
   b. Lowered blood pressure and central venous pressure
   c. Increased respirations
   d. Decreased urinary output
   e. Skin cool, diaphoresis
   f. Restlessness, anxiety
   g. Decrease in hematocrit
   h. Abdominal symptoms, *e.g.,* cramping, nausea, vomiting

A. *Is achieving control of life-threatening hemorrhage*

2. Assess and document location and extent of blood loss.
   a. Measure and record amount and character of vomitus, wound drainage, nasogastric drainage, and rectal drainage.
   b. Note characteristics of bloody drainage relating to its origin, *i.e.,* bright, brisk bleeding from arterial sites; darker red with clots from venous sites; bright red vomitus from upper gastrointestinal tract; dark, coffee ground vomitus and tarry stools from lower gastrointestinal tract.

INTERVENTION:
1. Intervene to stablize the patient who is massively bleeding.
   a. Assist/start large bore IV lines (central and/or peripheral)
   b. Begin infusion of volume expanders such as saline, plasma protein fraction and/or blood when available.
   c. Assist/draw baseline blood studies: Type and cross match, chemistries, coagulation studies.
   d. Assist/insert large bore nasogastric tube—may need 24 to 28 French tube for aspiration of large clots.
   e. Perform iced saline lavage for active bleeding.
   f. Insert indwelling catheter for urine monitoring.
   g. Request as ordered:
      • Chest radiograph to check for aspiration
      • EKG (hypotension may cause painless myocardial infarction)
   h. Assess continuously hemodynamic status, *i.e.,* vital signs, serial hematocrits, blood loss.
2. Provide general care measures.
   a. Prevent aspiration of gastric contents by frequent suction, proper position, and adequate drainage of gastric contents.
   b. Keep n.p.o.
   c. Continue monitoring vital signs and assessing further bleeding.
   d. Administer medications as ordered such as vitamin K, antacids, laxatives (lactulose), sedatives.
   e. Provide supportive nursing measures, including careful attention to skin and mouth.
   f. Observe respiratory status continuously. Note the effect of abdominal distention, nasogastric tube, vascular studies, and blood administration.
   g. Provide comfortable and quiet environment.
3. Provide emotional support for patient/family. Be aware that:
   a. The patient who is actively bleeding and receiving acute treatment is extremely anxious and frightened and in need of close personal contact and reassurance.
   b. The family's response can favorably or unfavorably influence the patient's progress depending on anxiety level. Provide careful explanation of patient's cares and response to therapy and listen to concerns.

Patient Outcome	Process

B. *Is prepared for and experiences safe and comfortable diagnostic studies*	4. Explain/answer questions and listen to concerns about diagnostic studies and care. See Chapter 3 Guidelines for the patient undergoing diagnostic studies p. 33. Possible studies include:
	  a. Esophagoscopy and gastroscopy
	  b. Femoral arteriogram
	  c. Hepatitis associated antigen
	5. Provide preparation for study and postprocedure care as indicated.
	  • In order to assess continuously and to intervene as needed, accompany patient to Radiology Department.

C. *Is prepared for and experiences no/minimal complications or discomfort from modes of treatment*
 	
• *Sengstaken-Blakemore tube*
	6. Prepare patient, assist during insertion, provide continuous surveillance and postprocedure care for the patient requiring Sengstaken-Blakemore tube for control of esophageal hemorrhage. (Fig. 5-7.)
	  a. Reinforce physician's explanation of treatment.
	  b. Prevent complications, *e.g.,* aspiration, occlusion of airway, mucosal erosion, displacement of tube.
	    • Suction frequently.
	    • Elevate head of bed 30° unless contraindicated.
	    • Maintain desired air pressure and traction of esophageal and gastric balloons.
	    • Label the lumen of each balloon.
	    • Provide emergency measures if gastric balloon deflates:
	      Keep scissors at bedside.
	      Cut tube or deflate esophageal balloon to prevent asphyxiation.
	    • Remain aware that patient cannot swallow with tube in place.
	    • Maintain function of gastric lumen of tube.
	  c. Keep n.p.o. No ice chips.

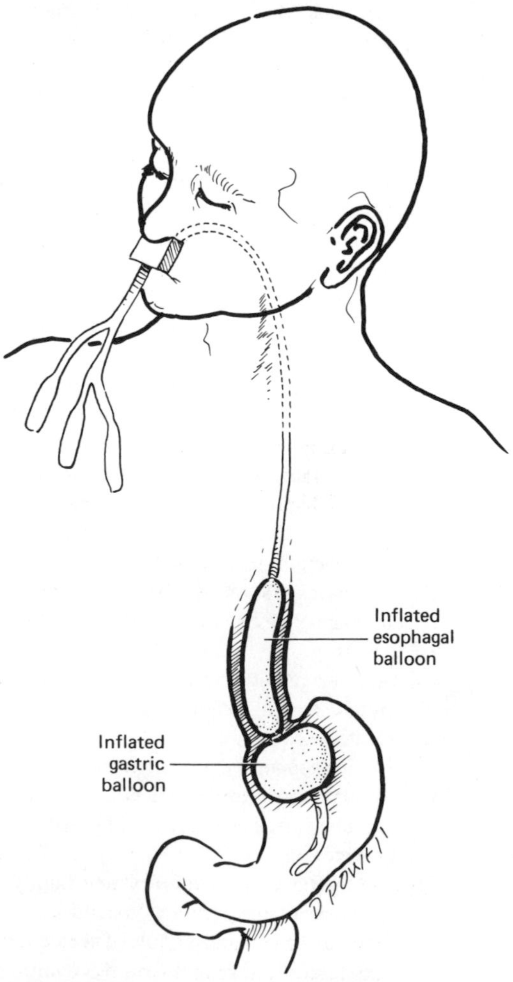

Fig. 5-7.   Sengstaken-Blakemore Tube.

Patient Outcome	Process

• *Pitressin infusion*	7. Provide care for patient receiving arterial vasopressin (Pitressin) infusion.
	   a. Check for history of coronary artery disease vasopressin (Pitressin) contraindicated.
	   b. Check for signed consent for procedure per hospital policy.
	   c. Reinforce physician's explanation of treatment.
	   d. Accompany patient to Vascular Radiology for catheter placement. Continue to provide treatment and support.
	   e. Begin prescribed vasopressin (Pitressin) infusion using intravenous infusion pump (not controller). A usual rate is 0.4 units per minute. This rate may be increased to 0.8 units per minute per physician's order.
	   f. Observe for side effects of vasopressin (Pitressin) and report to physician:
	     • Facial pallor • Arterial emboli to legs
	     • Abdominal discomfort • Oliguria and hyponatremia
	     • Sudden bowel evacuation • Aggravation of hepatic encephalopathy
	     • Hypertension with reflex bradycardia • Cardiac arrhythmias
	   g. Notify physician if bleeding does not decrease.
	   h. Maintain adequate fluid volume to minimize chances of renal impairment.
	   i. Assess circulation in extremity with catheter. Refer to Chapter 3 p. 38 for specific guidelines for the patient who has an arteriogram.
	   j. Provide catheter insertion site care daily using povidone-iodine.
	   k. Prevent hip flexion of affected site.
	   l. Monitor electrolyte balance, intake and output. Provide replacement as indicated.

• *Artificial clotting therapy*	8. Provide care for patient receiving artificial clotting therapy (Gelfoam).
	   a. Reinforce physician's explanation of treatment.
	   b. Accompany patient to Vascular Radiology. Continue to provide treatment and support during insertion of clot into bleeding artery.
	   c. Notify physician if further evidence of bleeding is observed.

D. *Is prepared for surgery*	9. Provide care for patient requiring surgical intervention. Summarize usual preoperative preparation and provide care as needed per hospital routine and physician's orders. See Chapter 5 Preoperative Phase of Hospitalization, p. 129.

E. *Is free of or has minimal discomforts or postoperative complications*	10. Provide postoperative care. See Chapter 5 Postoperative Phase of Hospitalization, p. 130.
	11. Intervene in the critical elements of patient care following surgery. Emphasize the following:
	   a. Continue assessment for bleeding:
	     • Monitor all vital signs parameters q 15 minutes until stable, then hourly.
	     • Measure all output, *i.e.,* urine, drainage from rectum, wounds and nasogastric tube.
	     • Monitor results of clotting factor studies and hematocrit.
	   b. Maintain fluid and electrolyte balance.
	     • Transfuse blood, blood products as ordered. Observe for untoward reaction.
	     • Maintain fluid replacement volume as indicated.
	     • Monitor results of electrolyte determinations.
	   c. Maintain nutritional status.
	     • Assess bowel sounds.
	     • Begin 30 cc hourly clear liquids with or without carbonation and progress to amounts as tolerated. Advance to full liquids to soft diet with frequent feedings as indicated.
	     • Determine caloric intake.
	     • Weigh daily.
	     • Modify diet according to patient's underlying disease state.
	     • Give diet supplements as indicated.

F. *Is knowledgeable about nature of illness, self-care, and resources for continuity of care*	12. See Chapter 5 Predischarge Phase of Hospitalization, p. 132. Include additional elements of preparation for discharge.
	   a. Reinforce physician's explanations and instructions.
	   b. Promote patient/family's understanding of preventive care:
	     • Avoidance of smoking; alcohol; excessive caffeine intake; irritating drugs such as salicylates; and foods which cause distress.
	     • Sufficient rest and sleep
	     • Medical assistance for any illness including return of symptoms of gastrointestinal bleeding
	     • Avoidance of undue stress and tension
	     • Maintenance of prescribed nutritional and medication regimen
	   c. Inform patient and family of community resources which may assist in continuity of care, *e.g.,* alcoholic rehabilitation centers.
	   d. Initiate interagency referral as appropriate.

Patient Outcome	Process

The patient experiences informed, comfortable, and safe preoperative, postoperative, and predischarge phases of hospitalization. This includes:

DESCRIPTION: Gynecological surgery involves procedures performed for evaluation and/or therapy for alteration of the female reproductive system. This surgery is performed for malignant and nonmalignant processes. Some of the most common surgical procedures include:

Vaginal hysterectomy: Removal of uterus through the vagina

Abdominal hysterectomy:
1. Routine—removal of the uterus through an abdominal incision
2. Radical—Panhysterectomy with wide excision of parametric tissue including removal of a wide vaginal cuff

Salpingo-oophorectomy, bilateral or unilateral: Removal of fallopian tube(s) and ovary(ies) either vaginally (colpotomy) or abdominally

Dilatation and Curettage; Dilatation of the cervix and scrapping or suctioning the contents of the uterus

Conization: Cone-shaped incision of cervical tissue for evaluation

Tubal sterilization (cauterization or ligation): Either burning or cutting the fallopian tubes for sterilization purposes, this procedure may be done through laparoscopy, laparotomy, colpotomy.

Vulvectomy:
1. Simple: Surgical excision of the vulva with a wide margin of skin
2. Radical: Tissue is excised from the anus to a few centimeters above the symphysis pubis. The inguinal and iliac nodes may be resected also. The extent of surgery varies with the location and size of the lesion and the condition of adjacent skin.

Laparoscopy: Insertion of lighted tube through a small abdominal incision

Laparotomy: (See Laparotomy Guideline, p. 179)

Pelvic Exenteration: (See Pelvic Exenteration Guideline, p. 199)

NURSING ASSESSMENT: In addition to the general admission assessment, the following information is especially important.
1. Assess and document physical status.
   a. Signs and symptoms of advanced stage of cancer
   b. Special problems which may affect status for surgery and/or recovery, *e.g.,* diabetes, obesity, anemia
   c. Other problems/disabilities, *e.g.,* fractures
2. Assess and document patient's response to information about the disease process, treatment, and anticipated surgery.
   a. Diagnostic and/or status evaluation
   b. Reasons for studies/surgery
   c. Patient's self-assessment of:
      • Personal strengths in coping with stresses, previous crises
      • Support people, *e.g.,* family, chaplain
3. Assess and document life-style including:
   a. Physical demands, *e.g.,* homemaking, occupation, recreational activities
   b. Position in family unit, *i.e.,* marital status, children
4. Assess and document patient's understanding of the disease process, treatment, and anticipated surgery.

A. Is prepared for surgery and possible body image change

INTERVENTION:
1. Reinforce understanding of patient and family regarding the disease process, implications and treatment.
2. Summarize usual preoperative preparation and provide care per hospital routine and physician's orders. See Chapter 5 Preoperative Phase of Hospitalization, p. 129.
   Emphasize specific postoperative expectations:
      • Abdominal and/or perineal dressing
      • Foley catheter for several days
      • Possible closed-wound drainage system
      • Possible vaginal packing with some kinds of surgery
      • IV fluids and n.p.o. Duration will vary with kind of surgery and individual postoperative progress.
      • Pad count with special attention to drainage, color, odor, and amount
3. Provide assistance to patient coping with altered body image.
4. Provide postoperative care. See Chapter 5 Postoperative Phase of Hospitalization, p. 130.
5. Intervene in the critical elements of care following gynecological surgery.
   a. Observe for signs and symptoms of cuff abscess and report to physician.
      • Elevation in temperature

B. Is free of or has minimal discomfort or postoperative complications

Patient Outcome	Process
	• Increase of lower abdominal pain
	• Color, odor, and consistency of vaginal discharge
• *Urinary*	b. Minimize chance of urinary tract infections. See Chapter 2 Bladder Care Guideline When There is Deviation From Normal Bladder Function, p. 23, Key points include:
	• Fluids—2500 cc unless contraindicated
	• Sterile catheterization and maintenance
	• Position catheter at least 1 foot below bladder at all times
	• Request removal of catheter as soon as possible.
	• Use techniques to initiate independent voiding.
	• Voiding schedule q 2 to 4 hours during waking hours
	• Perineal care
• *Respiratory*	c. Provide good pulmonary toilet.
	• Turn, cough, and deep breathe every 2 hours $\times$ 12 times or while immobilized
	• Incentive spirometry after first 24 hours
	• Ambulate q.i.d. starting first postoperative day (exception: vulvectomy).
	• Discourage smoking.
• *Circulatory*	d. Minimize chance of clot formation.
	• Antiembolic stockings
	• Elevate feet while sitting.
	• Ambulate 4 times a day: possible exception vulvectomy patient.
	• Observe for symptoms of swelling, heat, redness, pain in lower extremities; notify physician as necessary.
	• Encourage leg exercises.
• *Gastrointestinal*	e. Provide good bowel care: Refer to Chapter 2 Bowel Care Guideline, When There is Deviation From Normal Bowel Function, p. 25.
	• Encourage patient to drink hot liquids, ambulate.
	• Assess need for laxative, stool softener, rectal tube, or enema; request order from physician if indicated:
	f. Provide for special needs of patient if receiving chemotherapy/radiotherapy.
	• Prepare patient for therapy. See Chapter 4 Choriocarcinoma Guideline, p. 87.
	• Relieve mouth soreness.
	Give soft foods and nonacid food and drinks.
	Secure anesthetizing preparations to reduce soreness.
	• Intervene to relieve nausea.
	Administer antiemetrics as ordered.
	Give fluids as tolerated.
C. *Is able to cope wtith surgical alterations and life-threatening disease (oncology patient)*	g. Support patient's ability to cope with surgery and prognosis.
	• Assess support systems of patient/family: strengths and weakness, previous patterns of coping.
	• Employ "active listening" using verbal and behavioral clues indicating patient/family concerns.
	• Observe and document appetite and sleep patterns. Provide instruction, assistance, and comfort measures.
	• Supply verbal and written information suited to the patient's current capacity to understand.
	• Help patient accept self/body by demonstrating acceptance. Be kind but honest in preparing patient for change in body image and functioning.
	• Collaborate with physician, chaplain, oncology clinician and others in support of patient's emotional status.
D. *Is knowledgeable about nature of illness, self-care, and resources for continuity of care*	6. Chapter 5 Predischarge Phase of Hospitalization, p. 132. Include additional essential elements of preparation for discharge such as
	a. Teach and reinforce understanding of the care of the surgical wound, resumption of physical and sexual activities, and any dietary modifications.
	b. Provide needed dressings and medication and explain how a supply of these can be obtained.
	c. Clarify any written instructions and return appointment.
	d. Explain services and availability of public health nurse.
	e. Assist patient to obtain services as needed for continuity of care.

Patient Outcome

The patient experiences informed, comfortable, and safe preoperative, postoperative, and predischarge phases of hospitalization. This includes:

DESCRIPTION: An ileal conduit is the construction of a permanent urinary diversion using a 6 to 7 inch segment of ileum selected close to the junction of the small and large bowl. The ileum is resected without being disconnected from the mesentery, which supplies its blood.

The small bowel ends from which the segment is taken are anastomosed to re-establish normal bowel function. One end of the ileal segment is closed with sutures and attached to the peritoneum to avoid herniation. The other end of the ileal segment is everted and sutured to the skin to form the stoma. The ureters are anastomosed to the ileal segment and peristalsis propels the urine through the stoma. (Fig.5-8)

If the surgery is performed because of carcinoma, it may be done in combination with another surgical procedure.

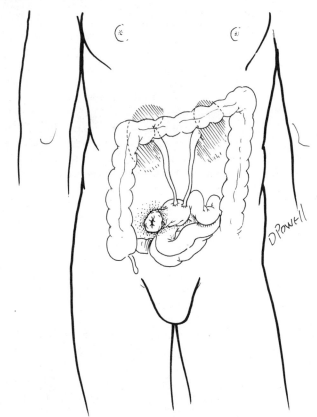

Fig. 5-8.   Ileal conduit.

NURSING ASSESSMENT: In addition to general admission assessment, the following information is important.

1. Assess and document physical status.
   a. Symptoms relating to underlying disease:
      • Pain: location, character, duration, effectiveness of relief measures
      • Current method of urinary drainage
      • Abdominal skin condition
      • Presence of urinary tract infection
   b. Risk factors:
      • Neurological status, *i.e.,* deficits
      • Previous radiation therapy
2. Assess and document patient's response to information about the disease process, treatment, and anticipated surgery.
   a. Apparent anxiety level
   b. Previous experience with surgery
3. Assess and document health habits prior to admission.
   a. Potential for self-care or need for supportive care
   b. Home health supervision/support
4. Assess and document patient's understanding of the disease process, treatment, and anticipated surgery.

Patient Outcome	Process

A. *Is prepared for surgery and body image change*	**INTERVENTION:**
	1. Reinforce understanding of patient and family regarding the disease process, implications, and treatment.
	2. Plan with patient and physician the placement of stoma considering skin folds, scars, appliance, usual activity, clothing. Mark chosen site on skin clearly.
	3. Provide assistance in coping with future altered body function and image.
	   a. Be alert to expression of feelings about stoma and handling of urinary excretion.
	   b. Contact support persons, *i.e.,* clinician, chaplain.
	4. Summarize features of preoperative preparation and provide care as needed per hospital routine and physician's orders. See Chapter 5 Preoperative Phase of Hospitalization, p. 129. Include additional explanations and needs
	   a. Need for urine drainage bag to stoma.
	   b. Need for Foley indwelling catheter and nasogastric drainage.

B. *Is free of or has minimal discomfort or postoperative complications*
 	
• *Wound healing*
	5. Provide postoperative care. See Chapter 5 Postoperative Phase of Hospitalization, p. 130.
	6. Intervene in the critical areas of patient care following ileal conduit procedure.
	   a. Check drainage bag for stoma bleeding when checking urine output.
	     • Q 1 hour progressed to 2 to 4 hours.
	     • First 8 hours expect 0 to minimal amount of blood-tinged drainage from stoma.
	     • If any blood-tinged urine comes from ureteral stent, notify physician.
	   b. Check for adequate stomal circulation q 8 hours; document signs of poor circulation.
	     • Use clear plastic bag for visibility.
	     • Check bag for proper fit allowing 1/16 to 1/8-inch space to permit free circulation around stoma.
	     • The stoma should be red and is usually edematous. Be alert to ischemic areas.
	   c. Observe skin during each bag change; document signs of skin deterioration.
	   d. Apply bag properly. See Colostomy, Ileostomy, Abdominoperineal Resection Guidelines, p. 149.
	   e. Assess for signs and symptoms of small bowel obstruction: nausea, vomiting, abdominal distention and absent bowel sounds. Cease feeding patient and notify physician.
	   f. Assess for signs and symptoms of pelvic abscess: Fever 38.5° C, pelvic pain, tenderness. Notify physician.

C. *Is knowledgeable about nature of illness, self care and resources for continuity of care*	7. Chapter 5, Predischarge Phase of Hospitalization, p. 132.
	8. Include additional essential elements of preparation for discharge of patient such as:
	   a. Assess the acceptance by the patient and his family of the changes in body function and self-image, the colostomy and its care.
	   b. Discuss personal and social adjustment such as:
	     • Odor control
	     • Clothing
	     • Sexual adjustment (confer with physician for patient concerns about impotence)
	     • Colostomy Club.
	   c. Reinforce self-care activities emphasizing:
	     • Skin care around stoma
	     • Bag application
	     • Connection to night drainage system
	     • Wound care
	     • Diet modification as ordered
	   d. Discuss functions of public health nurse and assist patient and family to secure services if needed.

Patient Outcome

The patient experiences informed, comfortable, and safe preoperative, postoperative, and predischarge phases of hospitalization. This includes:

Process

DESCRIPTION: Jejuno-ileal bypass surgery is performed for extreme obesity. By bypassing a major portion of the small intestine, absorption of calories is decreased resulting in weight loss. Patients are carefully screened and some may by rejected for the surgery. The abdomen is entered through a transverse buckethandle incision, and the jejunum is resected 8 to 12 inches from the ligament of Treitz and the ileum is resected 2 to 4 inches from the ileoceal valve. The two ends are joined (jejuno-ileal anastomosis) leaving approximately 20 feet of bypassed bowel. The remaining ileal segment end of the jejunum is closed. (Fig. 5-9.) This permits drainage of the excluded segment and reconnection of the bypassed bowel if necessary.

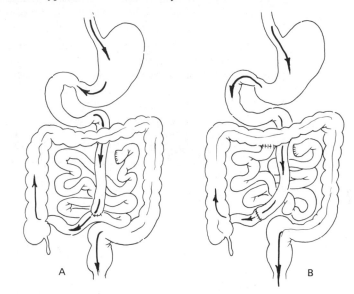

Fig. 5-9. Jejuno-ileal bypass.

NURSING ASSESSMENT: In addition to general admission assessment, the following information is especially important.
1. Assess and document physical status:
   a. Information relating to obesity:
      • Current weight
      • Skin condition, particularly around skin folds
   b. Risk factors/disease states including those resulting from obesity:
      • Pulmonary status, *i.e.,* shortness of breath, smoking, Pickwickian syndrome
      • Cardiovascular status, *i.e.,* hypertension, symptoms of cardiac disease, edema
      • Presence of other disease states including diabetes
2. Assess and document patient's response to information about disease process and anticipated surgery:
   a. Apparent anxiety level
   b. Previous experience with surgery
   c. Understanding of postoperative expectations such as weight loss, side effects, *e.g.,* diarrhea; and risks, *e.g.,* infection.
3. Assess and document patient's understanding of disease process, treatment, and anticipated surgery.
4. Assess and document health habits prior to admission:
   a. Potential for self-care or need for supportive care including the ability:
      • To reach perineal area for cleaning
      • To move self in bed
      • To wear hospital gown and use hospital chairs
   b. Nutritional history
   c. Home health supervision/support
   d. Psychological stability

A. *Is prepared for surgery*

INTERVENTION:
1. Plan for patient's general care needs.
   a. Provide for hygiene needs.
   b. Obtain suitable chair.
   c. Use personal clothing if hospital gown does not fit.

Patient Outcome	Process
	2. Institute preparation for diagnostic studies. See Chapter 3 Guidelines for the Patient Undergoing Diagnostic Studies p. 35. Studies may include: a. Barium enema b. Upper GI series and small bowel follow-through c. Blood studies d. Oral cholecystogram e. Psychological evaluation
	3. Reinforce physician's explanation about surgical procedure and postoperative effects. • Stress that postoperative diarrhea is a common occurrence and will be treated with medications and diet.
	4. Prepare patient for postoperative expectations, including: a. Pulmonary routines • Collaborate with physician for physical therapy evaluation and instruction. • Instruct patient in coughing, deep breathing and using incentive spirometry exercises. Observe return demonstrations. b. Leg exercises, maintenance of activity • Patients are high risk for thrombophlebitis leading to pulmonary embolus. • Encourage ambulation. • Instruct in leg exercises and observe return demonstrations. c. Diet resumption • Patient will be started on clear liquid diet when bowel activity returns (3 to 7 days). • Diet will be advanced per physician's orders. • Restrictions may include: fluid limit, low flat, high protein, low calories. d. Hygiene • Stress that patient should feel free to ask for assistance in maintaining good body cleanliness.
	5. Collaborate with physician to obtain preoperative order for fitting of abdominal binder. Explain purpose to patient. Send with patient to operating room.
	6. Summarize usual features of preoperative preparation and provide care per hospital routine and physician's order. See Chapter 5 Preoperative Phase of Hospitalization, p. 129.
B. *Is free of or has minimal discomfort or postoperative complications* • *Pulmonary*	7. Provide postoperative care. See Chapter 5 Postoperative Phase of Hospitalization, p. 130. 8. Intervene in the critical areas of patient's care following surgery. a. Stress preventive measures to avoid pulmonary complications. • Position patient with head of bed elevated at 30° angle. Do not allow patient to slide down in bed. Raise foot of bed for elevation of feet. Avoid jackknife position. • Encourage patient to deep breathe and cough each hour: support incision with pillow or folded towel. • Turn patient side to side q 2 hours. • Obtain postoperative order for physical therapy follow-up. • Encourage early ambulation as ordered.

• *Gastrointestinal*	b. Maintain fluid/electrolyte/nutritional status.
	• Accurate record of I and O—including:
	    Nasogastric drainage
	    Diarrhea—number of stools per day.
	• Monitor serum electrolytes.
	• When patient is started on oral fluids, they may be restricted. Explain rationale, amount of restriction, and measurement procedure.
	• Diet ordered per physician—have dietician explain any dietary restrictions.
	c. Control diarrhea to 3 to 5 stools per day.
	• Administer diphenoxylate (Lomotil) as ordered. Explain mechanism of action and side effects to patient.
	• Explain other methods of control to patient, *i.e.,* low fluid intake, avoidance of food causing diarrhea.

• *Circulatory*	d. Inspect lower extremities for symptoms of thrombophlebitis.
	• Encourage leg exercises q 4 hours while in bed.
	• Encourage early ambulation when allowed.
	• Position patient to maximize blood return, and decrease venous stasis.
	    Raise foot of bed to elevate feet.
	    Don't allow legs to hang in dependent position.

Patient Outcome	Process
	e. Inspect and document wound status. • Report signs of infection/eviseration/bleeding. • Keep binder on patient at all times, if ordered.
C. *Is realistic regarding postoperative course and weight loss*	9. Assess patient's understanding and reinforce information when necessary. Expectations are: a. Weight loss approximates 100 pounds first year after surgery; then stabilizes. b. Alterations in taste and food preferences are normal. c. Need for continuation of diet. d. Malaise for a period of time after surgery. e. Diarrhea may continue over a period of time but should decrease.

D. *Is knowledgeable about self-care and resources for continuity of care*	10. See Chapter 5 Predischarge Phase of Hospitalization, p. 132. Include additional essential elements of preparation for discharge of patient. These include:
	a. Teach dietary modifications:
	 • Collaborate with physician concerning diet.
	 • Explain rationale for special diet to patient and indicate usual restrictions, *i.e.,* calorie, liquids, fat and need for protein.
	 • Consult dietician for patient/family instruction. It is important to include the person responsible for cooking in the patient's home.
	 • Stress foods to avoid, *i.e.,* fruit juices, milk, fatty foods if they cause diarrhea; also avoid overeating.
	 • Discourage excessive use of alcoholic beverages (may contribute to liver changes/damages).
	b. Teach regarding prescribed medications.
	 • Diphenoxylate (Lomotil)—instruct patient when to take and possible side effects.
	 • Potassium—may be necessary depending on serum potassium levels; instruct patient regarding symptoms of low potassium:
	  Weakness
	  ''Skipped'' heart beats
	  Confusion
	  Lethargy
	  Nausea
	  Diarrhea
	c. Plan resumption of activity with patient.
	 • Anticipate malaise at first.
	 • Gradually resume work activity—advisable to begin with part-time activity.
	 • Avoid lifting heavy objects.
	d. Plan for follow-up care with patient.
	 • Stress importance of follow-up visits as scheduled.
	 • Remain aware that postoperative problems may involve electrolyte imbalance, especially potassium, and vitamin deficiencies.

Laparotomy

Patient Outcome	Process

The patient experiences informed, comfortable, and safe preoperative, postoperative, and predischarge phases of hospitalization. This includes:

DESCRIPTION: Exploratory laparotomy may be performed for a wide variety of reasons, *i.e.,* staging of a cancer, bowel perforation, diagnosis for cause and treatment of bleeding, peritonitis. The following guidelines are written for general care of patients undergoing abdominal laparotomies for any reason. Refer to guidelines for specific procedures, *e.g.,* jejuno-ileal bypass, abdominal aortic aneurysm, colostomy, ileostomy.

NURSING ASSESSMENT: In addition to general admission assessment, the following information is especially important.

1. Assess and document physical status.
   a. Symptoms related to underlying disease process:
      • Pain—location, character, duration and effectiveness of pain relief measures.
      • GI symptoms—nausea and vomiting, gastrointestinal bleeding, loss of appetite, diarrhea, constipation
      • Stool character, weight change, assessment of abdomen, *i.e.,* size, shape, presence of distention, organ enlargement, masses
      • Fever
   b. Risk factors:
      • Pulmonary status, *e.g.,* smoking history, abnormal breath sounds, chronic obstrusive pulmonary disease, shortness of breath
      • Cardiovascular status, *e.g.,* hypertension, symptoms of cardiac disease, edema
      • Presence of other disease states, e.g., diabetes.
2. Assess and document patient's response to information about the disease process, treatment, and anticipated surgery:
   a. Apparent anxiety level
   b. Previous experience with surgery
   c. Understanding of postoperative expectations
3. Assess and document health habits prior to admission:
   a. Potential for self-care or need for supportive care
   b. Nutritional history
   c. Medications—especially those relating to underlying disease process, *e.g.,* laxatives, antacids, chemotherapy
   d. Home health supervision/support
4. Assess and document patient's understanding of the disease process, treatment, and anticipated surgery.

A. *Is prepared for surgery*

INTERVENTION;
1. Reinforce understanding of patient and family regarding the disease process, implications, and treatment.
2. Summarize features of preoperative phase and provide care as needed per physician's orders and hospital routine. See Chapter 5 Preoperative Phase of Hospitalization, p. 129.

B. *Is free of or has minimal discomfort and postoperative complications*

3. Provide postoperative care. See Chapter 5 Postoperative Phase of Hospitalization, p. 130.
4. Intervene in the critical areas of patient care following laparotomy. These include:
   a. Be aware that wound healing will be determined in part by factors such as whether wound is open or closed, clean or contaminated, superficial (skin, subcutaneous tissue, sometimes fascia) or deep (fascia, omentum, possibly visceral organ). Most laparotomy incisions are deep and, therefore, are more prone to infection, dehiscence, and evisceration.

• *Wound healing*

   b. Monitor and document wound drainage every 4 hours × 24 hours; then at least q 8 hours. Expectations include:
      • Closed clean incision: minimal or no drainage
      • Common bile duct exploration: bile drainage from T-tube
      • Cholecystectomy: moderate amount serosanguineous drainage first 24 hours.
      • Gastrostomy: initially blood-tinged drainage for 24 hours, only gastric contents thereafter.
      • Contaminated wound (open) purulent drainage.
   c. Provide strict aseptic care for all wounds. Write time and date on dressing at each change.
      • First 24 hours:
         Clean, draining wounds may need dressings reinforced. Complete dressing change only with physician order. Contaminated wounds with purulent drainage require p.r.n. dressing changes.
      • After first 24 hours:
         Intact wounds may need no dressing. Check for signs and symptoms of wound complications: odor, edema, excessive pain, erythema.
         Send specimen for culture and sensitivity for suspected infection.

Patient Outcome	Process
	• Wounds with drains: Write note on outside of dressing indicating presence of drain. For copious drainage, apply sterile drainage bag for accurate collection and measurement. Expect physician to advance drains on about fourth postoperative day and remove drain before discharge.
• *Gastrointestinal*	d. Monitor and record gastric drainage including emesis. Report amount over 400 cc per 4-hour period. • Nasogastric drainage replacement may be ordered for excessive amount with loss of electrolytes. Amount and frequency of replacement determined by volume loss. • Test gastric drainage as needed: Guaiac test for suspected bleeding • pH test for hyperacidity (patients with history of ulcerative disease, potential stress ulcers). If pH is less than 5 consult physician for antacid order.
• *Comfort*	e. Anticipate moderate to severe incisional pain in first 48 hours. Factors to consider: • Patient's inability to splint or immobilize wound • Pulmonary regimen and early mobilization accentuate pain. f. Institute measures for comfort such as: • Offer analgesics as frequently as ordered during first 48 hours: coordinate with pain-producing activities. • Employ activities to alleviate pain and anxiety, *i.e.,* backrubs, repositioning, splinting.
C. *Is knowledgeable about nature of illness, self-care, and resources for continuity of care*	5. See Chapter 5 Predischarge Phase of Hospitalization, p. 132. Include additional essential elements of preparation for discharge of patient with a laparotomy such as: a. Reinforce understanding of care of the surgical wound, resumption of activities and any dietary modification. b. Provide needed dressings, medications, and explain how a supply of these can be obtained. c. Discuss return appointment and availability of public health nurse if needed.

Lumbar hemilaminectomy

Patient Outcome

The patient experiences an informed, comfortable, and safe preoperative, postoperative and predischarge phases of hospitalization. This includes:

Process

DESCRIPTION: Lumbar hemilaminectomy is most often done for patients with nerve root compression (Fig. 5-10) as a result of disc rupture (herniated nucleus pulposus—HNP). A more extensive laminectomy is carried out on patients with spondylolisthesis, spondylolysis, and tumor. The patient may be having this surgery for the first time or may have had a previous laminectomy. Many of the patients with ruptured discs have severe pain that has incapacitated them; they often have had a trial of conservative therapy prior to hospitalization for surgery. The content of these guidelines is applicable to but not comprehensive for patients with chronic low back pain.

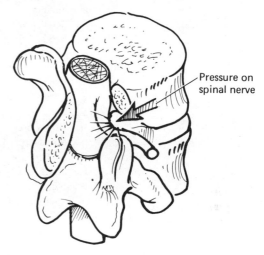

Pressure on spinal nerve

Fig. 5-10. Nerve root compression.

NURSING ASSESSMENT: In addition to the general admission assessment, the following information is especially important.
1. Assess and document physical status.
   a. Symptoms related to disease process, *e.g.,* herniated disc or tumor
      • Lower extremity motor or sensory weakness and/or sensory changes
      • Gait, any assistive devices required
      • Loss of bladder or bowel function
      • Posture
   b. Pain:
      • Location, character, and duration
      • Activity which produces or increases pain, *e.g.,* coughing, sneezing, straining at stool, bending, turning in bed
      • Positions that diminish pain
      • Activities of daily living that patient cannot perform independently due to pain
      • Medications that patient finds effective, *e.g.,* analgesics, antispasmodics, sedatives
      • Changes, if any, in normal bowel habits due to pain
      • Changes in previous life-style due to pain.
   c. Duration of activity prior to admission:
      • Symptomatology
      • Bed rest.
   d. Risk factors:
      • Urinary system problems which may affect postoperative course, *e.g.,* borderline prostatic hypertrophy, prior or current urinary tract infection
      • Pulmonary status, *i.e.,* history of heavy smoking or asthma
      • Cardiovascular status, *e.g.,* cardiac disease
      • Obesity
      • History of thrombophlebitis; consider duration of bed rest prior to hopsitalization.
      • Degree of constipation
2. Assess and document patient's understanding of disease process, anticipated surgery, and specific fears of surgery.
   a. Apparent anxiety level
   b. Previous experience with surgery
   c. Previous experience with persons who have had back surgery, *i.e.,* fears of paralysis, disability, and recurrence
   d. Understanding of postoperative expectations
   e. Fears of loss of job and physical strength

Patient Outcome	Process

	3. Assess and document health habits/life-style prior to admission.
	   a. Occupation, *e.g.,* heavy physical labor, homemaker, sedentary
	   b. Potential for self-care and/or need for supportive care after discharge
	   c. Previous participation in regular exercise program
	   d. Current and long-standing poor posture habits

A. *Is relatively free of pain preoperatively*	**INTERVENTION:**
	1. Formulate plan for dealing with pain, incorporating measures that have worked previously. This may include:
	   a. Bed rest with commode or bathroom privileges only
	   b. Bed board for all patients
	   c. Analgesics, muscle relaxants, sedatives
	   d. Positioning: Supine or lateral—moderate degree of leg flexion with pillows under knees when supine; between knees when lateral.
	   e. Turning: Log rolling—assist as needed; side rails and/or turning sheets may be helpful.
	   f. Place bed so patient will turn to nonaffected side to get up
	   g. Bowel program as needed
	   h. Moist or dry heat applications
	   i. No bending at waist or lifting heavy objects

B. *Is prepared for surgery*	2. Reinforce understanding with patient and family regarding the disease process, implications, and treatment including the operative procedure. Information about the procedure and operating room activities includes:
	   a. Type of anesthesia. Check with physician about selected anesthesia.
	     • Spinal anesthetic:
	       Will have varying levels of wakefulness in operating room. Encourage patient to inform anesthetist if he can't tolerate being awake of if he is feeling sensation.
	       May feel pressure during procedure.
	       Will remain in recovery room until sensation and movement in lower extremities return.
	     • General anesthetic for longer, more complex procedures and/or physician's preference.
	   b. Position:
	     • Usually patient is prone during surgery.
	   c. Time estimate until return to unit: Five hours (including anesthesia, OR, and recovery room)
	   d. Progression of activity
	     • Routine hemilaminectomy—progresses within 24 hours to standing and short walks. Restrict sitting to brief periods.
	     • Total laminectomy—bed rest with limited activity 1 to 2 days postoperatively
	     • If dura opened—on flat bedrest for 3 days. Delay vigorous coughing and straining.
	3. Institute preparation of patient for diagnostic studies. Refer to Chapter 3 Guidelines for the Patient Undergoing Diagnostic Studies, p. 35. Studies may include:
	   a. Spine radiography
	   b. Myelography
	   c. Electromyography
	   d. Minnesota Multiphasic Personality Inventory
	4. Summarize usual preoperative preparation and provide care per hospital routine and physician's orders. See Chapter 5 Preoperative Phase of Hospitalization, p. 129. Include additional elements of preoperative care relating to laminectomy. Emphasize specific aspects:
	   a. Pulmonary routine: Cough and deep breathe
	   b. Activity program immediately postoperative
	     • Log rolling: Back to side and into sitting position without back flexion
	     • Leg exercises: Recognize that a patient with radicular pain will not practice with affected leg.
	   c. Bowel program: Consider degree of constipation and pain level before obtaining order for suppository or enema.
	5. Collaborate with physical therapist for preoperative evaluation and teaching and especially with patient who has chronic lung disease.

C. *Is free of or has minimal discomfort or post-operative complications*
• *Respiratory*
	6. Provide postoperative care. See Chapter 5 Postoperative Phase of Hospitalization, p. 130.
	7. Intervene in critical elements of patient care following lumbar hemilaminectomy.
	   a. Provide pulmonary toilet.
	     • Log roll when turning
	     • Splint incision when coughing

Patient Outcome	Process
	• If dura opened: Delay vigorous coughing, IPPB, and incentive spirometry. Ultrasonic nebulizer to liquefy secretions
• *Comfort*	b. Anticipate that patient will require frequent consistent monitoring of pain status and effectiveness of pain relief measures. • Offer analgesic, muscle relaxant, antiemetic as often as ordered especially during first 72 hours. Most patients require narcotics for 24 to 72 hours. • Administer analgesics prior to increased activity. • Place bed in room so patient will turn to nonaffected side to get up. • Be aware leg pain may not be resolved immediately postoperatively because of time needed for gradual nerve root healing.

• *Elimination*	c. Facilitate normal bowel and bladder function. See Bladder and Bowel Care Guidelines, Chapter 2, pp. 23–25.
	• Use fracture bedpan until out of bed.
	• Assure adequate fluid intake.
	• Encourage patient to void as soon as possible after surgery. Patient often has difficulty voiding. Obtain order from physician for patient to sit or stand to void.
	• Provide for early detection and treatment of urinary tract complications.
	    Check for urinary retention, burning, frequency. Physician may order straight catheterization.
	    Encourage early removal of an indwelling catheter. Male patients with prostate problems may require longer duration of catheter drainage and attention to return to normal function.
	    Collect specimen for and monitor results of urinalyses and urine cultures.
	• Provide bowel regimen incorporating diet, stool softeners, laxatives, and suppositories. Prevent constipation to avoid straining at stool.
	    Encourage early mobilization.
	    Check for abdominal distention and absence of bowel sounds.
	    Continue to monitor bowel function.

• *Activity*	d. Plan progressive activity program as discussed preoperatively providing for adequate rest periods and pain relief. • Consider previous immobility, age, other factors affecting resumption of activities. • Assure that patient is fitted for corset by fourth postoperative day; generally, corset will not be required until sutures are removed. • Check with physician for physical therapy consult and discharge exercise instruction. e. Provide preventive measures for thrombophlebitis. • Antiembolic hose • Check for calf tenderness and leg pain at least once daily. • Active and passive leg exercises, q 2 hours • Early mobilization
• *Wound healing*	f. Check dressing q 8 hours for drainage and possible sources of contamination. • Report any drainage noted to physician; reinforce loosened dressing. • Sutures removed usually 6 to 10 days postoperative. • Prevent spillage of urine from bedpan onto dressing.

D. *Is knowledgeable about nature of illness, self-care, and resources for continuity of care*	8. See Chapter 5 Predischarge Phase of Hospitalization, p. 132. Include additional elements of preparation for discharge. Provide written instruction regarding specifics of home care.
	a. Discuss gradual resumption of activity related to patient comfort, energy level, vocational activities, and the physical demands of the activity.
	• Corset should be worn for out-of-bed activities during first 1 to 3 months as prescribed by physician.
	• Certain activities are temporarily restricted. In general, they are:
	    Prolonged sitting, *i.e.,* for 2 to 3 hours at a time (2 to 3 weeks)
	    Dressing (2 to 3 weeks)
	    Tasks involving stretching, straining, or bending at the waist (6 weeks)
	
	    Climbing into tub without assistance (2 weeks)
	    Lifting of objects greater than 5 pounds (6 weeks)
	    Strenuous sports requiring bending or twisting—ask physician before resuming.
	    Strenuous occupations which require physical labor—ask physician before resuming.

Patient Outcome	Process
	b. Emphasize good health practices: • Proper posture • Avoidance of back strain in everyday activities by using proper body mechanics • Sleep on extra firm mattress or use bedboard (½ inch plywood). • Avoidance of becoming overweight or set weight-loss goal. If patient wants diet consult, call dietician. c. Reinforce explanation of exercise program given by physical therapist. d. Instruct patient to report the following symptoms immediately to physician. • Redness, oozing, or swelling of surgical wound (check daily although infections are rare) • Onset of new or increased pain, particularly in lumbar region, or radicular leg pain. e. Provide patient with prescription for moderate pain relief. Encourage use of mild analgesic prior to pain producing activity. f. Emphasize importance of follow-up medical care as prescribed.

Mandibular or maxillary fractures (resulting in wired jaws)

Patient Outcome	Process
The patient experiences informed, comfortable and safe preoperative, postoperative and predischarge phases of hospitalization. This includes:	**DESCRIPTION:** Jaws may be wired as treatment for fractures of the mandible and maxilla which may be traumatic or elective. Elective fracture is for the purpose of correcting congenital bone deformities, *e.g.,* prognathia (protrusion of the mandible) and retrognathia (retrusion of the mandible). Tumors or cysts in either of these areas can cause destruction of the bony tissue and result in pathological fractures. The treatment for this begins with surgical removal of tumor or cyst and stabilization of bone until granulation occurs and bone is healed. In each of these conditions the wiring of jaws is most often the preferred treatment.

NURSING ASSESSMENT: In addition to the general admission assessment, the following information is especially important.
1. Assess and document physical status.
   a. Ability to breathe through nose
   b. Presence of other trauma
   c. Ability to communicate, *e.g.,* reading, writing
2. Assess and document patient's response to information about the disease process/trauma, treatment, and anticipated surgery.
   a. Apparent anxiety level
   b. Previous experience with surgery
3. Assess and document health habits/life-style prior to admission.
   a. Potential for self-care or need for supportive care
   b. Home health supervision/support
   c. Medications
4. Assess and document patient's understanding of disease process/trauma and anticipated surgery.

A. *Is prepared for surgery*

INTERVENTION:
1. Reinforce understanding of patient and family regarding anticipated surgery.
2. Summarize usual preoperative preparation and provide care per hospital routine and physician's orders. See Chapter 5 Preoperative Phase of Hospitalization, p. 129. Include additional elements of preoperative care.
   a. Emphasize postoperative expectations:
      • Teeth will be wired in closed-jaw position.
      • Head may be covered with large, bulky dressing.
      • Endotracheal tube in place overnight, if indicated
      • Close monitoring during first 24 hours
      • Specific discomforts: Lips and cheeks will be numb and swollen; gums will be sore.
      • Increased oral secretions will be removed by suction. Patient will be taught to suction when alert and ready to learn.
   b. Establish with patient and family alternatives to verbal communication and method *e.g.,* writing on pad.

B. *Is free of or has minimal discomfort or postoperative complications*
• *Respiratory*

3. Provide postoperative care. See Chapter 5 Postoperative Phase of Hospitalization, p. 130.
4. Intervene in the critical areas of patient care following procedure.
   a. Assess for signs and symptoms of airway obstruction. Critical time extends to 24 hours after endotracheal tube removed.
      • Cerebral hypoxia (restlessness, confusion, personality change, lethargy)
      • Decreased quality of breathing (rate, rhythm, depth)
      • Consistent inability to control secretions
   b. Control secretions and maximize lung function.
      • Keep wire cutters taped at head of bed at all times
      • Deep breathe, cough, and oral suction q 1 to 2 hours first 24 to 48 hours, then p.r.n.
      • Teach patient use of oral suction when appropriate: May use either wall, portable, or bulb suction.
   c. Control vomiting:
      • Maintain function of nasogastric tube to prevent vomiting.
      • Give antiemetics as needed.
      • If vomiting occurs:
         • Stay with patient.
         • Position on side.
         • Suction.
         • Have physician called who may cut wires. Learned staff may cut wires if indicated.
   d. Instruct patient to keep teeth clenched if wires are cut.

Patient Outcome	Process

• *Nutrition*	e. Maintain adequate nutritional intake.
	  • Begin with clear liquids (no gelatin) and progress to full liquid blenderized meals.
	  • Encourage patient to keep trying as feeding is difficult.
	  • Try various methods: bulb syringe, straw, spoon, or sipping from cup at side of mouth.

• *Wound healing*	f. Maintain cleanliness of mouth and incision area.
	  • Use 3 percent hydrogen peroxide for cleansing incision.
	  • Rinse mouth with mouthwash frequently.
	  • Do not use toothpaste due to foaming action.
	  • Use oral irrigating device, if appropriate.

C. *Is knowledgeable about self-care and resources for continuity of care*	5. See Chapter 5 Predischarge Phase of Hospitalization, p. 132. Include additional elements of preparation for discharge of patient with jaws wired.
	  a. Reinforce information given by physician.
	  b. Teach self-care measures:
	    • Mouth care:
	      Apply any lubricant cream to lips for dryness.
	      Apply wax obtained in oral surgery clinic to ends of wire that are irritating to mucous membranes. Remove wax before brushing teeth.
	      Rinse mouth after clear liquids.
	      Brush teeth and gums after meals and snacks. Use small bristle brush using small circular motions.
	  c. Provide diet instruction (include person who prepares patient's food).
	    • Include any foods that can be blended to thinned consistency that will go through a straw. Assist patient/family to secure blender as needed.
	    • Suggest liquid diet supplements that are available at drug or grocery stores, which should be used for between-meal nourishment.
	  d. Instruct in safety measures to prevent aspiration.
	    • Patient should wear wire cutters visibly around neck on string which is long enough to permit easy use.
	    • Show patient and family where, how, and when to cut wires:
	      Cut *only* if patient vomiting or having difficulty in breathing.
	      Pull lips back and use mirror to see wires.
	      Maintain position to facilitate breathing or drain vomitus.
	      If wires are cut, keep teeth clenched and return immediately for wires to be reset by physician.
	  e. Teach care of incision area.
	    • Use one-half strength peroxide, rinse with water, and dry if sutures are present.
	    • Wash with soap and water, and dry following suture removal.
	    • Use antibiotic ointment after cleansing until incision completely healed.
	    • Report any signs of infection to physician, *e.g.,* pain, swelling, redness, increase in drainage.
	  f. Assist patient to obtain services as needed for continuity of care.
	    • Initiate interagency referral if appropriate.
	  g. Give return appointment.

Patient Outcome	Process

The patient experiences informed, comfortable and safe preoperative, postoperative, and predischarge phases of hospitalization. This includes:

DESCRIPTION: Most women are admitted for diagnosis of a breast mass and scheduled for biopsy and possible mastectomy under general anesthesia. Types of mastectomy include:

Radical Mastectomy: Through an incision, the entire breast is removed along with a margin of skin around the nipple, areola and the tumor. The pectoral major and minor muscles are removed, axillary vein is dissected, and axillary nodes are removed. Depending upon the amount of skin removed, grafting may be necessary.

Modified Radical Mastectomy: Through an incision, the breast tissue including the nipple, skin, tissue, and lymph nodes are removed. Skin grafts are not necessary.

Simple Mastectomy: Through an incision the skin, nipple, and breast tissue are removed.

Subcutaneous Mastectomy: Through an incision under the nipple, the subcutaneous breast tissue is removed. Implants are then placed in the resulting cavity. See Bilateral Subcutaneous Mastectomy with Implants Guideline, Chapter 5, p. 141.

NURSING ASSESSMENT: In addition to the general admission assessment, the following information is especially important.

1. Assess and document physical status.
   a. Symptoms relating to underlying disease:
      • Breast skin care needs
      • Symptoms of advanced stage of cancer
   b. Risk factors:
      • Presence of other disease states, *e.g.,* diabetes, CVA
2. Assess and document patient's response to information about the disease process and anticipated surgery.
   a. Apparent anxiety level
   b. Previous experience with surgery and/or diagnostic studies
   c. Patient's self-assessment of:
      • Personal strengths in coping with stress or previous crises.
      • Support people, *e.g.,* family, chaplain
3. Assess and document health habits/life-style prior to admission.
   a. Physical demands, *e.g.,* homemaking, occupation, recreational activities
   b. Position in family unit, *i.e.,* marital status, children
4. Assess and document patient's understanding of disease process, treatment, and anticipated surgery.

A. *Is prepared for surgery and body image change*

INTERVENTION:

1. Reinforce understanding of patient and family regarding the disease process, implications, and treatment. Information given may include:
   a. Procedure for biopsy and possible mastectomy if mass is malignant.
   b. The physician will discuss part to be surgically removed.
   c. Postoperative expectations:
   Biopsy:
      • Dressings dependent upon size and kind of mass removed
      • Discharge usually day after surgery
      • Expect incisional soreness and/or tightness
   Mastectomy:
      • Large, pressure dressing
      • Skin catheter(s) attached to closed wound drainage
      • Affected arm will be elevated
      • Up *ad lib*, day of surgery
      • Usual length of hospitalization, 7 to 10 days
      • Resume p.o. nutrition first postoperative day
      • Most masectomy patients experience incisional pain which usually diminishes to soreness on second postoperative day.
2. Assess patient's general coping ability and the uses of coping mechanisms in the current situation.
   a. What has helped patient cope with difficult situations in the past?
   b. How can the nursing staff initiate measures that may assist the patient in this situation? Examples:
      • Be present to provide emotional support and communicate emotional needs to other staff.
      • Contact and communicate with identified support people, *e.g.,* family chaplain, clinicians.

Patient Outcome	Process

- Allow support people to remain with patient.
- Collaborate with physician to obtain order for tranquilizer or sedative as needed.

3. Assess patient's awareness and emotional readiness for surgery. Examples of questions which may be helpful:
   a. "What has the doctor told you about your operation?"
   b. If the patient discusses biopsy but does not mention the possibility of a mastectomy, "Has the doctor mentioned anything else?"
   c. If the patient mentions mastectomy without emotional expression, "How do you feel about that?", or "What do you think about that?"
   d. "Have you ever known anyone who has had a mastectomy?"

4. Provide opportunity for patient/family members and significant others to discuss concerns, or ask questions. Usual concerns involve potential threat of surgical findings (cancer), disfigurement, and change in function and/or relationships. Resource people may be chaplains, nurse clinicians, former mastectomy patients.

5. Provide information which may include:
   a. When participating in ordinary daily activities, people will not be able to tell that patient has had a mastectomy.
      - A temporary lightweight postoperative prosthesis is available after dressing is removed and until incision has healed enough to use a permanent prosthesis.
      - After incision is healed (about two months) a heavier, permanent prosthesis may be worn.
   b. After healing is complete, patient will be able to resume most daily activities.
   c. Surgical reconstruction is a later possibility and should be discussed with the physician prior to surgery if patient is interested.
   d. Importance of postoperative exercises, *e.g.,* "wall climbing".

6. Summarize usual preoperative preparation and provide care per hospital routine and physician's orders. Chapter 5 Preoperative Phase of Hospitalization, p. 129.

7. Provide postoperative care. See Chapter 5 Postoperative Phase of Hospitalization, p. 130.

B. *Is free of or has minimal discomfort or postoperative complications*
- *Wound healing*

8. Intervene in the critical elements of patient care following a mastectomy
   a. Observe and record signs of bleeding.
      - Check vital signs q 4 hours.
      - Observe drainage on dressing.
      - Empty closed drainage system q 8 hours, record on I and O sheet. Check for clots and maintain patency of drainage by milking tubing, q 4 hours. System will be removed when drainage subsides.
   b. Note no blood pressures, blood drawn, or injections in affected arm. Place sign over bed with this information.

- *Rehabilitative*

   c. Begin progressive exercises:
      - Explain exercises to resume function in affected arm—forward and lateral motion.
      - Encourage patient to squeeze object, *e.g.,* gauze roll in hand while in bed to increase lymph drainage.

- *Body image*

   d. Assist patient to cope with feelings associated with body image change, threat of cancer, change of life-style.
      - Emotional support measures in early postoperative period may include:
         Providing time and opportunity for patient to talk about her feelings regarding changes brought about by surgery and disease implications
         Providing time and opportunity for family/significant others to verbalize feelings and concerns
         Meeting immediate informational needs of patient/family.
         —Explain and reinforce surgical procedure performed.
         —Clarify meaning of lymph node report. The physician will explain results which are usually available 2 to 4 days later.
         —Provide explanation for sensations patient may experience which include numbness/hypersensitivity under affected arm (caused by bruising of nerves during operation and will resolve); "phantom breast" (cause unknown).
         Explaining "Reach to Recovery" program: Group sponsored by American Cancer Society whose members have had mastectomies. They provide patient with kit containing temporary breast form, information for family members and patients, and

Patient Outcome	Process

other equipment. Patient and physician consent needed before volunteer can be contacted.

C. *Is knowledgeable about nature of illness, self-care and resources for continuity of care*

9. See Chapter 5 Predischarge Phase of Hospitalization, p. 132. Include additional essential elements of preparation for discharge to patient and family such as
   a. Wound care:
       • Expect patient and/or family to look at incision before discharge.
       • Explain appearance of wound.
           Location of incision
           Sutures will be removed 10 to 14 days.
           Swelling, bruising, redness, will gradually resolve.
       • Offer to be present when patient first looks at wound.
       • Explain and give written information regarding signs and symptoms of wound infection.
       • Advise patient she may resume shower (preferred) or bathe 2 to 3 days after discharge unless contraindicated by physician.
       • Instruct patient not to shave or use deodorant under affected arm until wound has healed completely (about two months). May use light application of talcum powder.
       • Advise patient not to use lotions, medications, or other topical preparations on wound.
       • Cover with light gauze dressing and paper tape if incision needs some protection.
   b. Exercises/activity:
       Goal: To restore full range of motion.
       Exercises should be done two to three times daily using the affected arm, gradually increasing the range of motion.
       • Squeeze object in hand to increase lymph drainage.
       • Face wall with feet apart and forehead against wall. Start with hand at shoulder level and slowly "walk" fingers up the wall. Slide hands back and repeat.
       • Lift arm straight in front and raise until "pulling" or pain is felt under arm or incisional area.
       • Lift arm straight to side and raise until pulling or pain is felt under arm or in incision.
       • Encourage to resume normal posture especially during ambulation, *i.e.,* head up, shoulders back, arms at side.
       • Resume normal activity at home with exception of strenuous exercises and lifting, until physician gives permission.
           Car driving: Resume when patient feels strong enough (about two weeks).
           Resume sexual activity as soon as patient feels comfortable doing so. Common fears include trauma to incision area and acceptance by spouse.
   c. Care of affected arm:
       • Carry heavy objects with nonaffected hand and arm.
       • Do not wear tight garments, watches, etc. on affected arm.
       • Take care not to cut or burn arm or hand. In event of cut or burn, wash immediately and protect from dirt. Precautions include:
           Wear gloves when gardening, washing dishes, or using strong detergents.
           Wear a mitt-type holder when using oven.
           Wear a thimble when sewing.
       • Protect arm from sunburn.
       • Do not allow injections, vaccinations, blood samples, or blood pressures to be taken in affected arm.
       • Use lanolin based creams to keep cuticles soft instead of cutting.
       • Call physician if swelling or infection develops in arm or hand.
   d. Wearing of prosthesis:
       • Temporary lightweight prosthesis (breast form) can be obtained from brace shop or "Reach to Recovery" volunteer.
       • Also pad bra with dressing material, soft cloth or material, *e.g.,* clean hose or sanitary pads.
       • Bra should be loose fitting, nonbinding, without wires, *e.g.,* an old bra, sleep bra, or bra purchased 2 inches larger than usual.
       • Should wear temporary form until incision healed and physician gives prescription for permanent form (about six weeks).
       • Permanent form may be obtained from facility or store which has a fitting specialist, *e.g.,* department store, brace shop, lingerie shop. The forms are expensive but most insurance policies cover a large portion of the cost for the first form purchased.

Patient Outcome	Process

e. Breast examination:
   * Inform patient that like any other woman, she should perform a monthly breast examination by:
     - Gently sliding fingers over breast and axillae while in shower or bath to check for lumps, knots, or thickening
     - Inspecting the appearance of her breast if front of a mirror for swelling, dimpling, changes in the nipple, or changes in the shape of the breast; This may be done by raising arms over head and also by placing hands on hips.
     - Lying down and putting a pillow under the shoulder of the same side. Press gently in a circular motion from the outer edge of the breast to and including the nipple.
     - Inspecting the incision line for any abnormalities (lumps, redness, etc.)
   * Instruct patient to inform physician of any abnormal findings.

f. Avoid use of hormone preparation, *e.g.*, birth control pills, vaginal creams, postmenopausal medications.

g. Follow-up care:
   * Instruct patient regarding the importance of returning for regular appointments.
   * Instruct patient that she will be given specific information by physician regarding any follow-up therapy that may be recommended depending upon age of patient and state of disease. For example:
     - Chemotherapy
     - Radiation therapy
     - Hormonal manipulation by medication or surgery (oophorectomy, adrenalectomy)
   * Initiate visiting nurse referral as indicated.

Patient Outcome

The patient experiences informed, comfortable, and safe preoperative, postoperative, and predischarge phases of hospitalization. This includes:

Process

DESCRIPTION: Occlusive vascular disease is a disease which involves the large and medium-size arteries supplying the extremities, usually the lower extremities. The symptoms are caused either by dilation or by blockage of the artery (Fig. 5-11). The symptoms include claudication (pain, cramping, fatigue in the extremity brought on by exercise), sensitivity to cold, change in color, and impotence. As the disease progresses, the patient may experience rest pain and changes in the feet which include loss of hair from toes; brittle, opaque nails; atrophy of the skin; and rubor (redness) when the foot is in a dependent position. The patient and family must understand the importance of the prescribed medical regimen as the foot is extremely susceptible to ulceration from even minor trauma which may lead to gangrene and subsequent amputation. The aim of management is avoidance of trauma leading to ulceration and improvement of blood supply to the extremity. Diagnostic studies include arteriography to determine location of occluded vessels. If vascular by-pass surgery is indicated, incisions are made above and below the occluded area. A vein graft of dacron is sewn to the vessel above and below the occlusion thus allowing blood to bypass the occlusion resulting in increased blood supply to the extremity. Small occluded areas may be "cleaned out"

NURSING ASSESSMENT: In addition to general admission assessment, the following information is especially important:

1. Assess and document physical status.
   a. Signs and symptoms related to involved extremity(ies) including:
      - Pulses (Fig. 5-12)
      - Temperature—Identify level of any temperature change.
      - Color and condition of skin and nailbeds: lesions, edema, ulceration, infection
      - Subjective symptoms: numbness, tingling, muscular aches (after exercises), and pain—including location, precipitating factors, and relief measures.
   b. Risk factors/disease states:
      - General health status—Identify pathophysiological conditions.
      - Nutritional status, *i.e.,* obesity, malnutrition, dehydration

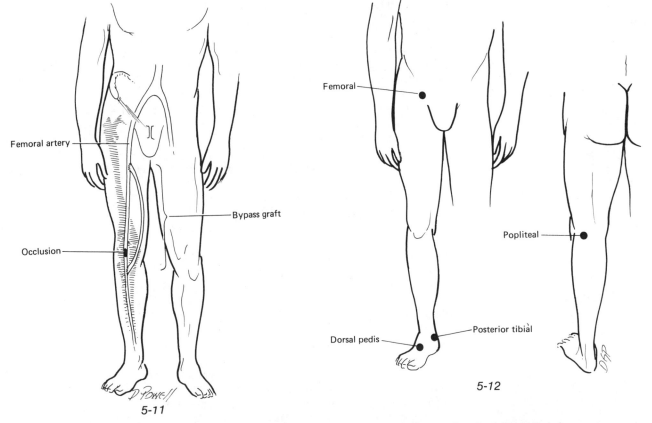

Fig. 5-11. *Bypass graft.*

5-11

Fig. 5-12. *Peripheral Pulses.*

5-12

Patient Outcome	Process

2. Assess and document patient's response to information about the disease process and possible surgery.
   a. Apparent anxiety level
   b. Previous experience with surgery
3. Assess and document health habits/life-style prior to admission.
   a. Home remedies and medications
   b. Foot care and precautions
   c. Activity, exercise program
   d. Smoking
   e. Diet
   f. Home health supervision/support
   g. Occupation
   h. Potential for self-care or need for supportive care
4. Assess and document patient's understanding of the disease process, treatment, and possible surgery.

A. *Understands nature of illness and participates in treatment plan*

INTERVENTION:
1. Reinforce understanding of patient and family regarding the disease process, implications, and treatment. Include:
   a. Causes
   b. Symptoms
   c. Aims of therapy
   d. Medications
2. Teach care of the involved extremities.
   a. Foot care:
      • Wash feet daily with warm soap and water.
      • Dry feet gently with a soft clean cloth and avoid drawing cloth vigorously between toes.
      • Apply lanolin to feet after cleansing.
      • Inspect feet for pressure areas and wounds daily.
      • Clip toe nails straight across and above the level of the quick. Do not cut into the corners or make V-cut into the nail.
   b. Foot precautions:
      • Wear clean, nonrestrictive socks. Change daily. Wool socks are appropriate in the winter and cotton in the summer. Avoid synthetics.
      • Consult podiatrist for removal of corns, callouses, or warts.
      • Avoid use of strong disinfectants, compounds, or corn cures which contain strong acids that can injure skin.
      • Wear properly fitting shoes.
         • Leather should be pliable.
         • When "breaking in" a new pair of shoes, wear initially for a half hour daily and increase by one hour daily.
      • Avoid temperature extremes. Test water with hand before applying to foot. A hot water bottle or heating pad should never be applied directly to the skin. Loose fitting socks may be worn at night to keep feet warm. Avoid prolonged exposure to cold.
      • Do not soak feet for longer than 10 minutes.
      • Protect from possible trauma, *e.g.,* do not walk barefoot.
      • Consult doctor for treatment of athletes foot.
      • Report sudden pain, paleness, coldness, or numbness to physician.
      • Also report change in exercise tolerance or character of pain.
   c. Hand care:
      • Inspect daily for breaks in skin, *e.g.,* blisters.
      • Apply lanolin after washing.
      • Avoid use of strong disinfectants or detergents.
      • Avoid temperature extremes, *e.g.,* hot water, exposure to cold.
      • Protect from trauma, *e.g.,* use gloves.
      • Report pain, coldness, paleness, or numbness to physician.
   d. General precautions and care measures:
      • Smoking is forbidden.

Patient Outcome	Process

	• Avoid restrictive garments such as girdles and garters.
	• Avoid body positions which hinder circulation, *e.g.,* crossing legs.
	• Carry out regular exercise/walking program according to physical ability or physician's instructions.
	• Diet recommendations may include:
	    Restriction of cholesterol and saturated fats
	    Achievement or maintenance of desired weight goal
	• Daily alcohol intake may be recommended (dilates peripheral vessels).
	• Take medications as prescribed, knowing frequency, dose, effects, and side effects.

B. *Is prepared for surgery*	3. Summarize usual preoperative preparation and provide care per hospital routine and physician's orders. See Chapter 5 Preoperative Phase of Hospitalization, p. 129. Include additional elements of preoperative care relating to vascular bypass surgery.
	  a. Assess extremities for pulses, color, temperature, and sensation. Mark pulse sites on skin.
	  b. Provide information about postoperative expectations:
	    • Pulses will be checked frequently.
	    • May spend night in recovery area
	    • Restrictions on certain positions temporarily
	    • Smoking will not be permitted.

C. *Is free of or has minimal discomfort or postoperative complications*
• *Circulation*
 	
• *Wound healing*
	4. Provide postoperative care. See Chapter 5 Postoperative Phase of Hospitalization, p. 130.
	5. Intervene in the critical areas of patient care following vascular bypass surgery.
	  a. Assess and document circulation in extremity:
	    • Check pulses, color, warmth, sensation q 15 minutes for first 2 hours, q 1 to 2 hours for 24 hours; and with routine vital signs after 24 hours.
	    • Notify physician immediately for loss of pulse.
	  b. Provide positioning to promote circulation.
	    • Sitting may be restricted.
	    • Crossing legs is prohibited.
	    • Consider placing sheepskin under feet.
	    • Place blanket between legs when patient lies on side.
	    • No acute flexion of hips or knees when lying
	  c. Inspect incision site for bleeding and hematoma. Expect small amount of sanguineous drainage.
	  d. Maintain surveillance for signs of infection.
	    • Check with physician regarding first dressing change.
	    • Inspect incision site for redness, swelling, drainage. Send any drainage for culture and sensitivity and notify physician.
	    • Monitor temperature.
	    • Continue to monitor incision site for bleeding, since infection may cause leakage of graft.

D. *Is knowledgeable about self-care and resources for continuity of care*	6. Provide patient/family with information and support in making decisions regarding necessary life-style changes.
	  a. Assist patient to consider alternatives in employment situation if job requires exposure to cold or prolonged standing or walking.
	  b. Inform patient that participation in sports with prolonged exposure to cold or prolonged standing or walking may be restricted.
	  c. Be aware the male patient may become or continue to be impotent postoperatively. Give patient/family explanation regarding cause and emotional support. Physician can discuss medical intervention (penile prosthesis by urologist).
	7. Teach specific aspects of care:
	  a. Avoid periods of prolonged sitting, standing, or walking.
	  b. Continue foot and hand care and exercise regimen as well as general precautions.
	  c. Perform wound care consistent with condition of incision, *e.g.,* open to air, dry dressings, wet-to-dry dressings. Report problems to physician.
	  d. Avoid smoking.

Opthalmologic care for patients needing medical treatment and/or surgical intervention

Patient Outcome

The patient functions comfortably within limitations due to opthalmologic disorder. This includes:

Process

DESCRIPTION: Opthalmologic care involves medical treatment and surgical procedures performed for evaluation and/or therapy for eye disorders. Some of the most common disorders include:

Cataract (opacity of the lens): Treatment is surgical extraction.

Retinal detachment (due to a hole, tear, or peeling of retinal membrane): Treatment includes bed rest, laser therapy, cyclocryotherapy, and surgical reattachment.

Intra- and extraocular tumors (malignant and nonmalignant): Surgical treatment may include: enucleation (removal of eye and tumor), Krönlein procedure (removal of extraocular tumor), and exenteration (removal of eye and contents of orbital cavity).

Corneal disorders such as congenital abnormalities, abrasions, and ulcers: Treatment may be medical or surgical including corneal transplant.

Ptosis (drooping lid) and strabismus (squint): Treatment is surgical correction of muscle dysfunction.

Retinopathy (degenerative changes of the retina due to diabetes, arteriosclerosis, etc.): Treatment may be laser therapy, cyclocryotherapy or vitrectomy (removal of vitreous).

Glaucoma (elevated intraocular pressure): Treatment may be medical or surgical to allow proper outflow of aqueous.

Traumatic injuries (hyphema, foreign bodies, lacerations, orbital fractures (blowout): Treatment may be bed rest or surgical repair.

NURSING ASSESSMENT: In addition to the general admission assessment, the following information is especially important.

1. Assess and document physical status.
   a. Degree of visual impairment/loss
   b. Ability to perform self-care activities
   c. Presence of other disease states, *e.g.,* diabetes, hypertension
2. Assess and document health habits/life-style prior to admission.
   a. Physical demands, *e.g.,* occupation
   b. Position in family unit, *e.g.,* marital status, dependent children.
3. Assess and document patient's emotional response to visual impairment/loss.
   a. Apparent anxiety level
   b. Expectation of outcome of treatment
   c. Patient's self-assessment of:
      • Personal strengths in coping with stress, crisis
      • Support persons, *e.g.,* family, friends
4. Assess and document patient's understanding of the eye disorder, implications, and treatment.

A. *Is prepared for therapy and/or surgery*

INTERVENTION:

1. Reinforce understanding of patient and family regarding eye disorder, implications, and treatment.
2. Summarize usual preoperative preparation and provide care per hospital routine and physician's orders. See Chapter 5 Preoperative Phase of Hospitalization, p. 129.
   a. Emphasize specific postoperative expectations.
      • Treated eye will be covered. Length of time depends on procedure and physician's orders:
         Strabismus: 24 hours or less
         Cyclodialysis, cyclocryotherapy, laser treatment: 24 hours or less
         Ptosis: 24 hours or more
         Evisceration (Krönlein): 3 to 5 days or more
         Enucleation: 5 days
         Retina, vitrectomy: 5 to 7 days
      • Nonoperative eye may be covered.
      • Discomforts will be minor.
      • Bed rest: 3 to 24 hours as ordered
      • Activity: Move arms and legs about while in bed. May not stoop, bend, or strain.
   b. Preoperative medication may include osmolytic glycering "cocktail" (glycerine, lime juice, and water over ice) to reduce intraocular pressure prior to and during surgery.

Patient Outcome	Process

B. *Is free of or has minimal discomfort or posttherapy complications*	3. Provide postoperative care. See Chapter 5 Postoperative Phase of Hospitalization, p. 130.
	4. Intervene in the critical elements of care following surgery/therapy.
	   a. Minimize chance of infection.
	     • Use good hand washing techniques.
	     • Instruct patient not to touch operative eye.
	     • Change dressing as ordered after initial change by physician.
	     • Give antibiotics (systemic or topical) as ordered.
	     • Observe for signs and symptoms of infection such as fever, drainage from eye, and increased eye pain. Report to physician.
	   b. Provide measures to prevent/treat hyphema.
	     • Maintain bed rest with or without bathroom privileges as indicated.
	     • Elevate head of bed 20° to 45° as ordered
	     • Observe for sudden increase in severity of pain and report to physician.
	   c. Provide therapeutic measures if enzyme glaucoma occurs (serious complication which can occur within 12 hours postsurgery).
	     • Observe for signs and symptoms: headache, pain not relieved by usual medication, nausea, and vomiting. Report to physician.
	     • Administer medications as ordered, *e.g.,* acetazolamide (Diamox), glycerine "cocktail".
	   d. Observe for symptoms of corneal abrasion.
	     • Report to physician complaints of pain during movement of eye.
	   e. Intervene to prevent disorientation.
	     • Remain aware of patient at risk (*i.e.,* elderly) for disorientation.
	     • Assist patient preoperatively to become familiar with environment of room, *e.g.,* bed, bedpan.
	     • Keep call bell within reach.
	     • Reorient patient to environment as needed.
	     • Identify self upon approaching patient.
	     • Provide periods of uninterrupted sleep.
	     • Provide sufficient sensory stimulation, *e.g.,* radio, "talking books", touch.
	     • Encourage family member to remain with confused patient.
	   f. Assist patient to cope with disability and treatment.
	     • Provide opportunities for patient to express feelings, fears, and concerns about future.
	     • Identify coping strategy and reinforce successful attempts.
	     • Consult resource persons, *e.g.,* chaplain.
	     • Provide diversional activities, *e.g.,* radio, "talking books".
	     • Observe for unusual behavior indicating need for further support, *e.g.,* depression.
	   g. Provide a safe environment.
	     • Keep side rails up.
	     • Assist patient in and out of bed and while ambulating.
	     • Keep call light within reach.
	     • Supervise smoking if necessary.
	     • Minimize disorientation.
	     • Do not rearrange contents of room and bedside unit.
	   h. Prevent urinary retention.
	     • Assist patient to void as needed. If unable to void, check for distention and report to physician.
	   i. Prevent thrombophlebitis.
	     • Encourage leg exercises q 2 hours.
	     • Ambulate three times daily as soon as possible.
	     • Observe for signs and symptoms, *e.g.,* calf pain, and report to physician.
	   j. Prevent respiratory complications. Refer to Chapter 2 Pulmonary Care Guidelines, p. 29.
	     • Turn q 2 hours until ambulating.
	     • Promote deep breathing and nonvigorous coughing exercises q 2 hours as ordered.
	   k. Maintain bowel function. Refer to Chapter 2 Bowel Care Guidelines, p. 25.
	     • Assess bowel habits.
	     • Plan bowel program as indicated.
	     • Record bowel movement.
	     • Caution patient not to strain.
	     • Do not give enemas unless absolutely necessary.

Patient Outcome	Process

C. *Is knowledgeable about nature of illness, self-care, and resources for continuity of care*	1. Provide skin care. Refer to Chapter 2 Skin Care Guidelines, p. 31.
	5. See Chapter 5 Predischarge Phase of Hospitalization, p. 132. Include additional essential elements of preparation for discharge such as:
	  a. Instruct regarding resumption of activity as ordered:
	    • Cataract, retina, corneal graft and hyphema: Caution patient against bending, stooping, swimming, and lifting heavy objects. Check with physician for permission for showers and shampoos before first return visit.
	  b. Instruct regarding eye care as ordered.
	    • Surgical patients should cleanse area with cotton ball and Dacriose or clean cloth and warm water.
	    • Use sun glasses in bright light.
	    • Wear eye shield during rest periods and at night.
	    • Administer eye solution/ointment according to prescriptions.
	    • Reinforce physician's instructions for care of eye socket after enucleation/exenteration, *e.g.*, use sterile saline and hydrogen peroxide for cleansing.
	    • Reinforce instructions for care of contact lens and the prosthesis.
	    • Provide specific instructions for diabetic patients. Refer to Chapter 4 Diabetes Mellitus Guidelines, p. 105.
	  c. Instruct to notify physician of symptoms of swelling, increased pain, drainage, or change in vision.
	  d. Inform patient of community resources which may assist in continuity of care.
	  e. Initiate interagency referral if appropriate.

Patient Outcome	Process

The patient experiences informed, comfortable, and safe preoperative, postoperative, and predischarge phases of hospitalization. This includes:

DESCRIPTION: Pelvic exenteration is indicated for gynecological cancers that are locally destructive and capable of growth but do not tend to metastasize; for tumors that have not responded to radiotherapy; or tumors incurable by less radical surgery. Extent of surgery is determined during operative procedure. A total pelvic exenteration involves the removal of the pelvic contents (uterus, adnexae, bladder, vagina, bilateral lymph nodes, rectum, and diseased portion of bowel) creating urinary and bowel diversions. An anterior pelvic extenteration involves the removal of pelvic contents as indicated above with the exception of the rectum and bowel. A posterior pelvic exenteration involves the removal of pelvic contents as indicated above with the exception of the bladder.

NURSING ASSESSMENT: In addition to the general admission assessment, the following information is especially important.
1. Assess and document physical status.
   a. Signs and symptoms of advanced stages of cancer
   b. Special problems which may affect status for surgery and/or recovery, *e.g.,* diabetes, obesity, anemia
   c. Other problems/disabilities, *e.g.,* fractures, poor dental hygiene
2. Assess and document patient's response to information about disease process and anticipated surgery.
   a. Diagnostic and/or status evaluation
   b. Reasons for studies/surgery
   c. Patient's self-assessment of:
      • Personal strengths in coping with stresses and previous crises
      • Support people, *e.g.,* family, chaplain
      • Resource people, *e.g.,* cancer clinician, former patients who have had similar surgery.
3. Assess and document life-style including:
   a. Physical demands, *e.g.,* homemaking, occupation, recreational activities
   b. Position in family unit, *i.e.,* marital status, children.
4. Assess and document patient's understanding of disease process and anticipated surgery.

A. *Is prepared for surgery, and body image change*

INTERVENTION:
1. Reinforce understanding of patient and family regarding the disease process, implications, and treatment. Include these special considerations:
   a. Faced with diagnosis of cancer, patient may need time to work through fears before she can "free her mind" for anything else.
   b. Sexually active patients will be concerned with body image and sexual alternatives available if total vaginectomy is performed.
   c. The psychosocial and sociocultural background of the patient and her knowledge of body function may make explanation of surgical procedures difficult.
2. Consult resource persons, *e.g.,* chaplain, or clinician as needed.
3. Summarize usual preoperative preparation and provide care per hospital procedure and physician's orders. See Chapter 5 Preoperative Phase of Hospitalization, p. 129. Include additional elements of care relating to pelvic exenteration.
   a. Reinforce physician's explanation regarding removal of organs; change in bowel, bladder, and sexual function.
   b. Emphasize preoperative expectations.
      • Clear liquid diet usually beginning as soon as possible preoperatively
      • Medicated douche per physician's order
      • Bowel preparation per physician's order
      • Cantor tube before surgery as ordered
      • Antiseptic skin scrub by patient or nurse b.i.d. for two days prior to surgery
      • IV begun prior to surgery
      • Daily weights pre-and postoperatively
   c. Emphasize postoperative expectations.
      • Length of time in recovery room varies: ranges from several hours to overnight.
      • Possible equipment in addition to usual:
         Central Venous Pressure
         Closed wound drainage system
         Colostomy and/or urine drainage bag
         Drainage tube into perineal cavity and vaginal packing around tube
         Long term IV therapy and n.p.o status (1 to 3 weeks)

Patient Outcome	Process

	d. Emphasize patient participation.
	    • Ambulate first postoperative day.
	    • Nurse will care for drainage bags for several days and patient will gradually assume care.
	4. Provide assistance to patient coping with altered body image.

B. *Is free of or has minimal discomfort or postoperative complications*
 	
C. *Is able to cope with surgical alteration and life-threatening disease*
	5. Provide postoperative care. See Chapter 5 Postoperative Phase of Hospitalization, p. 130. Ileal Conduit, p. 173 and Colostomy Guidelines, p. 149 for specific intervention.
	6. Consider additional specific needs if patient is receiving radiation therapy or chemotherapy.
	7. Support patient's ability to cope with surgery and prognosis.
	    a. Assess current support systems of patient/family: strengths and weakness, previous patterns of coping.
	    b. Employ "active listening" using verbal and behavioral clues indicating patient/family concerns.
	    c. Observe and document appetite and sleep patterns. Provide instruction, assistance, and comfort measures.
	    d. Supply verbal and written information suited to the patient's current capacity to understand.
	    e. Help patient accept self/body image by demonstrating acceptance. Be kind but honest in preparing patient for change in body image and functioning including sexual limitations.
	    f. Collaborate with physician, chaplain, oncology clinician and others in support of patient's emotional status.

D. *Is knowledgeable about nature of illness, self-care, and resources for continuity of care*	8. See Chapter 5 Predischarge Phase of Hospitalization, p. 132.
	9. Include additional essential elements of preparation for discharge of the patient such as
	    a. Reinforce understanding of the care of the colostomy and ileal conduit, care of the surgical wound, resumption of physical and sexual activities, and any dietary modification.
	    b. Provide needed equipment, supplies, and medications and explain how a supply of these can be obtained.
	    c. Clarify any written instruction and return appointment.
	    d. Explain services and availability of public health nurses, colostomy clubs.
	    e. Assist patient to obtain services as needed for continuity of care.

Radical neck dissection

Patient Outcome	Process

The patient experiences informed, comfortable, and safe preoperative, postoperative and predischarge phases of hospitalization. This includes:

DESCRIPTION: Radical neck dissection is indicated for treatment of carcinoma of the neck, nose, throat, and mouth. The procedure involves removal of all affected areas and the lymph nodes. Usually the jugular vein is removed; the carotid artery is left intact along with the vagus nerve. When a radical neck dissection is combined with a hemiglossectomy or mandibulectomy, a tracheostomy may be performed; if combined with a laryngectomy, a tracheostomy must be performed. Skin grafting is occasionally required.

NURSING ASSESSMENT: In addition to the general admission assessment, the following information is especially important.

1. Assess and document physical status.
   a. Preexisting respiratory problems, *e.g.,* asthma
   b. Any physical limitations which might interfere with ability to carry out self-care, *e.g.,* arthritis
   c. Healing capacity, *e.g.,* previous irradiation to affected area
   d. Ability to communicate, *e.g.,* reading, writing skills
   e. Risk factors, *e.g.,* alcoholism

2. Assess and document patient's response to information about the disease process, treatment, and anticipated surgery.
   a. Apparent anxiety level
   b. Previous experience with surgery
   c. Expectations of outcome of surgery
   d. Patient's self-assessment of:
      • Personal strengths in coping with stress
      • Self-concept and body image
      • Support persons, *e.g.,* family, friends

3. Assess and document health habits/life-style prior to admission.
   a. Potential for self-care or need for supportive care
   b. Medications
   c. Diet
   d. Position in family unit, *e.g.,* homemaker

4. Assess and document patient's understanding of disease process and anticipated surgery.

A. Is prepared for surgery

INTERVENTION:
1. Reinforce understanding of patient and family regarding anticipated surgery.

2. Summarize usual preoperative preparation and provide care per hospital routine and physician's orders. See Chapter 5 Preoperative Phase of Hospitalization, p. 129. Include additional elements of preoperative care such as
   a. Emphasize postoperative expectations:
      • Close monitoring for several days
      • Endotracheal tube overnight at least
      • Tracheostomy is permanent for patient with laryngectomy and temporary otherwise— usually removed in 5 to 7 days.
      • Frequent suctioning of mouth, nose tracheostomy
      • Bulky head dressing
      • Skin catheters attached to suction
      • Nasogastric tube
      • May have donor site (thigh) for skin grafts
      • Expected discomforts: sore throat, swollen numb tongue, headache, incisional pain, inability to talk
      • Permanent loss of voice for laryngectomy patient
      • Alterations in senses of smell and taste
      • Use of antiembolic hose
      • Turning, coughing, deep breathing exercises
   b. Secure physician's order for speech therapy consultation as indicated.
   c. Provide sufficient opportunity for expression of feelings regarding surgical intervention and its implications for changes in physical appearance, ability to communicate.
   d. Establish with patient and family alternatives to verbal communication and method, *e.g.,* writing on pad.

201

Patient Outcome	Process

B. *Is free of or has minimal discomfort or complications following surgery*	3. Provide postoperative care. See Chapter 5 Postoperative Phase of Hospitalization, p. 130.
	4. Intervene in the critical elements of patient care following surgery. This includes:
	  a. Maintain respiratory function.
	    • Monitor vital signs q 1 hour for first 24 to 48 hours, then q 4 hours.
	    • Administer oxygen as needed.
	    • Provide humidity.
	    • Position to facilitate ease of respiration.
	    • Turn, cough, deep breath q 2 hours until ambulating.
	    • Percuss as needed.
	    • Ambulate as soon as possible.
	    • Report any signs and symptoms of hypoxia, *e.g.,* shortness of breath, cyanosis, lethargy, anxiety, or headache which may be due to increased intracranial pressure from venous congestion.
	    • Provide oral hygiene as needed.
	    • Suction mouth and nose as needed.
	    • For the patient with tracheostomy and/or laryngectomy,
	      Suction mouth, nose, laryngectomy and tracheostomy tubes q 1 hour × 8 hours; then q 2 hours ×48 hours; then as needed.
	      Perform tracheostomy care q 2 hours × 24 hours, then q 4 hours thereafter.
	  b. Promote adequate circulation.
	    • Encourage leg exercises q 2 hours until ambulating.
	    • Apply antiembolic hose.
	    • Ambulate as soon as possible.
	    • Observe and report evidence of excessive wound drainage.
	      Monitor q 1 hour × 4 hours, then q 4 hours.
	      Skin catheter drainage:
	        First to second day: Expect no greater than 100 cc per 8 hours.
	        Third day: Expect no greater than 10 to 15 cc per 8 hours.
	        Fourth to sixth day: Expect less than 10 cc per 8 hours.
	    • Observe for and respond to signs and symptoms of extreme swelling in areas of wounds.
	      Check that dressing is loose enough to permit finger under edge.
	    • For the patient with tracheostomy and/or laryngectomy,
	      Remain aware that rupture of carotid artery is a potential complication.
	      Report immediately:
	        Bleeding from incision, tracheostomy
	        Bloody sputum with clots
	      Check for complaints of "can't breathe", "dressing too tight".
	      Check with physician before cutting dressing.
	      Keep tracheostomy tray at bedside.
	  c. Maintain neurological status.
	    • Assess for and report to physician signs and symptoms of nervousness, shakiness, hypoxia, and sleep deprivation, *e.g.,* confusion, restlessness.
	    • Provide periods of undisturbed sleep.
	    • Administer medications as ordered to promote rest and comfort.
	  d. Facilitate communication.
	    • Establish plan with patient and family for nonverbal communication, *e.g.,* writing, use of flash cards.
	    • Keep call bell within easy reach.
	    • Provide reassurance.
	    • For the patient with tracheostomy, and/or laryngectomy,
	      Reinforce fact that there are electronic devices that may enable the patient to communicate.
	      Reinforce possibility of learning esophageal speech techniques.
	  e. Promote adequate nutrition.
	    • Progress diet as ordered.
	      Day 1 to 2: nothing via nasogastric tube (NG) until bowel sounds are heard, then 30 to 60 cc clear fluids hourly via NG tube.
	      Day 3 to 7: Give tube feeding q 2 hours when awake. Keep patient in upright position during and for 30 minutes after feeding. Check for residual; if more than half of previous feeding, report to physician.

Patient Outcome	Process

	Full liquids by mouth supplemented by tube feeding until intake reaches 2400 cc daily. Then clamp NG tube.
	Remove NG tube and give soft diet.
	Initiate referral to dietician as indicated.
	• For the patient with tracheostomy and/or laryngectomy;
	  Progression of dietary intake for tracheostomy patient may be delayed.
	  Begin instruction in tube feedings as early as possible, if indicated.
	  Supervise all feeding to minimize chance of aspiration.
	  Observe and report signs of esophageal fistula, *e.g.*, secretions from area other than suture line or established opening.
	  f. Assess for signs and symptoms of infection and report findings to physician.
	    • Blood-tinged, purulent drainage
	    • Wound edema, redness, warmth, pain
	    • Temperature elevation to 38.5° C

C. *Is coping with illness*	5. Assist patient/family to cope with body image change, threat of cancer, and change of life-style.
	  a. Provide opportunity for patient and family to express fears, concerns, and questions.
	  b. Identify with patient current coping strategy and support appropriately.
	  c. Demonstrate acceptance of patient and patient's appearance.
	  d. Identify resource persons for assistance in counseling, *e.g.*, social worker.
	  e. Expect patient to participate in daily self-care activities as soon as possible.
	  f. Help patient to set realistic goals.

D. *Is knowledgable about self-care and resources, for continuity of care*	6. See Chapter 5 Predischarge Phase of Hospitalization, p. 132. Include additional essential elements of preparation for discharge of patient.
	  a. Teach self-care skills.
	    • Oral hygiene:
	      Use equal parts of water and 3 per cent hydrogen peroxide as mouth wash after meals and at bedtime.
	      Brush teeth regularly.
	    • Suture area:
	      Cleanse area b.i.d. with soap and water.
	      Apply antibacterial ointment if prescribed.
	    • Fistula care:
	      Give instructions about dressing changes.
	      Supervise until performed independently by patient/family.
	    • Laryngectomy site care:
	      Remove and clean inner and outer tubes daily and p.r.n. using powdered cleansing agent. Reinsert tubes after stoma care.
	      Wash area of stoma with soap and water and dry well.
	      May apply thin layer of antibacterial ointment to prevent irritation.
	      Supervise until performed independently by patient/family.
	      Prevent dust, dirt, water from entering tube; no swimming, provide protection while bathing.
	  b. Provide dietary instruction. Consult dietician as needed.
	    • Emphasize importance of nutrition for wound healing.
	    • Suggest soft diet until regular foods can be tolerated.
	    • Give instructions for tube feeding if indicated. Supervise feeding until performed independently by patient/family.
	    • Assist patient/family to secure blender as needed.
	  c. Discuss resumption of normal activities.
	  d. Instruct patient to report signs and symptoms of complications to physician. These include:
	    • Difficulty swallowing
	    • Increased pain
	    • Production of bloody and or purulent sputum.
	  e. Stress need for continuous humidity; assist patient/family to obtain appropriate equipment.
	  f. Arrange referral to speech therapist as indicated.
	  g. Assist patient to obtain other services as needed for continuity of care.
	    • Initiate interagency referral.
	  h. Discuss Lost Chord associations.
	  i. Give return appointment.
	  j. Suggest use of medical identification, *e.g.*, bracelet, wallet card.

Patient Outcome

*The patient experiences
informed, comfortable,
and safe preoperative,
postoperative, and
predischarge phases
of hospitalization.
This includes:*

Process

DESCRIPTION: Transplantation is performed on children and adults as one mode of therapy (in conjunction with dialysis) for end-stage renal disease in an attempt to restore renal function. Donor source may be family member (sibling or parent) or unrelated (cadaver). Selection of donor/recipient pairs is based on immunogenetic histocompatibility testing. There is a high rate of kidney loss, both acutely and chronically, due to the immunologic rejection phenomenon, recurrence of disease process, and other complications. The patient may require long hospitalization period of three weeks to three or more months.

The procedure includes placing the kidney in either iliac fossa retroperitoneally through a six-inch incision. The renal artery is anastomosed to the hypogastric artery; the renal vein is anastomosed to the external iliac vein, and the ureter is anastomosed to the bladder. (Figure 5-13). The operation requires about 3½ to 5 hours to complete.

NURSING ASSESSMENT: In addition to general admission assessment, the following information is important.
1. Assess and document physical status.
    a. Symptoms/situations relating to underlying disease states:
        * Condition of arteriovenous fistula/shunt including patency (Figure 5-14.)
        * Visual impairment
        * Signs and symptoms of any infection, acute or chronic
        * Amount and character of urine output from native kidneys
        * "Dry" weight on dialysis
        * Hepatitis associated antigen/antibody status (whether positive or negative)
    b. Risk factors;
        * Cardiovascular status, *e.g.*, hypertension, edema, cardiac disease
        * Pulmonary status, *e.g.*, smoking history, recent infections, tuberculosis history
        * Presence of other pathophysiological states, *e.g.*, diabetes
2. Assess and document patient's response to information about the disease process and implications of planned surgery.
    a. Apparent anxiety level
    b. Previous experience with surgery
    c. Expectations regarding outcome of transplantation
    d. Patient's self-assessment of:
        * Personal strengths in coping with stress or crises

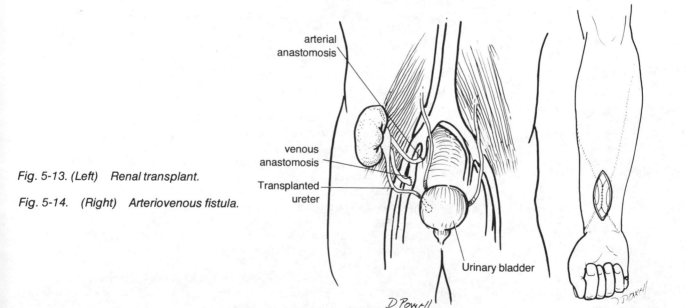

Fig. 5-13. (Left)   Renal transplant.

Fig. 5-14.   (Right)   Arteriovenous fistula.

Patient Outcome	Process
	• Support persons, *i.e.*, family, spouse, chaplain e. Adherence to chronic regimen. 3. Assess and document patient's understanding of the disease process, treatment and anticipated surgery. 4. Assess and document health care needs/habits prior to admission. a. Potential for self-care or need for supportive care b. Medications, especially those relating to renal disease, *e.g.*, antihypertensives, antacids, anticonvulsants, laxatives c. Diet, *i.e.*, restrictions, patient's knowledge and adherence d. Home health supervision/support

A. *Is prepared for surgery*	**INTERVENTION:**
	1. Reinforce understanding of patient and family regarding the disease process, implications, and planned treatment. Include donor if appropriate.
	• Provide assistance in the patient's coping strategy such as
	  • Encourage verbalization about surgery and recognize patient's concerns.
	    Attempt to determine patient's expectations of the outcome of transplantation.
	    Help him accept that some degree of threatened rejection of graft is expected.
	  • Listen and observe for misconceptions and for signs of anxiety.
	  • Include family members in nursing interventions (especially if donor is a family member).
	  • Use identified support people such as renal transplant clinician and chaplain.
	  • Provide contact with other transplant recipients if appropriate.
	  • Assure patient and family that they will be kept informed regarding progress during long hospitalization.
	2. Summarize usual features of preoperative preparation and provide care per hospital routine and physician's order. See Chapter 5 Preoperative phase of hospitalization, p. 131.
	3. Include additional elements of preoperative care due to transplantation surgery:
	a. Begin immunosuppressive therapy (steroids and azathioprine [Imuran]) two days preoperatively for living related donor recipients.
	b. Document body weight after last dialysis completed.
	c. Alert patient and family about postoperative expectations:
	  • Patient returns directly to special care area (patient's private room) from OR.
	  • Supplies necessary postoperatively include: CVP, IV, suction, O_2, and possible peritoneal dialysis equipment.
	  • Frequent observations by nursing staff
	  • Progressive diet changes from clear liquids to regular 1 gm sodium diet if normal renal function is achieved.
	  • Fluids will be regulated on a daily basis; no restriction if adequate renal function present.
	  • Changes in bowel function
	  • Progression of activity is begun first postoperative day. Patient must be either lying or ambulating. No sitting for more than five minutes at a time during first 10 postoperative days—then for no longer than 15 minutes at a time until discharge.
	  • Patient must lie on transplant side or back for 72 hours postoperatively.
	  • Protective precautions to minimize hazard of infection
	  • Daily collection of blood and urine specimen
	  • Patient participation:
	    Make feelings and needs known to nursing staff
	    Turn, cough, deep breathe, and incentive deep breathing exercises
	    Leg exercises until ambulating well
	    Progression of self-care, personal hygiene, measurement of I and O, daily weight, and other activities of daily living
	    Smoking is discouraged.
	d. Discuss with patient and family the following points on immunotherapy:
	  • Produces increased risk of infection, therefore, need for protective precautions.
	  • Steroid side effects: changes in physical appearance, *i.e.*, moonface; muscle wasting and weakness; gastric irritation; sodium and fluid retention; abnormal weight gain; mental reactions, *e.g.*, irritability, euphoria.

C. *Is free of or has minimal discomfort or postoperative complications*	4. Provide postoperative care. See Chapter 5 Postoperative phase of hospitalization, p. 132. 5. Intervene in the critical elements of patient care following transplantation as summarized into immediate (1 to 48 hours) and intermediate (24 to 96 hours) phases.

Patient Outcome

Process

	IMMEDIATE Postoperative Period (1 to 48 hours)	INTERMEDIATE Postoperative Period (24 to 96 hours)
• *Neurological*	a. Observe and record levels of consciousness to verbal and physical stimuli as patient recovers from general anesthesia.	

• *Circulatory*	b. Monitor vital signs (first 24 hours): check and record P, R, BP, q 15 minutes until reacted fully from anesthesia, q 30 minutes until stable and then q 1 hour.
	• Rectal temperature immediately postop. and then q 4 hours.
	• CVP q 1 hour.
	• Monitor vital signs (second 24 hours): take BP, CVP q 1 hour; P,R,T, q 4 hours.
	• Treat symptoms of shock. See Chapter 5 Postoperative Phase of Hospitalization, p. 130.
	• Observe, protect arteriovenous fistula/shunt.
	  No blood pressure or venipuncture in fistula arm
	  Check for patency by palpating fistula thrill or absence of clots in shunt.
		• Check BP q 2 hours until 96 hours then q 4 until discharge.
		
		• Check CVP q 1 hour until CVP catheter removed.
		
		• Continue to observe patency of fistula or shunt.

	c. Identify patient susceptible to cardiovascular complications.	• Remain alert to high-risk patient.
• *Respiratory*	d. Maintain respiratory status: • Apply O_2 mask (4 to 6 liters/minute) upon arrival to ward. • Discontinue when vital signs are stable and patient is reacted from anesthesia. • Maintain patent airway. • Check respirations and encourage good pulmonary toilet. • Incentive deep breathing exercises *p.r.n.*	 • Administer analgesic *p.r.n.* prior to coughing exercises. • Continue pulmonary toilet. See Chapter 5 Postoperative Phase of Hospitalization, p. 130. • Incentive deep breathing exercises until ambulating independently.
	e. Identify patient susceptible to respiratory complications.	• Remain alert to high-risk patient.

• *Urinary/Fluid Balance*	f. Remember: Urinary output in a transplant recipient is a *vital* sign; maintain constant awareness of urinary output.
	• Measure and record q 1 hour
	  Volume: Polyuria of 75 to 130 cc per hour is desirable.
	  Specific gravity: 1.003 to 1.015 is desirable in this phase.
	  Appearance: Clear to blood-tinged with few clots is expected.
	• Report to physician any sudden increase or decrease in volume.
	• Collect all urine per protocol/physician's orders.
	• Observe/maintain patency of ureteral and Foley catheters.
	  Irrigate Foley with 30 cc sterile saline *p.r.n.*
	  Ureteral catheter may be irrigated by physician or nurse clinician.
	  No catheter clamping
		
		• Continue q 1 hour urine measurements until catheters removed (7 to 10 days postop.); then q 2 hours during waking and sleeping hours.
		• Check specific gravity q 2 hours; then q 8 hours after catheter removed.
		
		• Continue until catheter removal.

Patient Outcome	Process	
	IMMEDIATE Postoperative Period (1 to 48 hours)	**INTERMEDIATE** Postoperative Period (24 to 96 hours)

	Make sure catheters and tubing are properly positioned and secured.
	  • Provide for routine catheter maintenance.
	  • Do not change or remove catheter without physician's order.
	 g. Maintain fluid and electrolyte balance:
	  • Replace fluids and electrolytes q 1 hour per physician's order.
	  • Do not allow replacement deficit of over 200 cc per hour. Notify physician or clinician for assistance with any problems.
	  • Obtain accurate daily weight every a.m. using same scales.
	  • Demand accurate recording of I and O from *all* members of the health team.
	  • Note daily blood and urine electrolyte determinations as performed per protocol.
		
		• Include oral fluids as part of replacement volume.
		• Provide fluid intake of 2500 to 3000 cc daily when adequate renal function achieved.
		• Continue daily weights until discharged.
		
		• Instruct and encourage patient to participate in recording I and O as soon as possible.

• *Musculoskeletal*	h. Maintain proper positioning:
	  • First 72 hours:
	     Supine or on side of transplanted kidney; change position q 2 hours.
	  • Elevate head of bed no more than 45°.
	  • Permit no flexing of hip on side of transplanted kidney except for routine leg exercises and ambulation.
	  • Permit no sitting for more than 5 minutes at a time.
	 i. Encourage leg exercises q 1 hour.
	 j. Ambulate in room b.i.d. first postop. day.
		• May also lie on opposite side after 72 hours.
		
		• Elevate head of bed no more than 45°.
		• Permit no flexing of hip on side of transplanted kidney except for routine leg exercises and ambulation.
		• The first 10 days permit no sitting for more than 5 minutes at a time.
		• Continue leg exercises q 2 hours until ambulating.
		• Ambulate in hallway q.i.d. and p.r.n.

• *Skin*	k. Be aware that patient with chronic renal failure has generalized itching, dryness, and/or peripheral neuropathy resulting in decreased sensation. • Provide for special skin care needs.	• Remain alert to skin and neuromuscular problems.

• *Wound healing*	l. Provide wound care:
	  • Expect minimal drainage.
	  • Change soiled dressing using sterile technique; *do not reinforce.*
		• Continue observation of wound and drainage until healed.

• *Comfort and rest*	m. Anticipate and evaluate patient's need for analgesics.
	  • Administer medication prior to required activity which produces discomfort.
	  • Consider use of other pain relieving measures.
	 n. Provide periods of undisturbed sleep.
	  • Be aware that sleep deprivation is a common complication during first several days of intensive care environment.
		• Continue evaluation of need for analgesic. Adjust type of medication according to need and nurse and/or physician judgment.
		
		• Remain aware that high dose steroid therapy can contribute to sleep deprivation.
		• Continue to provide periods of undisturbed sleep.

• *Immunological*	o. Observe continuously for the following signs and symptoms which herald threatened kidney rejection:	

Patient Outcome	Process

- Decrease in urine volume, hypertension, sustained temperature elevation, edema, weight gain, swelling and tenderness over transplant site, malaise
- Laboratory values: elevated serum creatinine and blood, urine, nitrogen, decreased creatinine clearance and urinary sodium

p. Expect to give massive daily doses of IV methylprednisolone (Solu-Medrol) if threatened rejection is diagnosed in addition to maintenance immunosuppressant therapy. Additional renal function studies, radiation therapy, antithymocyte globulin, diet and fluid changes, and dialysis may be ordered by physician.

q. Remain aware of special nursing considerations because of immunotherapy:
- Administer drugs per physician order without deviation (azatheoprine [Imuran], cyclophosphamide [Cytoxan], steroids, antithymocyte globulin).
- Be aware that patient has lowered resistance and is particularly vulnerable to the following infections:
    Urinary tract
    Pulmonary
    Wound
    Skin (herpes simplex, staphlococcal)
    Oropharyngeal (herpes simplex, monilial)
    Central nervous system (fungal, bacterial)
    Generalized sepsis
- Provide the cleanest possible environment and care to minimize chance of infection.
    Strict hand washing and aseptic technique
    Restrict visitors to immediate family.
    Exclude staff and visitors with communicable diseases from room.
    Establish special mouth care routine.

• Side effects

r. Remain aware that the following problems may occur as side effects of therapy:
- Gastric irritation. Therapy: preventive antacids; no steroids on empty stomach
- Sodium and fluid retention. Therapy: diet restriction, diuretics
- Abnormal mental reactions. Therapy: adequate sleep and rest, emotional support
- Glucose intolerance. Therapy: diet control
- Changes in body appearance—skin, hair, facial skin oiliness, abnormal weight gain. Therapy: frequent washing, good general hygiene, appetite control
- Myopathy of lower extremities. Therapy: daily exercise programs
- Constipation. Therapy: dietary, stool softeners, exercises, enema

D. *Is coping with impact of surgery and threat of graft rejection*

s. Approach patient and family in supportive ways.
- Be aware that patients with chronic renal disease have multiple concerns. Help patient to identify significant problems and work through appropriate solution.
- Accept the fact that patient is usually well informed about renal disease and expects honesty and factual information concerning care and condition.
- Be supportive by approaching the patient with consistency, firmness, and understanding.
- Explore patient's concerns about graft rejection and support appropriate coping strategies.
- Help patient adjust to change in physiological function caused by transplant (from no renal function to hopeful resumption of renal function) and understand implications of new therapeutic plan of care.
- Include family as participants in care when appropriate.

E. *Is knowledgeable about nature of illness, self-care, and resources for continuity of care*

6. See Chapter 5 Predischarge Phase of Hospitalization, p. 132. Include additional essential elements of preparation for discharge of a renal transplant recipient.
a. Assess continuously need for teaching and counseling.
b. Teach skills/knowledge related to:
- Intake and output measurement
- Twenty-four-hour urine collection
- Clean-catch urine specimen collection
- Urine sugar testing
- Daily weight
- Daily temperature
- Wound care if healing incomplete at discharge
c. Emphasize and reinforce knowledge about diet and fluid modifications.

Patient Outcome	Process
	d. Provide written information and instruction about: • Signs and symptoms of rejection, infection, and urinary tract obstruction • Medication: therapeutic and toxic effects; dosages and times; measures to minimize side effects • Importance of infection prevention measures, *e.g.*, good personal hygiene, early reporting of any symptoms to transplant team member. • Importance of reporting illness or significant symptom to physician. e. Discuss importance of continued monitoring of renal function by blood and urine chemistries and radiographs. f. Discuss gradual resumption of normal activities of daily living (exception: contact sports). g. Assess level of understanding and acceptance of health-illness state. • Include family in teaching when appropriate. h. Provide: • Dressing supplies, medications/prescriptions and explain how new supply can be obtained. • Return appointment. Discuss importance of follow-up care on frequent basis (weekly until stable renal function achieved). • Information about health agencies which might assist in continuity of care. i. Initiate interagency referral as needed.

Patient Outcome	Process

The patient experiences informed, comfortable, and safe preoperative, postoperative, and predischarge phases of hospitalization. This includes:

DESCRIPTION: Replantation is a microvascular surgical procedure for reattaching amputated extremities, usually fingers and hands. The procedure must be done soon (within 12 to 24 hours) after the amputation. Candidates are selected according to which digit is amputated, age, physical condition and condition of severed part. The procedure can be 4 to 23 hours in length and the postsurgical outcome for the replanted part is uncertain. Close observation is crucial during the postoperative period.

NURSING ASSESSMENT: In addition to general admission assessment, the following information is important. Informant may be family member.
1. Assess and document physical status.
   a. Smoking, drinking, drug history
   b. Significant health problems, especially note hypertension
   c. Prescribed medications
2. Assess and document psychosocial status.
   a. Notification of family
   b. Circumstances of amputation
   c. Occupation—determination if accident was job related
   d. Other accidents involving patient
   e. Anticipated reaction of patient to prolonged postoperative bed rest and hospitalization
   f. Information family would like staff to consider

A. *Is prepared for replantation experience*

INTERVENTION:
1. Provide essential emergency care if appropriate. Patient may be referred from other facility where initial care given.
   a. Protect amputated part:
      • Cleanse obvious dirt from amputated part (do not ligate, perfuse, or shorten vessels or bone.)
      • Place in plastic bag with sterile Lactated Ringer's solution or normal saline.
      • Place bag on ice and in insulated container, *e.g.,* styrofoam cup.
   b. Apply bulky compression dressing to stump.
   c. Transport as soon as possible to appropriate medical facility if necessary.
   d. Keep n.p.o. prior to surgery.
2. Summarize features of preoperative phase and provide care as needed per hospital routine and physician's orders. See Chapter 5, Preoperative Phase of Hospitalization, p. 129.
3. Include additional elements of preoperative care due to trauma and need of replantation. This includes:
   a. Provide additional information:
      • Surgery will be prolonged.
      • Patient will be given axillary block in emergency room or operating room. In operating room the procedure will be made more tolerable by being given an IV analgesic and tranquilizer. Exception: Children may be given general anesthesia.
   b. Give additional physical care prior to surgery which includes:
      • Tetanus injection may be given, if not within past 5 years.
      • Antibiotics given IV or IM
      • Polaroid pictures usually taken
      • IV inserted
      • Axillary block started by anesthesia. Lidocaine (Xylocaine) and bupivacaine (Marcaine) will be injected into axillary nerve sheath causing motor and sensory anesthesia for about 12 hours.)
   c. Support the family/responsible person during the wait for the patient in surgery:
      • Provide occasional progress reports from the operating room.
      • Listen to family/responsible person as they need to talk about the accident.
      • Make sure family needs are being met: waiting place, food, medication.

B. *Is free of or has minimal discomfort and post operative complications*

• *Circulatory*

4. Provide postoperative care. See Chapter 5 *e.g.,* Postoperative Phase of Hospitalization, p. 130. (For any problems, notify replant team.)
5. Intervene in the critical areas of patient care following replantation surgery:
   a. Assess and document circulation in replantation area q 1 hour.
      • Describe skin color, which should be pink; report paleness or blue color.
      • Assess temperature.
         Subjectively (warm, cool, cold)
         Objectively (temperature probe). Make sure probe is taped securely to replant part.

Patient Outcome	Process

Temperature of normal extremity is about 30°C. Report anything less than 29°C or more than 5°C difference between normal and replanted extremity(ies).

Be aware of other factors influencing temperature, *e.g.*, room temperature, patient's baseline temperature.

- Check capillary refill by gently compressing and releasing tip of extremity. Expect blanching, sluggish response.

b. Do not ask patient to demonstrate movement or sensation. (Bone is fixed with a wire and movement may damage surgical repair. Numbness is expected.)

c. Elevate replanted extremity above level of heart, using IV pole and canvas arm elevator which supports entire arm. In case of arterial insufficiency, physician may order extremity to be lowered for short periods of time.

d. Assess for venous congestion in replantation area and report immediately:
- Symptoms: "full", "tight" hand, may throb
- Color: dark, cherry red or purple
- Lack of blanching; capillaries remain filled on pressure

e. Check fit of bandage to avoid constriction. Dried drainage may increase tightness of bandage.

f. Be aware of other measures that may be used to improve circulation:
- Physician may perform axillary block to relieve vasoconstriction in the extremity.
- Caution patient not to smoke and explain rationale (vasoconstriction).
- Physician's orders may include:
  "Milk fingertips" to improve venous return
  Bolus of heparin to reduce clotting
  Other drugs which affect circulation directly or indirectly, *e.g.*, chlorpromazine (Thorazine), polyanhroglucose (Dextran), aspirin.
  Maintain bed rest, then gradual resumption of activity, taking care to avoid orthostatic hypotension. Maintain arm elevation when ambulating.

g. Monitor heparin infusion carefully. Excessive bleeding or clotting due to improper administration is a major postoperative complication.
- Use infusion controller and mini-drip infusion set.
- Check that pharmacist member of replant team or appropriate person regulates heparin administration.
- Check q 8 hours for proper dosage, rate.

h. Check for bleeding q 1 hour. Report any fresh bleeding immediately.
- Observe dressing around fingers; check under elbow and back for hidden bleeding.
- Be alert to patient reports of "dripping", "warm", "soggy", or "sticky" sensations.
- Have hand dressing tray at bedside for immediate dressing changes.
- Monitor for signs, symptoms indicating excessive or internal bleeding, *e.g.*, nose bleeds, hematuria, blood in stools or emesis, headaches.

i. Provide special precautions to prevent accidental injury.
- Caution patient not to use razor blade; use electric shaver instead.
- Avoid activities that might cause bruising, *e.g.*, IM injections may cause subcutaneous hematoma.

• *Pulmonary*

j. Encourage coughing, especially first postoperative day, because the patient has remained stationary during the extremely long operation.

• *Gastrointestinal*

k. Assess bowel history for constipation. Provide preventive bowel program and check progress daily. See Chapter 2 Bowel Care Guideline, p. 25.

• *Urinary*

l. Consult with physician to discontinue indwelling catheter as soon as possible. See Chapter 2 Bladder Care Guideline, p. 23.

m. Encourage fluids 3000cc per day unless restricted.

• *Wound healing*

n. Check for signs of infection. Report:
- Temperature greater than 37.5°C (after third postoperative day)
- Unusual amount of redness, tenderness, swelling
- Foul odor

C. *Is emotionally able to cope with traumatic experience*

6. Be aware that patient is usually in good health except for injury and may find it difficult to accept prescribed regimen. Difficulties may involve:

a. Frustration in not being able to care for self using two hands. (Patient will also have IV in nonaffected arm or hand).

b. Lengthy hospitalization keeps patient away from job and family.

Patient Outcome	Process

| | c. Altered body image is dependent upon the patient's self-concept, life-style, prognosis, loss of function and change in appearance. In children, parent's adjustment can favorably or unfavorably affect child's response. |

7. Allow patient to verbalize concerns and express feelings and be accepting of them.
8. Individualize care to meet patient's needs such as
   a. Place bedside table and needed items within reach of nonaffected hand.
   b. Adjust care plan to incorporate reasonable patient requests.
   c. Plan for diversional activities to change focus from affected extremity. Examples: TV, conversations with visitors, staff, other patients.

D. *Is knowledgeable about self-care, and resources for continuity of care*

9. See Chapter 5 Predischarge Phase of Hospitalization, p. 132.
10. Include additional essential elements of preparation for discharge of patient. These include:
    a. Teach care of limb/bulky dressing.
       • Maintain elevation; may use sling.
       • When sleeping use pillow to keep arm elevated.
       • Protect from moisture; for shower, may use plastic bag completely surrounding dressing and taped securely. *Do not immerse*.
       • May need to alter shirt armhole due to size of bulky dressing.
       • Avoid direct or indirect causes of trauma to limb, *e.g.*, contact sports, tennis.
    b. Teach and supervise patient to do active and passive range of motion exercises to each joint of each unaffected finger at least four times daily. Rationale: Joints may become stiff if immobilized for long periods of time.
    c. Teach symptoms to report immediately to physician if they occur in affected extremity:
       • Bleeding
       • Change in color towards dusky shade
       • Decreased temperature
       • Increase in pain level
    d. Teach regarding prescribed medications which include:
       • Aspirin b.i.d. used for anticoagulation
       • Analgesic p.r.n.
       • Sedative p.r.n.
       • Tranquilizer p.r.n.
11. Include family/responsible person in all homegoing preparations of patient.
12. Be aware that the patient may have questions about home care that should be answered by physician in charge:
    a. When may I return to work; smoke?
    b. May I remove my dressing?
    c. Will I need further surgery?
13. Explain services and availability of agencies such as: Vocational Rehabilitation; Social Services for financial or job related assistance; and public health nurse and assist family in making contact with agency identified for needed assistance.
14. Provide needed dressings and medications and explain how a supply of these can be obtained.
15. Alert patient to date of return appointment—usually 10 days after discharge.

Rhinoplasty: including surgery to the nasal septum and turbinates

Patient Outcome	Process

The patient experiences informed, comfortable, and safe preoperative, postoperative, and predischarge phases of hospitalization. This includes:

DESCRIPTION: A rhinoplasty is plastic surgery of the nose usually involving reshaping of the tip, hump, septum, and narrowing of the bony base. A septoplasty is surgery of the nasal septum usually to repair a deviation or to correct the nasal septum. In a submucous resection, an incision is made at the edge of the nasal septum to correct deviation by removing cartilage causing obstruction.

NURSING ASSESSMENT: In addition to the general admission assessment, the following information is especially important.
1. Assess and document physical status.
   • Include any risk factors which might affect postoperative course such as pulmonary disease.
2. Assess and document patient's response to information about disease process and anticipated surgery.
   a. Apparent anxiety level
   b. Previous experience with surgery
3. Assess and document patient's understanding of the disease process and anticipated surgery.
   • Understanding of postoperative expectations, *e.g.*, change in appearance and function (immediate and long range).

A. *Is prepared for surgery and body image change*

INTERVENTION:
1. Reinforce understanding of patient and family regarding the disease process, implications, and treatment.

2. Summarize usual preoperative preparation and provide care per hospital routine and physician's orders. See Chapter 5 Preoperative Phase of Hospitalization, p. 129. Include additional elements of preoperative care.
   • Emphasize postoperative expectations.
     • Nasal packing for 2 to 3 days
     • Nasal splint covered with dressing and tape across forehead and cheeks
     • Drip pad underneath nose
     • Discomforts including sore throat; dry mouth; choking sensation due to inability to breathe; difficulty hearing, talking, smelling, and tasting
     • Generalized discoloration and swelling about face
     • Nausea

B. *Is free of or has minimal discomfort or postoperative complications*

• Respiratory

3. Provide postoperative care. See Chapter 5 Postoperative Phase of Hospitalization, p. 130. Intervene in the critical areas of patient care following surgery.
   a. Observe for signs of obstructed airway resulting from posterior slippage of nasal packing and/or swelling.
     • Check position of packing by looking in patient's throat. Packing should not be visible in back of throat. Patient may complain of gagging.
     • Elevate head of bed 45°, provide humidity as necessary, and have O_2 available.
     • Call physician to remove and replace packing if needed.
   b. Observe and record symptoms of bleeding. Call physician as necessary.
     • Change drip pad frequently as needed—usually q 15 minutes first hour and then depending upon the amount of drainage and patient preference.
     • Expect nausea and vomiting to occur immediately after surgery; vomitus may contain old blood tinged with bright blood.
     • Encourage patient to cough up secretions; measure and record vomitus.

• Comfort

   c. Provide comfort measures according to source of discomfort.
     • Apply ice packs to sides of nose and under eyes to decrease swelling.
     • Give sufficient oral fluids to keep throat moist.
     • Reinforce eventual improvement of appearance and decrease of discomfort.

C. *Is knowledgeable about self-care and resources for continuity of care*

4. See Chapter 5 Predischarge Phase of Hospitalization, p. 132. Include additional elements of preparation for discharge of patient.
   a. Teach self-care measures.
     • Dressing:
       • Dressing remains approximately seven days.
       • Caution not to get dressing wet (no swimming; take baths, not showers).

Patient Outcome	Process
	• Teach patient to change drip pad.
	• When dressing removed, may have initial increase in swelling and discoloration which should subside within 24 hours.
	• Comfort:
	• May want to use home humidifier, particularly at night to keep nose moist.
	• A Neosporin ointment to dry skin around nostril
	• Elevate head by using pillows to ease breathing.
	• Numbness and swelling may take 4 to 6 months to resolve.
	b. Instruct patient to apply ice pack if nose bleed occurs and see physician.
	c. Instruct patient about activity.
	• All normal activities may be resumed except the following:
	• No contact sports or activities in which nose might be easily injured until allowed by physician.
	• Do not blow nose during time packing is in place and for 3 to 4 days after removal.
	• Attempt to avoid sneezing.

Patient Outcome	Process

The patient experiences informed, comfortable, and safe preoperative, postoperative, and predischarge phases of hospitalization. This includes:

DESCRIPTION: A skin graft is the transplantation of tissue from the original site (donor) to another area (recipient). Grafts are classified by similarity between host and recipient, *e.g.*, isograft, autograft, allograft and by the layers of tissue included in the graft, *e.g.*, split thickness, full thickness.

A skin flap is skin and subcutaneous tissue that is moved from one part of the body to another with a vascular attachment being maintained for nourishment. The "pedicle" is the base or stem of a flap.

NURSING ASSESSMENT: In addition to the general admission assessment, the following information is especially important.

1. Assess and document physical status.
   a. Condition of graft site, *e.g.*, infection
   b. Circulation in area to be grafted
   c. Joint mobility and muscle strength in affected area
   d. Nutritional status
   e. Any other disease state, *e.g.*, diabetes, peripheral vascular disease
2. Assess and document patient's response to information about the disease process, treatment, and anticipated surgery.
   a. Apparent anxiety level
   b. Previous experience with surgery
3. Assess and document health habits/life-style prior to admission.
   a. Potential for self-care or need for supportive care.
      • Use of specific assistive devices such as bed cradle, sheepskin, cane, walker
   b. Medications
   c. Diet
   d. Home health supervision/support.
4. Assess and document patient's understanding of disease process and anticipated surgery.

A. *Is prepared for surgery*

INTERVENTION:
1. Reinforce understanding of patient and family regarding anticipated surgery.
2. Summarize usual preoperative preparation and provide care per hospital routine and physician's orders. See Chapter 5 Preoperative Phase of Hospitalization, p. 129. Include additional elements of preoperative care.
   • . Emphasize postoperative expectations:
      • Bulky dressing to donor and recipient sites
      • Bed rest for several days which is determined by condition of graft and location
      • Restricted movement of graft site for prolonged period determined by condition of graft and location
      • Graft site may have closed drainage system.
      • Donor site will be exposed and dried beginning the day of surgery if graft is superficial. Donor site may be more painful.

B. *Is free of or has minimal discomfort or postoperative complications*

• *Circulatory*

• *Wound healing*

3. Provide postoperative care. See Chapter 5 Postoperative Phase of Hospitalization, p. 130.
4. Intervene in the critical areas of patient care following surgery.
   a. Maintain circulation at surgical sites.
      • Check circulation (color, appropriate blanching, warmth) per physician orders q 1 hour × 8 to 12 hours, then q 4 hours. Record and report if deviates from normal.
      • Observe and record wound drainage q 1 hour × 4; then q 4 hours.
         Outline drainage on dressing, date, and time of observation.
         Skin catheter drainage: Break suction q 1 hour × 4; then q 2 hours.
         Check for clots. Empty drainage and measure q 8 hours.
      • Do not allow wall suction pressure to exceed 150 mm unless otherwise ordered.
   b. Provide donor site care.
      • Use hair dryer as ordered by physician.
         Remove outside dressing and leave protective gauze layer on wound.
         Place hair dryer on "cool" setting 12 inches from site for 20 minutes q 4 hours until site dry and then p.r.n.
      • Do not wash site.
      • Protect from injury.
      • Place bed cradle to keep sheets off wound.
   c. Observe for signs and symptoms of infection and report to physician.

Patient Outcome	Process
• *Activity*	d. Be alert for complications of prolonged bed rest: • Thrombophelbitis (use below-the-knees antiembolic hose if unable to use regular size) • Pulmonary embolus • Skin breakdown • Constipation • Urinary retention e. Establish exercise routine with physician, physical therapist, and patient.

C. *Is knowledgeable about self-care and resources for continuity of care*	5. See Chapter 5 Predischarge Phase of Hospitalization, p. 132. Include additional elements of preparation for discharge of patient.
	 a. Teach care of donor site:
	 • Wash with soap and water in or out of tub or shower.
	 • Pat dry with clean towel; finish drying with hair dryer at ''cool'' setting.
	 • Trim loose edges of gauze over donor site.
	 b. Teach care of graft site:
	 • Wash with soap and water and apply prescribed cream t.i.d.
	 • Report any change in appearance or sensation to physician:
	     Redness
	     Drainage, openings
	     Numbness, tingling
	 c. Reinforce instruction by physical therapist for home exercises.
	 d. Emphasize importance of maintaining balance nutritional intake with increased protein intake.
	 e. Discuss possibility of some pigmentation changes.

Patient Outcome	Process

The patient experiences informed, comfortable, and safe preoperative, postoperative, nad predischarge phases of hospitalization. This includes:

DESCRIPTION: Patients with idiopathic scoliosis (lateral curvature of spine) are usually adolescent females (age 9 to 16) who may have worn a brace or body cast for long periods of time. At adolescence, due to rapid growth, the curve of the spine becomes more severe and noticeable. Patients with congenital malformations such as myelomeningocele, spina bifida, and cerebral palsy may also develop scoliosis and require this surgery. The purpose of the procedure is to reduce the curve, prevent progression of the scoliosis, prevent pulmonary complications, and improve cosmetic appearance. This surgery involves a spinal fusion and insertion of a Harrington Rod to maintain stability.

NURSING ASSESSMENT: In addition to general admission assessment, the following information is especially important.
1. Assess and document physical status.
   a. Motor and sensory function of extremities
   b. Peripheral pulses
   c. Bowel function
   d. Activity pattern and problems impairing normal activity, *e.g.*, neurological deficit related to spinal cord dysfunction
   e. Menstrual history (cycle likely to be disrupted by surgery)
2. Assess and document patient and family's response to information about the disease process and anticipated surgery.
   a. Apparent anxiety level
   b. Behaviors that reflect emotional needs
   c. Patient's self-assessment of:
      • Concept of body image
      • Support people and objects
3. Assess and document patient's understanding of the disease process, treatment and anticipated surgery.

A. *Is prepared for surgery*

INTERVENTION:
1. Explain and answer questions about scheduled diagnostic studies which might include:
   a. Stress radiographs
   b. Pulmonary function
   c. Blood gases
   d. Medical photograph
   e. EKG
   f. Consults which may include cardiology, pulmonary, and neurosurgery
2. Reinforce understanding of patient and family about disease process and anticipated surgery.
3. Summarize usual preoperative preparation and provide care per hospital routine and physician's orders. See Chapter 5 Preoperative Phase of Hospitalization, p. 129. Include additional elements of preoperative care relating to spinal fusion.
   a. Make clear specific care expectations and rationale. Reinforce physician information.
      • May go to operating room in hospital bed
      • May have bowel preparation
      • May have preoperative evaluation by various therapists, *e.g.*, physical therapist, respiratory therapist
      • May stay overnight in recovery area and return to special care unit
      • May have compression dressing over incision or partial cast (full cast over back from shoulders to buttocks, cast strips over chest and abdomen)
      • Closed wound drainage system
      • Usually have indwelling urinary catheter
      • Flat in bed; log-rolling; position with pillows at back and between legs
        Practice log rolling; turn with shoulders and hips in same line.
      • Antiembolic measures: support hose, ankle exercises
      • Practice coughing, deep breathing, use of incentive spirometry, leg exercises
      • Incisional pain is severe for first few days; pain medication will be available. Patient may need to initiate request.
      • May have bone graft from iliac crest; may have increased hip pain.
      • Keep n.p.o. for 2 to 3 days, then gradually progress to ice chips and fluids.

Patient Outcome	Process

b. Anticipate need for diversional activity/studies.
- Alert play therapist, hospital school teacher.
- Consider obtaining clock, calendar, radio, magazines, prism glasses.
- Arrange care schedule to assure privacy for classes.

B. *Is free of or has minimal discomfort or postoperative complications*

4. Provide postoperative care. See Chapter 5 Postoperative Phase of Hospitalization, p. 130.
5. Intervene in the critical areas of patient care following spinal fusion.

• *Circulatory*
• *Respiratory*

a. Remain alert that shock is a major immediate postoperative complication. Call physician for:
- Decreased BP
- Pulse greater than 120
- Urine output less than 60 cc per 2 hours.

b. Assess pulmonary status and provide preventive pulmonary routine.
- Pain may hinder ability to take deep breaths or cough.
- Assess for pulmonary complications.
    Listen to audible breath sounds with stethoscope (with vital signs).
    Check for temperature elevation greater than 38.5°C.
- Consider using humidifier continuously to liquify secretions and for comfort.
- Log-roll at least q 2 hours to promote pulmonary drainage and ventilation.
- Compare blood gases with baseline data.
- Report symptoms of pulmonary embarrassment.

• *Neurological*

c. Assess neurological status. Paralysis is dreaded complication of spinal surgery.
- Check movement, sensation, strength and pulses in lower and upper extremities, dorsiflexion, plantar flexion, and quadriceps setting at least q 2 hours for first 24 hours and compare with preoperative status. Then check with vital signs q 4 hours.

• *Skeletal*

d. Maintain proper positioning to prevent rod displacement.
- Strict bed rest on either side or back
- No head elevation
- No trapeze, no transfer to stretcher
- All studies must be done at bedside with nurse assisting to log roll patient.
- Reinforce log-roll instruction. Assist patient and observe as patient gradually assumes increasing independence in correct turning.

e. Be aware of symptoms which may indicate displacement of rod:
- Popping sound
- Sudden onset of pain
- Patient may feel something slip

• *Wound healing*

f. Provide wound care:
- Monitor closed wound drainage q 2 to 4 hours. Amount should gradually decrease. Notify physician for quantity greater than 100 cc per hour.
- Check dressing for bleeding. Outline drainage on dressing upon return to ward and q 8 hours.
- Be alert for signs of infection:
    Elevated temperature
    Foul odor and/or drainage—observe under cast if possible.
    Patient may complain of gurgling or "mushy" sounds.

• *Comfort*

g. Keep patient as clean and dry as possible.
- Remove excess particles of plaster from bed.
- Use hair dryer on cool setting for itching.
- Use alcohol on skin to relieve itching; do not use powder.
- Dry thoroughly after urination or bath.
- Protect lower edge of cast with plastic material.
- Wash axilla carefully and use deodorant.
- Wash hair as needed; use in-bed rinser.
- Wash perineum as a part of daily care. Provide privacy; be matter-of-fact.
- For females: Be prepared that menstrual cycle may occur. Suggest tampons or sanitary pads attached to panties.
- Cast may have rough edges and be uncomfortable to patient when turned to side. Use discretion with padding—too much padding will increase pressure.

h. Look for pain cues, *e.g.*, requests to be turned frequently, restlessness, increased pulse.
- Give analgesics as ordered.
- Patient may need encouragement to take injectable analgesics. Children and adolescents dislike "shots"

• *Elimination*

i. Monitor output via indwelling catheter for first 24 hours; then patient will need fracture bedpan.

Patient Outcome	Process
	• Be careful when removing bedpan not to spill urine which could cause wound contamination.

        • Be careful when removing bedpan not to spill urine which could cause wound contamination.

        • Patient may have difficulty voiding in prone position and need assistance. Be resourceful.

        • Patient must log-roll onto bedpan.

        • Observe for symptoms of urinary tract infection.

    j. Listen for return of bowel sounds and passing of flatus.

        • Determine date of last bowel movement (check chart and ask patient).

        • Request stool softener and suppository.

        • Observe for abdominal distention; paralytic ileus is common.

        • As diet progresses, encourage fruit, vegetables, and bulk.

C. *Is prepared for application of body cast*

6. Provide factual and physical perparation for suture removal and cast application (usually applied on tenth postoperative day).

    a. Institute immediate preparation for cast application:

        • Give laxative several days prior to ensure minimal distention.

        • On day of application:

            Light meals to minimize distention

            Thorough cleansing bath and shampoo (it will be the last body bath for six months).

            Inspect skin for open wounds and areas of possible irritation.

            For females: Send to cast room with bikini panties if available.

            Premedicate if ordered.

    b. Review actual procedure and sensation patient will experience. Assess patient's anxiety level and give information which might include:

        • Instruct patient to lie very still during the procedure (approximately one hour). Although the table used for cast application may feel like "being on a tightrope" there is no danger of falling.

        • *Procedure:* Patient will go to cast room in hospital bed. If the patient is in a partial cast, this will be removed. The subcutaneous sutures will be removed, which will be momentarily uncomfortable but not painful. The back will be cleaned, which will feel cool. The nurse will place a body stocking from knees to ears and this will be only thing worn during procedure. Three doctors will lift patient off bed and place on Risser table. Chin strap and straps crossed over iliac crests will provide stability and traction. Felt padding is applied over bony prominences (iliac crests, shoulder blades); a thin layer of cast padding is applied. Stockinette is pulled over face and hair as protection from plaster and nose hole is made to permit easy breathing. Plaster is applied and body cast is molded tightly over entire torso, which requires pressure and rubbing. Plaster is at first cold and damp. Later it becomes very hot as the material reacts chemically; then it becomes cold for about 12 hours. The front of the cast is trimmed around arm holes, neck, and groin using cast knife or saw. The saw will sound very loud and may feel warm; reassure patient that the skin will not be cut. Patient is returned to bed. Then back of cast is trimmed around armholes, neck, groin. Any plaster noted on skin (arms and legs) after cast application will be removed with washcloth and warm water immediately. Plaster hardens quickly and would be more difficult and painful to remove when dry.

7. Provide postcast application care.

    a. Leave cast uncovered for 24 to 48 hours for complete drying and evaporation of water from plaster.

    b. Be aware that patient will be cold while cast is drying.

        • When drying do not cover cast with blankets to keep patient warm; this prolongs drying time. May cover other parts of the body with blanket.

    c. Keep patient stationary on back for four hours.

    d. Check under back of cast for large sheet wrinkles and/or foreign objects that would tend to dent cast.

    e. Provide comfort measures:

        • Wash off plaster from skin as soon as possible.

        • Cover patient with towel at neck and blanket over arms and legs.

        • Be alert to signs and symptoms of tightness of cast, at the neck, arm pits, shoulder, pelvis, buttocks, hips.

        • Using pillows, give full support of body when positioning patient on sides and abdomen.

    f. Provide skin care measures:

        • Observe for and remove any plaster "crumbs" on skin and/or bedding which may irritate skin and lead to eventual breakdown.

        • Observe for rough edges on cast, especially those areas which have been trimmed. "Petal" (cover) edges with moleskin or tape.

Patient Outcome	Process
	• Feel under edges of cast for areas of pressure, blisters, or tightness. Attempt to place 1 to 2 fingers between skin and cast to assess degree of tightness and areas of potential breakdown.

g. Be alert to symptoms of cast syndrome, which is a potentially fatal condition and thought to be caused when the superior mesenteric artery compresses the third portion of the duodenum resulting in high intestinal obstruction.
  • Report to physician these signs and symptoms:
    Nausea, vomiting
    Vague abdominal pain
    Complaint of tightness of cast over abdomen

h. Assist with treatment of cast syndrome.
  • "Window" cut in front of cast to relieve pressure.
  • Cast may be removed.
  • Intestinal decompression by use of NG tube

i. Assist patient to resume normal body functions.
  • After cast is dry, attempt sitting with assistance. Progress as tolerated to walking. Remember patient has been on prolonged bedrest and will have orthostatic hypotension and will fatigue easily.
  • Assist in use of toilet. Remind patient to wipe from front to back. Use protective padding at back of cast.
  • Provide preventive constipation routine (stool softeners, diet).
  • Notify physician if cast interferes with sitting, standing, eating, as it may need to be trimmed.

D. *Is knowledgeable about nature of illness, self-care, and resources for continuity of care.*

8. See Chapter 5 Predischarge Phase of Hospitalization, p. 132. Include additional elements of preparation for discharge.
  a. Teach patient and family specific care skills:
    • Cast care:
      Keep cast clean and dry. May use small amount of white powder cleanser with damp (not wet) cloth.
      Do not take tub bath or shower.
      Do not scratch under cast. No objects are to be placed under the cast.
      Be aware that small objects may fall into cast which could cause irritation and infection, *e.g.*, bobby pins.
      Be alert to signs of infection:
        —Localized pain
        —Elevated temperature
        —Foul odor, drainage
        —Gurgling or mushy sounds
      Observe under edges of cast each day for pressure around arm holes, iliac crest, and sacral area. Use adhesive tape to cover rough edges of cast. Teach family how to check with fingers and have a return demonstration.
      Do not pull out padding which could alter fit of cast.
      Use plastic bag to protect cast when washing hair.
    • Hair washing suggestions include:
      Spray attachment to faucet
      Have patient lie on bed with head off bed, put bucket under the head, and pour water over.
      Go to beauty parlor.
  b. Assess nutritional needs and provide teaching as needed:
    • Stress need for foods high in protein, Vitamins C and D, calcium and phosphorus to aid in bone healing.
    • Encourage raw fruits, vegetables, fluids, and cereals with bulk.
    • Advise patient to maintain present weight. Significant weight gain or loss would alter fit of cast. Avoid pregnancy during the period when the cast is on.
  c. Assist patient with planning clothing selection. Suggestions may include:
    • Loose fitting tops and dresses, *e.g.*, smock, tent dresses, pants with elastic or drawstring waists, or clothing that fastens in front.
    • Slip-on shoes are best. Avoid high-heeled shoes.
    • Use of scarf at the neck helps decrease irritation from the cast.
  d. Instruct patient to report immediately to physician if nausea and vomiting occurs.

Subarachnoid hemorrhage resulting from ruptured cerebral aneurysm

Patient Outcome

The patient experiences informed, comfortable, and safe preoperative, postoperative and predischarge phases of hospitalization. This includes:

Process

DESCRIPTION: Persons who suffer subarachnoid hemorrhage as a result of a ruptured cerebral aneurysm often experience the acute onset of severe headache, neck stiffness, nausea, vomiting, and abrupt change in level of consciousness. Although the aneurysm is a congenital defect of a cerebral artery (Fig. 5-15.), the hemorrhage does not usually occur until middle age or later. There may or may not have been premonitory symptoms. After the initial bleed, there is a high risk of rebleed and death within several weeks. Subarachnoid hemorrhage patients are classified by a grading system with grade one being those who are alert and neurologically intact to those who are grade four or five being those who are in deep coma. The initial medical treatment includes adherence to a specific program which reduces the possibility of a recurrent hemorrhage. Once patients undergo surgery for repair of the aneurysm (Fig. 5-16.), their postoperative care becomes that of a routine craniotomy. After the aneurysm has been repaired, it is unlikely that the patient will have this problem again. There may or may not be permanent neurological deficits associated with this problem. An occasional patient may require a shunt for communicating hydrocephalus which has resulted from the effect of blood in the subarachnoid space.

NURSING ASSESSMENT: In addition to general admission assessment, the following information is important.
1. Assess and document baseline level of consciousness (LOC).
   a. Alert, awake, oriented to time, place, person, and self.
   b. Behaves and responds inappropriately to questions and situations
   c. Increasingly irritable to environment
   d. Drowsy, lethargic, decreased responsiveness to stimuli
   e. Able to follow simple commands only
   f. Responds to name verbally or nonverbally
   g. Pushes away or withdraws from painful stimulus
   h. Responds to pain or environmental stimulus by abnormal posturing (decorticate, decerebrate)
   i. No observable response to stimuli
2. Assess other neurological symptoms and signs including:
   a. Degree and type of headache
   b. Photophobia
   c. Neck rigidity
   d. Double or blurred vision
   e. Nausea, vomiting

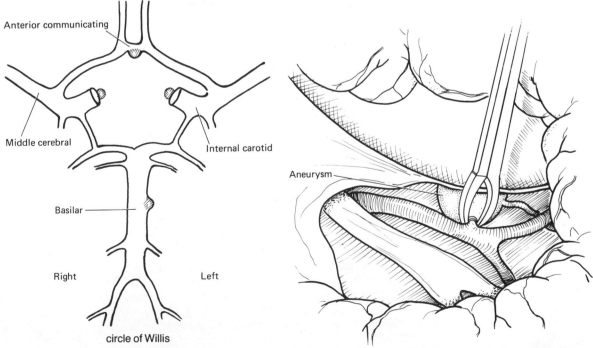

Anterior communicating

Middle cerebral

Internal carotid

Basilar

Right

Left

circle of Willis

Aneurysm

Fig. 5-15. Common sites of aneurysms.   *Fig. 5-16. Intracranial application of clip on aneurysm.*

Patient Outcome	Process

    f.   Pupil changes: size and reaction to light. Compare right to left.

    g.   Ptosis, abnormal eye movements

    h.   Strength and movement of extremeities. Compare right to left.

    i.   Abnormal motor tone—spastic or flaccid

    j.   Seizure activity

    k.   Vital signs, especially blood pressure

    l.   Speech

3. Report the folliwng changes immediately to physician:
   a. Decrease in LOC, pupil changes
   b. Elevation of blood pressure, usually in combination with other neurological signs
   c. Increase in headache and/or visual symptoms
   d. Seizure activity and/or motor weakness (Note: a to d may represent a rebleed of the aneurysm or cerebral vasospasm.)
   e. Increased respirations and complaints of chest pain
4. Assess and document risk factors/disease states which might affect pre- and postoperative care:
   a. Cardiovascular status: rate and rhythm of pulse, EKG, history of cardiac disease, blood pressure, history of thrombophlebitis/pulmonary embolus
   b. Pulmonary status: pulmonary disease, breath sounds, rate, expansion, and smoking history
   c. Renal status: voiding difficulties, and infections—renal disease
   d. Gastrointestinal status: bowel habits
5. Assess and document patient's health status and habits prior to admission.
   a. Potential for self-care or need for supportive care
   b. Medications
   c. Diet
   d. Home health supervision/support.

A. *Is benefiting from therapeutic environment to reduce possibility of aneurysm rebleed.*

INTERVENTION:

1. Maintain appropriate therapeutic environment (''Subarachnoid hemorrhage (SAH) Precautions'') for the patient. Avoid any Valsalva's maneuvers, sudden changes in position, sudden increases in environmental stimuli and/or psychological stimuli which may result in blood pressure elevation thereby increasing risk of rebleeding.
   a. Establish restful surroundings: quiet, private room with subdued lighting and limited visitors.
   b. Maintain strict bed rest with head of bed kept in constant position—usually flat and small pillow if permitted by physician.
   c. Give total supportive nursing care.
   d. Monitor neurological signs and vital signs q 1 hour until stable. No rectal temperatures.
   e. Avoid need for straining or enemas, by good bowel regimen. Avoid rectal stimuli.
   f. Give (IV) antifibrinolytic agent as ordered.
   g. Be aware that patient's impaired judgment requires special provisions for patient safety. Use appropriate restraints.
   h. Anticipate that patient may have several lumbar punctures and minimum of two cerebral angiograms and cerebral blood flow studies.
   i. Observe for change in psychological status due to sleep deprivation and stress. Request order for medication to reduce anxiety.
2. Depending on the patient's state of cerebral function, how long patient has been in the SAH environment, and pre-SAH personality, observe the patient's varying reaction(s) to the following:
   a. Lack of control over environment
   b. Loss of independence
   c. Sleep deprivation
   d. Social isolation
   e. Fears of rebleed, neurological deficit(s), death, surgery
   f. Family and staff anxieties
3. Recognize significant change in the patient's emotional behavior. Discuss this with physician, family, and health team members. Consider implementing the following:
   a. Make minor, individualized modifications in the SAH environment, *e.g.*, use of radio, TV.
   b. Extend visiting times for immediate family.
   c. Increase the patient's involvement in his care planning.

Patient Outcome	Process
	d. Take vital signs every 2 hours at night so patient can increase sleep time.
	e. Administer ordered pain medication and or mild sedation to facilitate patient comfort and relaxation.
	4. Provide continuing information and emotional support to patient and family throughout preoperative waiting period.
B. *Is maintaining body system function with out complications*	5. Provide care to assist early detection and treatment of acute problems. Collaborate with physician as necessary regarding the following:
	a. Respiratory distress: Patient may arrest with aneurysm rebleed.
	• Assess change in character, rate, and depth of respirations.
	• Have equipment available: airway, suction.
	b. Cardiac distress: Stress may exacerbate previous cardiac disease. Arrhythmia may be seen after SAH.
	• Assess changes in rate and thythm of pulse.
	• Be aware of previous existing cardiac problems.
	• Obtain 12-lead EKG.
	c. Emboli:
	• Be aware that drug therapy may have a potential side effect of thromboemboli.
	• Implement preventive program including antiembolic hose on admission.
	• Provide active/passive range of motion exercises to extremities q 2 hours during a day; q 4 hours at night.
	• Assess for signs and symptoms of phlebitis especially in calves and IV sites.
	d. Fluid and electrolyte balance:
	• Keep accurate intake and output because of constant IV therapy.
	• Check for signs and symptoms of dehydration and sodium imbalance, *i.e.*, hyponatremia
	• Anticipate orders for fluid restriction.
	6. Prevent or minimize effects of long-term bed rest.
	a. Establish pulmonary care regimen with exception of coughing.
	• Use nebulizer for patient with nasal stuffiness.
	• Refer to Chapter 2 Pulmonary Care Guidelines, p. 29.
	b. Establish bladder care regimen with special attention to possibility of urinary retention.
	• Refer to Chapter 2 Bladder Care Guidelines, p. 23.
	c. Maintain bowel care program.
	• Refer to Chapter 2 Bowel Care Guidelines, p. 25.
	d. Maintain skin integrity.
	• Refer to Chapter 2 Skin Care Guidelines, p. 31.
	e. Establish activity program.
	• Turn, reposition q 2 hours during day and q 4 hours at night.
	• Give range of motion exercises; active or passive depending upon patient's capability q 2 to 4 hours.
C. *Is prepared for surgery and post operative phase*	7. Facilitate patient's/family understanding.
	a. Provide accurate information to questions as they arise.
	b. Be aware of information given to patient and family; reinforce explanations.
	c. Defer specific questions about operative procedure, risks, and prognosis to surgeon.
	8. Summarize features of preoperative preparation and provide care as needed per hospital routine.
	a. Refer to Chapter 5 Preoperative Phase of Hospitalization, p. 129.
	b. Refer to Craniotomy Guidelines, p. 153 for specific aspects of preoperative care.
	c. Be prudent in appropriately providing realistic amount of information to patient; this is not the time to magnify patient anxiety.
	d. Emphasize necessity for adjustment to change from quiet, dark environment to frequently noisy, bright Intensive Care Unit.
D. *Is free of or has minimal post operative complications*	9. Provide postoperative care. Refer to Chapter 5 Postoperative Phase of Hospitalization, p. 130.
	10. Intervene in the critical areas of care following surgery. Refer to Craniotomy Guideline, p. 154 for specific aspects of care.
	11. Assess the impact of any neurological deficit on the patient and family.
	a. Consider such deficits as:
	• Mental status: impaired judgment, memory, loss of inhibitions
	• Ptosis
	• Hemiparesis
	b. Reinforce physician's explanation that deficit may be temporary.

Patient Outcome	Process
	c. Support and counsel patient/family.
	• Accept behavior and encourage positive coping mechanisms.
	• Reinforce positive signs of patient progress.
	• Utilize available inpatient services such as chaplain and/or clinician.
	• Discuss typical living situations and realistic modifications in family routines.
	• Prepare for emotional reactions patient/family may experience at home such as frustration, depression, dependence; suggest possible approaches to solve problems.
E. *Is knowledgeable about home care and resources for continuity of care*	12. Initiate and coordinate discharge planning.
	a. Refer to Chapter 5 Predischarge Phase of Hospitalization, p. 132.
	b. Collaborate with physician about tentative discharge date and medical plans.
	d. Identify patient/family needs and resources; problem solve with them using other resources as necessary.
	d. Provide teaching related to needed skills and knowledge. Check for accurate understanding and observe return demonstration of skills. Components include:
	• Patient's current mental status and ability to make judgments
	• Emotional considerations
	• Increasing independence in resumption of activities of daily living to include:
	Personal hygiene
	Ambulation
	Homemaking/occupation
	Recreation
	Sexual activities.
	• Bowel and bladder care
	• Use of assistive devices, *e.g.*, sling, walker, cane, commode chair
	• Care of scalp and head dressing
	e. Determine need to initiate interagency referral.
	f. Consider with family and health care team the possibility of referral to a rehabilitation facility if patient has sensory/motor deficit.
	g. Inform patient of available community resources which may assist in continuity of care.
	h. Write nursing discharge note to include the following:
	• Plan for dealing with any pain
	• Appearance of wound
	• Level of independent activity
	• Mode of travel when leaving ward and with whom
	• Patient outcomes met and unmet at discharge
	• Plan for home care
	• Referrals made.

Thyroidectomy

Patient Outcome	Process

The patient experiences informed, comfortable and safe preoperative, postoperative and predischarge phases of hospitalization. This includes:

DESCRIPTION: A thyroidectomy (removal of thyroid gland) may be total or partial. A total thyroidectomy is indicated for thyroid malignancy following which the patients must remain on thyroid hormone replacement. A subtotal thyroidectomy (removal of approximately ⁵⁄₆th of the gland) is performed to correct hyperthyroidism and simple goiter. The procedure is carried out through a midline low collar incision to expose the underlying thyroid gland. Following identification of the laryngeal nerve, the thyroid artery and vein are ligated and the thyroid tissue is removed from its attachment to the trachea. A Penrose drain may be inserted if the wound is not dry.

NURSING ASSESSMENT: In addition to the general admission assessment, the following information is especially important.

1. Assess and document physical and mental status.
   a. Signs and symptoms related to underlying disease:
      - Thyroid function studies
      - Nutritional status, *e.g.,* weight loss, appetite
      - Hoarseness
      - Changes in physical appearance, *e.g.,* skin, hair, protruding eyeballs
      - Cardiovascular status
      - Bowel function, *e.g.,* diarrhea
      - Activity and rest patterns, *e.g.,* mood swings from mild euphoria to hyperactivity to extreme fatigue and depression
   b. Risk factors:
      - Presence of other disease states, *e.g.,* diabetes, renal disease, blood dyscrasia, chronic obstructive pulmonary disease
      - Smoking history
2. Assess and document patient's response to information about the disease process, treatment, and anticipated surgery.
   a. Apparent anxiety level
   b. Previous experience with surgery
3. Assess and document health habits/life-style prior to admission.
   a. Potential for self-care or need for supportive care
   b. Medications
   c. Diet
   d. Home health supervision/support.
4. Assess and document patient's understanding of the disease process, treatment, and anticipated surgery.

A. *Is prepared for surgery*

INTERVENTION:

1. Reinforce understanding of patient and family regarding the disease process, implications, and anticipated surgery.
2. Summarize usual preoperative preparation and provide care per hospital procedure and physician's orders. See Chapter 5. Preoperative Phase of Hospitalization, p. 129.
   Include specific postoperative expectation that tracheostomy tray will be kept at bedside.

B. *Is free or has mini-discomfort or postoperative complications*

3. Provide postoperative care. See Chapter 5 Postoperative Phase of Hospitalization, p. 130.
4. Intervene in the critical areas of patient care following thyroidectomy.
   a. Prevent respiratory obstruction.
      - Elevate head of bed.
      - Observe for signs and symptoms of respiratory distress and report to physician.
      - Assist physician if necessary to open and evacuate hematoma from wound.
   b. Provide/teach wound care and precautionary measures.
      - Instruct patient to avoid flexion and hyperextension of neck.
      - Support head and neck when changing position.
      - Observe for swelling and bleeding.
         Check dressing q 1 hour × 8.
         Check for complaint of fullness and tightness.
   c. Relieve discomfort from sore throat and tracheal irritation.
      - Offer ice chips and soothing lozenges.
      - Place humidifier at bedside.
   d. Observe for hoarseness.
      - Expect some hoarseness the first few days (due to irritation from endotracheal tube, edema).

227

Patient Outcome	Process
	• Discourage overuse of voice during recovery phase. e. Assess for signs and symptoms of tetany (Parathyroids may be damaged or removed during surgery). • Numbness and tingling, especially around mouth • Cramping • Muscle twitching • Decreased serum calcium • Positive Chvostek's sign (contraction or spasm of facial muscles resulting from tapping the facial nerves against the bone just anterior to the ear) • Positive Trousseau's sign (carpal spasm induced by occluding the brachial artery for three minutes with inflated blood pressure cuff) f. Report abnormal responses to physician.
C. *Is knowledgeable about nature of illness, self-care, and resources for continuity of care*	5. See Chapter 5 Predischarge Phase of Hospitalization, p. 132. Include additional elements of preparation for discharge of patient such as a. Instruct patient to report signs and symptoms of tetany to physician immediately. b. Teach effects and side effects of any medications, *e.g.,* calcium. c. Assure that return appointment for evaluation is given.

Total hip replacement

The patient experiences informed, comfortable, and safe preoperative, postoperative, and predischarge phases of hospitalization. This includes:

DESCRIPTION: Patients are usually elderly and often have a long history of degenerative joint disease (usually arthritis) causing pain and decreased mobility. They may have had other hip surgeries. The surgical procedure replaces both ball and socket parts of the hip joint. The head of the femur (ball) is replaced by a stainless steel prosthesis and the acetabulum (socket) is replaced by a hard plastic component (Fig. 5–17). Parts are cemented into the bone.

NURSING ASSESSMENT: In addition to general admission assessment, the following information is especially important.
1. Assess and document physical and mental status.
    a. Functional limitations.
    b. Bowel and bladder problems.
    c. Baseline neurovascular status:
        • Pain, pulses, paralysis, paresthesia, pallor
        • History of phlebitis
        • Gait
    d. Signs and symptoms of infection:
        • Skin lesion
        • Fever
        • Sore throat or cold
        • Urinalysis.
    e. Mental clarity.

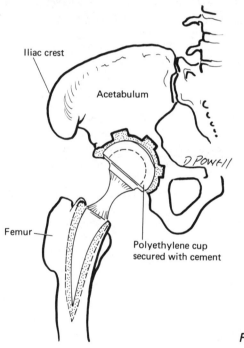

Fig. 5-17. Prosthesis —total hip replacement.

2. Assess and document patient's response to information about disease process and anticipated surgery:
    a. Apparent anxiety level
    b. Expectations regarding relief of pain and improvement in mobility
3. Assess and document patient's understanding of the disease process, treatment, and anticipated surgery.
4. Assess and document home environment to which patient will return.
    a. Physical layout
    b. Steps into house and stairs within house
    c. Others at home to provide help

A. *Is prepared for surgery*

INTERVENTION:
1. Eliminate possible sources of infection.
    a. Do not give injections in affected hip.
    b. Give antibacterial scrub to operative area evening before and morning of surgery.

Patient Outcome	Process
	2. Summarize usual preoperative preparation and provie care per hospital routine and physician's orders. See Chapter 5 Preoperative Phase of Hospitalization, p. 129. Include additional elements of preoperative care relating to hip replacement.

a. Make clear specific care expectations and rationale. Reinforce patient's understanding of:
- Spica dressing: soft, bulky compression dressing around waist and operative leg
- Closed wound drainage system
- Antiembolic measures may include: support hose, anticoagulants, intermittent compression boots, and ankle exercises.
- Thorough pulmonary routine due to age and immobility
- Careful positioning to avoid extreme adduction; abduction pillow to keep legs apart; no crossing ankles or knees
- Use of urinal and bedpan; possibility of catheter
- Use of overhead frame with trapeze and knee exerciser to assist in moving and exercises

b. Answer common questions which arise:
- Length of surgery (2 to 4 hours)
- Recovery Room (2 to 4 hours)
- Pain is considerable for about three days; patient to ask for available medication.
- Bed rest 3 to 5 days, then gradual, progressive ambulation under physical therapist supervision

c. Emphasize to patient and family that it requires time (about six weeks) to achieve the expected great relief from pain and improvement in mobility.

B. *Is free of or has minimal discomforts or postoperative complications*

3. Provide postoperative care. See Chapter 5 Postoperative Phase of Hospitalization, p. 130.
4. Intervene in the critical areas of patient care following hip replacement.

a. Provide thorough pulmonary care.

• *Respiratory*

- Turn, cough, deep breathe q 2 hours during first 24 hours and q 4 hours thereafter.
- Use incentive spirometry or IPPB as needed.
- Check for symptoms or complications:
  - Embolus: dyspnea, chest pain, tachycardia, decreased pO_2
  - Fluid overload: dyspnea, rapid short breaths, wet breath sounds
  - Pneumonia: congested cough, fever, pleuritic pain

• *Neurovascular*

b. Check and compare with baseline neurovascular data: q 2 hours × 24 hours; then q 8 hours:
- Peripheral circulation: color, capillary filling, temperature, sensation
- Peripheral pulses: dorsalis pedis (top of foot), posterior tibial (behind interior aspect of ankle) (Fig. 5–12.)

c. Test for intact motor and sensory nerves when checking vital signs:
- Motor:
  - Sciatic: dorsiflexion (upward movement) to toes and foot
  - Femoral: tightening of quadriceps (thigh muscle)
- Sensory to foot and toes: Check by response to finger touch.

• *Musculoskeletal*

d. Provide careful positioning:
- Keep leg abducted (legs apart); maintain neutral position of knees and toes (toward ceiling).
  - May use abduction pillow
  - Turn only to operative side, using pillow between legs
  - Strict bed rest for three days
  - All radiographs portable
- Do not adduct (bring legs toward midline) nor allow legs to cross or internally rotate foot.
- Check for symptoms of dislocation:
  - Pain in groin (operative side)
  - May hear or feel "popping" of dislocation
  - Position of leg: abduction, external rotation
  - Change in leg length (shortening)
- Do not elevate head of bed more than 45° to avoid acute flexion.

• *Circulatory*

e. Prevent thrombophlebitis.
- Check signs and symptoms of thrombophlebitis, q 8 hours: Homan's sign—pain in calf on dorsiflexion; localized warmth; swelling; pain.
- Be sure anticoagulant agent is ordered and observe for side effects.
- Provide antiembolic hose as ordered.
- Position: Semi-Fowlers. Maximize venous drainage from legs; avoid acute flexion of hips.

Patient Outcome	Process
	f. Minimize adverse reaction to anticoagulant agent, dextran.
	• Observe patient for rash generalized itching which may occur within first hour after infusion is started.
	• Infuse no faster than 50 cc per hour to prevent fluid overload and maximize anticoagulant effects.
• *Skin*	g. Check skin especially over body prominences during bath and while turning.
	• Remove elastic hose completely once daily during bath for skin inspection: (especially heels, ankles, top of foot).
	• Elevate heel slightly to relieve heel pressure when lying on back.
	• Change positions from back to affected side while coughing and deep breathing; massage back and sacrum gently.
	• Provide sheepskin for patients with special skin care needs.
• *Elimination*	h. Consider patient's response to immobilization; previous bowel, or bladder history.
	• Check daily and keep accurate record of I and O and bowel function status.
	• Obtain order for laxative of patient's choice as necessary.
• *Wound healing*	i. Check for signs of healing and provide wound care. Report excessive drainage to physician.
	• Check closed wound drainage system and dressing while checking vital signs during first 24 hours; then q 8 hours. Reinforce dressing p.r.n.
	• After dressing is removed, may spray once using a protective coating as ordered.
	• After 24 hours, check wound for warmth, swelling, redness, and drainage q 8 hours.
	• Be aware that some bruising around wound is normal.
	• Be sure antibiotics are ordered.
• *Comfort*	j. Promote comfort:
	• Help patient understand that preoperative joint pain will differ from postoperative incisional pain.
	• Teach patient that complete pain relief will not be attainable in immediate postoperative period but that it will be tolerable with analgesics.
	• Consider possible side effects of selected analgesics, *i.e.,* depressed respirations, effect on mental faculties, decreased mobility.
	• Make sure overhead frame is on bed to assist patient.
• *Activity*	k. Assemble and instruct patient in use of knee exerciser. Start three days postoperatively as ordered by physician. Consult physical therapy as needed.
	• Assure that equipment is assembled properly to include: two pulleys, handle, six-foot cord, spreader bar, knee sling, two side arm bars.
	• Supervise patient in proper use of knee exerciser: knee flexion, straight leg raising, abduction; use 5 minutes each waking hour.
	• Reinforce use of exerciser throughout entire postoperative period.
	l. Gradually progress activities per physician orders.
	• Third day postoperative out of bed, partial weight bearing 15 minutes, b.i.d.; increase time and frequency as tolerated.
	• Physical therapy is to see patient for partial weight bearing and progressive ambulation.
	• Assist patient with walking, using assistive devices prescribed (crutches, walker).
C. *Is knowledgeable about nature of illness, self-care, and resources for continuity of care*	5. See Chapter 5 Predischarge Phase of Hospitalization, p. 132. Include additional elements of preparation for discharge.
	a. Assess home environment considering limitations:
	• Hazards such as steps, bathroom facilities (shower, low toilet seats), distance between bath and bedroom, throw rugs, small children, dogs, electrical cords, highly waxed floor.
	b. Discuss resumption/restriction of activities.
	• Generally, partial weight bearing for six weeks (crutches, walker)
	• Avoid acute flexion for six weeks.
	Driving or riding in car for prolonged periods
	Low chairs
	Activities that would require stooping or squatting.
	• Elevate legs to help reduce swelling.
	c. Assure that patient and family understand exercise instructions given by physical therapist.
	• Hip flexion, extension, abduction, straight leg raising
	d. Provide prescription and drug information:
	• Analgesic
	• Anticoagulant: warfarin (Coumadin) or aspirin (never both)

Patient Outcome	Process

Coumadin: Patient must arrange to have regular blood tests at home. Contact physician for any symptoms of bleeding, *e.g.*, nose bleeds, blood in vomitus or stools, easy bruising.

Do not take aspirin or other over-the-counter drugs which contain salicylates, unless ordered.

Take acetaminophen instead, *e.g.*, Tylenol, Datril.

Aspirin: Dose must be prescribed by physician.

- Resumption of previously prescribed drugs must be checked by physician prior to discharge.

e. Instruct patient to report signs of infections:
  - Incision (hip joint): redness, heat, swelling, drainage, tenderness
  - Any other suspected infection which could result in hip joint becoming infected: sore throat, urinary tract infection, prostatitis, dental extractions

f. Assure that patient has return appointment and knows importantce of follow-up medical care.

g. Initiate interagency referral as indicated.

Patient Outcome	Process

The patient experiences informed, comfortable and safe preoperative, postoperative and predischarge phases of hospitalization. This includes:

DESCRIPTION: Patients receiving a total knee replacement are usually elderly and often have a long history of degenerative joint disease (usually arthritis) which causes pain and decreased mobility. The surgical procedure involves resurfacing the distal femur with a metal prosthesis and the proximal tibia with a hard plastic component (Fig. 5-18.). These parts are cemented into the bone. The patella may or may not be replaced. There are several kinds of prostheses available; the choice depends upon the patient's condition and the physician preference. Common names include: Guepar, Marmor, Spherocentric, Duopatella, Walldius, Townsend.

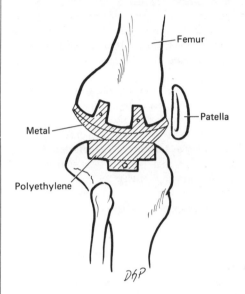

Fig. 5-18. *Prosthesis —total knee replacement.*

NURSING ASSESSMENT: In addition to the general admission assessment, the following information is especially important.
1. Assess and document physical status.
   a. Baseline neurovascular status:
      • Pain, pulses, paralysis, paresthesia, temperature, pallor
      • Range of motion
      • History of phlebitis, peripheral vascular disease
   b. Skin status: general condition of skin and any lesions
   c. Infection: skin and nails, oral cavity, urinary tract, respiratory system
2. Assess and document physical and mental ability including methods of coping with pain and disability.
   a. Level of independence
   b. Mental clarity, level of cooperation
   c. Functional limitations, *e.g.,* other arthritic joints which will affect activities of daily living
   d. Assistive devices used by patient
   e. Bowel and bladder habits, identify problems.
   f. Current drugs used, *e.g.,* to treat rheumatic disease processes; habit-forming medications (narcotics, sleeping pills, over-counter drugs)
3. Assess and document home environment.
   a. Physical layout, *e.g.,* multi-levels, indoor or outdoor plumbing
   b. Hazards, *e.g.,* throw rugs, floor coverings, steps
   c. Assistance patient will need at home and availability of same
4. Assess and document patient's response to information about the disease process and anticipated surgery.
   a. Apparent anxiety level
   b. Expectations regarding relief of pain and improvement in mobility
5. Assess and document understanding of disease process and anticipated surgery.

A. *Is prepared for surgery*

INTERVENTION:
1. Summarize usual preoperative preparation and provide care per hospital routine and physician's orders. See Chapter 5 Preoperative Phase of Hospitalization, p. 129. Include additional elements of preoperative care relating to knee replacement.

Patient Outcome	Process

	a. Eliminate possible sources of infection.
	  • Give antibacterial scrub to knee evening before and morning of surgery.
	b. Reinforce information given by physician.
	c. Emphasize postoperative expectations such as
	  • Dressing will be soft, bulky compression dressing with splint or knee immobilizer.
	  • Closed wound drainage system or Penrose drain.
	  • Antiembolic measures may include support hose: anticoagulant dextran, heparin sodium, (Heparin), aspirin; ankle exercises.
	  • Use of overhead frame with trapeze and knee exerciser to assist in moving and exercise
	  • No pillow under knee is permitted after the knee immobilizer is removed.

B. *Is free of or has minimal discomfort or postoperative complications*
 	
• *Neurovascular*
	2. Provide postoperative care. See Chapter 5 Postoperative Phase of Hospitalization, p. 130.
	a. Check affected leg and compare with baseline neurovascular data: q 2 hours × 24 hours, then q 4 hours:
	  • Peripheral circulation: color, capillary filling, temperature, sensation
	  • Peripheral pulses: dorsalis pedis (top of foot), posterior tibial (behind interior aspect of ankle) (Fig. 5–12.)
	b. Test for intact motor and sensory nerves when checking vital signs.
	  • Peroneal: Check ability to dorsiflex foot of affected leg.
	  • Sensory to foot, toes: Check response to finger touch.

• *Musculoskeletal*	c. Provide appropriate positioning/activity.
	  • Elevate foot of bed 30°.
	  • Place one pillow under splint to keep heel off bed.
	  • Turn as desired. Keep leg elevated. May use pillow between legs in side position for comfort.
	  • Out of bed in chair with leg elevated first day unless contraindicated.
	d. Assemble and instruct patient in use of knee exerciser as ordered.
	  • Assure that equipment is assembled properly to include: two pulleys, handle, six-foot cord, spreader bar, kneel sling, two side arm bars.
	  • Supervise patient in proper use of knee exerciser: knee flexion, straight leg raising, abduction; use 5 minutes each waking hour.
	  • Place sling directly under thigh just above knee. Avoid positioning sling under knee.
	  • Reinforce use of exerciser throughout hospitalization.

• *Wound healing*	e. Provide wound care.
	  • Check closed wound drainage system, dressing, and operative area for warmth, swelling, and redness when checking vital signs during first 24 hours, then q 8 hours.
	  • May spray wound once with protective coating as ordered when dressing is removed.
	  • Call physician for excessive drainage.
	  • Be aware that some bruising around wound is normal.

• *Circulatory*	f. Prevent thrombophlebitis.
	  • Check signs and symptoms of thrombophlebitis q 8 hours: Homan's signs (pain in calf on dorsiflexion), localized warmth, swelling, pain.
	  • Be sure anticoagulant agent is ordered and observe for for side effects.
	  • Provide embolic hose as ordered on unaffected leg.
	  • Maintain feet elevation.
	g. Minimize adverse reaction to dextran, an anticoagulant agent.
	  • Observe patient for rash or generalized itching which may occur within first hour of infusion.
	  • Infuse no faster than 50 cc per hour.
	h. Consider effects of immobilization on bowel and bladder function. See Chapter 2 Bowel Care Guidelines, p. 25.

C. *Is knowledgeable about nature of illness, self-care, and resources for continuity of care*	3. See Chapter 5 Predischarge Phase of Hospitalization, p. 132. Include additional elements of preparation for discharge.
	a. Discuss resumption/restriction of activities.
	  • Permit partial weight bearing usually with use of assistive devices, *e.g.,* walker, cane, crutches.
	  • Continue knee exercises as taught by physical therapy.
	b. Provide drug information and prescription.
	  • Analgesic
	  • Anticoagulant: warfarin (Coumadin) or aspirin (never both)

Patient Outcome	Process
	Coumadin: Collaborate with physician for arrangements to have prothrombin time monitored after discharge by referring physician or public health nurse.

Aspirin: Dose must be prescribed by physician.

Instruct patient to report any evidence of bleeding, *e.g.,* nose bleeds, blood in vomitus or stools, easy bruising.

- Do not take aspirin or other over-the-counter drugs which contain salicylates, *e.g.,* Bufferin, Alka-Seltzer. May take acetaminophen instead (Tylenol, Datril)
- Resumption of previously prescribed drugs must be checked by physician prior to discharge.

c. Instruct patient to report signs of infection.
- Incision: redness, heat, swelling, drainage, tenderness
- Any other suspected infection which could result in knee becoming infected, *e.g.,* urinary tract infection, prostatitis, dental extractions

d. Initiate interagency referral as needed.

e. Assure that patient has return appointment and knows importance of follow-up care.

Patient Outcome	Process

The patient experiences informed, comfortable, and safe preoperative, postoperative, and predischarge phases of hospitalization. This includes:

DESCRIPTION: Transurethral resection is a surgical procedure by which prostatic or bladder tissue is removed through an instrument passed through the urethra. Indications for such treatment includes prostate enlargement due to hyperplasia of normal tissue, malignant tumors, and bladder tumors. This procedure is most often performed on males in the older age group.

NURSING ASSESSMENT: In addition to general admission assessment, the following information is especially important.
1. Assess and document physical status.
   a. Signs and symptoms related to underlying disease state:
      • Present voiding pattern, *i.e.*, frequency, dribbling, hesitancy
      • Degree of urinary retention
      • Presence of hematuria, pyuria
   b. Risk factors:
      • Presence of older disease states, *e.g.*, diabetes, cancer, hypertension, cardiopulmonary disease.
2. Assess and document patient's response to information about the disease process, treatment, and anticipated surgery.
   a. Apparent anxiety level, *e.g.*, concern for body image, fear of loss of libido
   b. Previous experience with surgery
   c. Expectations of outcome and surgery
3. Assess and document health habits/life-style prior to admission.
   a. Potential for self-care or need for supportive care.
   b. Medications, especially those affecting clotting time, blood pressure, or cardiac function
   c. Diet modifications
   d. Home health supervision/support
4. Assess and document patient's understanding of the disease process, treatment, and anticipated surgery.

A. *Is prepared for surgery*

INTERVENTION:
1. Reinforce understanding of patient and family regarding the disease process, implications, and treatment. Discuss with physician possible outcomes of surgery, *i.e.*, impotence, continuation of symptoms.
2. Summarize usual preoperative preparation and provide care per hospital routine and physician's orders. See Chapter 5 Preoperative Phase of Hospitalization, p. 129. Include additional elements of preoperative care relating to transurethral resection.
   • Emphasize postoperative expectations:
      • Foley catheter in bladder
      • Urine will be bloody
      • Possible need for bladder irrigations
      • Discomforts due to surgery and bladder spasms

B. *Is free of or has minimal discomfort or postoperative complications*

• *Urinary*

3. Provide postoperative care. See Chapter 5 Postoperative Phase of Hospitalization, p. 130.
4. Intervene in the critical elements of patient care following transurethral resection.
   a. Promote adequate fluid balance.
      • Force fluids to 2000 to 3000 cc daily unless contraindicated.
      • Monitor intake and output and check for symptoms of imbalance, *i.e.*, edema, dehydration.
   b. Prevent urinary drainage system obstruction.
      • Provide urinary catheter care.
      • Check for symptoms of obstruction.
         Frequent, severe bladder spasms
         Passage of urine around catheter
         Suprapubic distention and discomfort
      • Irrigate urinary catheter as ordered or request physician's order if catheter becomes obstructed.
   c. Instruct patient in bladder and sphincter control techniques following removal of catheter.
      • Void no more frequently than q 2 hours, first 24 hours.
      • Void no more frequently than q 4 hours, second 24 hours.
      • Teach patient to start and stop stream voluntarily.

Patient Outcome	Process

• *Comfort*	d. Provide comfort measures.
	    • Position patient comfortably to relieve extreme tension on catheter. Do not loosen tape placed by physician to create tension on bladder.
	    • Maintain gravity flow of tubing to prevent distention.
	    • Provide analgesics as ordered and according to patient need.

C. *Is knowledgeable about nature of illness, self-care, and resources for continuity of care*	5. See Chapter 5 Predischarge Phase of Hospitalization p. 132. Include additional elements of preparation for discharge such as:
	    a. Teach patient to report signs and symptoms to physician immediately:
	      • Bloody urine
	      • Inability to urinate
	      • Prolonged uncontrollable dribbling (longer than one week)
	      • Burning on urination.
	    b. Teach self-care:
	      • Cleanse periurethral area with soap and water and rinse well.
	      • Continue to force ample fluid intake.
	    c. Discuss possible changes in sexual activity, *e.g.,* impotence.

CHAPTER VI
Guidelines for the patient with a psychiatric illness

INTRODUCTION: There are common features in the nursing care required by the hospitalized patient who needs psychiatric therapy. These are considered in the Psychiatric Patient General Care Guidelines, p. 241. In these guidelines, the described nursing interventions promote the patient's ability to participate in the treatment plan and benefit from the therapeutic environment.

Specific guidelines are described for the patient experiencing varying emotional difficulties in adjusting to life situations. Highly skilled nursing interventions are identified to facilitate the desired patient outcomes necessary for restoration and maintenance of mental health at an optimum level.

There is evidence of primary nursing care in the key activities which stress the critical aspects of the therapeutic relationships essential to the successful desired outcomes of care.

Electroconvulsant Therapy Guidelines are described in Chapter 11, p. 409.

Patient Outcome	Process

The patient is able to participate in treatment plan and benefit from thera- peutic environment. This includes:

A. *Experiences a sense of personal acceptance and worth in the environment*

B. *Identifies reason and goals for hospitalization*

C. *Understands and participates in treat- ment plan*

D. *Is receiving medi- cations safely*

1. Prepare for arrival of patient.
   a. Attempt to plan/schedule all admissions and transfers with the exception of the closed ward.
      - When the ward is notified of a scheduled admission, contact the physician and request information pertinent to the patient and admission.
      - When the ward is notified of a transfer:
        Request information from transferring ward nurse.
        Interview and discuss transfer plans with patient.
      - Each patient is assigned to a primary nurse, who works with the patient throughout hospitalization.
   b. Assess available information and consider this in preparation for patient arrival.
2. Convey a sense of concern and warmth on admission of patient and throughout hospitalization.
3. Orient patient/family to ward environment on admission. Include such activities as:
   a. Tour ward and explain facilities available to patient.
   b. Introduce him/them to other patients and staff available at time.
   c. Explain staff dress and identification by name tag.
   d. Discuss hospital routines with patient such as meal times.
   e. Question possession of drugs/alcohol/other restricted items and remove them from the patient's possession. (Patients admitted to closed ward will have possessions searched. This will be done as needed for patients admitted to other psychiatric units.)
4. Interview patient and family and obtain information.
   a. Patient problems
   b. Behavior of patient and family
   c. Family interactions
   d. Patient strengths
   e. Social and work history
   f. Sexual history
   g. Educational level
   h. Mental status
   i. Physical condition, including disabilities, aids, prostheses, recent injuries, special needs
   j. Diet modifications
   k. Allergies
   l. Medications (brought in or at home, previous history)
   m. Summary of previous hospitalization
5. Identify and record patient and/or family behavior which indicates level of adjustment to hospitalization (on admission and throughout).
6. Recognize and acknowledge patient requests. Assess the appropriateness of the request and respond accordingly.
7. Establish goals for care with patient and family.
   a. In initial interview, ask patient and family to identify why he/she is hospitalized in a psychiatric unit and document response. Identify problem areas and goals with patient and contract how to meet specific, realistic goals within stated time limits.
   b. Document in progress notes a weekly assessment of patient's progress in relationship to goals of hospitalization.
   c. Alter goals as necessary.
8. Facilitate patient's understanding and participation in treatment plan.
   a. Coordinate treatment plan with entire treatment team.
   b. Discuss treatment plan with patient and physician and modify as needed.
   c. Write nursing orders which reflect patient goals and nursing approaches.
   d. Document in progress notes a weekly assessment of patient's progress in relationship to goals in treatment plan.
9. Administer prescribed medications.
   a. Give drugs accurately according to hospital procedure.
   b. Be aware of desired effects, side effects, and drug interaction of drugs being dispensed.
   c. Check blood pressure prior to administering any medication which could alter blood pressure.
   d. Evaluate patient for mental status, physiological well-being, and appropriateness of designated route of administration before administering any drug.
   e. Document reasons for not giving a medication as ordered and notify physician.
   f. Be aware of specific considerations when p.r.n. medication is requested by patient.
      - Explore with patient precipitating factors and nature of need, *e.g.,* pain, anxiety, sleeplessness.

Patient Outcome	Process
	• Encourage patient to verbalize feelings, examine alternatives, and adjust to medications.
	• Document time medication is given and reason.

E. *Views self as a member of the community in which learning and growth are a part of daily living*

10. Facilitate community participation.
    a. Explain to patient what community means. Include such information as:
       • Purpose: to provide an atmosphere conducive to growth and learning
       • Members consist of:
         Patients
         Nursing staff
         Clerical staff
         Permanent housekeeping staff
         Dietician
         Physical therapist
         Recreation therapist
       • Opportunities for patient members within the community:
         Move toward autonomy and independence with respect for realistic dependence.
         Develop communication skills that result in recognizing needs and getting them met appropriately.
         Test new behaviors.
         Demonstrate appropriate consideration for onself and other members.
       • Responsibilities of all members:
         Regularly attend community meetings.
         Plan and participate in ward activities.
         Dress appropriately.
         Utilize community areas.
         Take responsibility for personal space and belongings.
         Observe responsibilities.
         Follow stated ward rules.
    b. Facilitate discussion at community meetings regarding issues of community living.
    c. Remind patient of various activities when appropriate and encourage him to become involved.
    d. Take part in community activities as much as possible.

F. *Utilizes members of various disciplines to reach goals appropriately*

11. Assist the patient to utilize treatment team members appropriately.
    a. Serve as coordinator of the treatment team specifically responsible for:
       • Ongoing communication with members of the team
       • Documentation of significant interactions between nurse and other members of the treatment team
    b. Assure that the patient knows the different categories of personnel and, in general, the roles of each as a resource person.
    c. Assess and document the therapeutic quality of the nurse-patient relationship using outside resources as needed to provide reality based expectations of oneself and patient.

G. *Begins to utilize improved modes of communication*

12. Assist patient to utilize improved modes of communication.
    a. Identify with patient difficulties in interactions and jointly set goals.
    b. Discuss with team previous information and collectively arrive at plan of care and assigned roles to assure productive movement.
    c. Document team planning in progress notes with plan reflected in nursing orders.
    d. Discuss with patient situations of difficulty and consider new behaviors.
    e. Elicit from patient fantasies of responses to new behaviors and feelings concerning these responses.
    f. Give positive feedback to patient for efforts toward wellness and appropriate new behavior.
    g. Help patient to recognize behaviors which do not get the desired positive response and discuss possible modifications.
    h. Strive continuously to:
       • Reinforce patient.
       • Assess effectiveness of treatment plan.
       • Communicate with team members.
       • Document progress and changes in plan.

H. *Recognizes self as an individual with abilities and responsibilities*

13. Support patient's ability to assume responsibility.
    a. Evaluate patient's ability to assume increasing responsibility for self through evidence of:
       • Verbalizing one or more new learned behavior(s) and exhibiting same within hospital
       • Identifying pre-existing personal and interpersonal problems and verbalizing realistic application of new learned behaviors

Patient Outcome	Process
	• Identifying potential problems which may arise in response to new behaviors and ways to deal with them
	b. Monitor patient's ability to use leisure time effectively and consult with recreational therapist as needed.
I. *Views self as a dynamic force within the family unit*	14. Facilitate patient's perception of self within the family unit.
	a. Assess the influence these factors may have on the patient.
	• Cultural
	• Social
	• Socioeconomic
	• Geographical
	• Religious
	• Educational
	• Age
	• Sex
	• Family composition
	• Vocational choices
	b. Explore with patient what expectations family and/or significant others hold for him.
	c. Identify appropriate and realistic needs for change in relation to self and family and/or significant others.
	• Assist patient with new behavior.
	• Review with patient experience with new behaviors in order to support positive feelings and to help problem solve.
	• Help patient deal with those situations which cannot be changed.
	d. Initiate patient/family interviews. Observe patient/family patterns of interaction for progress toward goals.
J. *Is aware of medications received and desired effects when appropriate*	15. Teach patient and family about prescribed drug therapy except in certain circumstances when the physician and/or nursing staff may deem it inadvisable to discuss medications with patient.
	a. Explain desired effects of each medication when it is given initially.
	b. Give and discuss medication information sheets for certain medications which have important precautions, *e.g.*, MAOIs, lithium carbonate. Document in chart.
	c. Evaluate patient's understanding and motivation to take medications as prescribed prior to leaving the hospital.
	d. Discuss with patient and family who will be responsible for dispensing the medication when the patient is unable to self-medicate.
	e. Teach patient and/or family the following information: dose, frequency, effects, route, possible untoward reactions.
K. *Terminates appropriately with significant treatment team members, members of the patient community, and hospital environment*	16. Assist patient in appropriate termination.
	a. Initiate discussion with patient concerning:
	• The significance and substance of the nurse-patient relationship
	• Feelings about leaving the community and the hospital environment
	• Methods and feelings regarding postterminations with significant people
	• How effects of the community and hospital environment have helped him to reach stated goals
	• How he plans to terminate with community members in a way that would be most self-satisfying
	b. Create opportunity at community meeting for patient to terminate with community members in the way that he has decided.

Patient Outcome	Process
The patient is able to participate in treatment plan and benefit from therapeutic environment. This includes:	**DESCRIPTION:** Acting-out patients use negativistic, challenging, limit-testing behavior in an attempt to communicate underlying feelings such as fear or anger which they are unable to express directly. This behavior may be physical, verbal, or sexual. Examples are scratching themselves or others, throwing tantrums, inappropriate seductive mannerisms or attire, verbal abuse on others, or misbehaving in group activities or meetings. Patient populations that have an increased tendency to act out are: adolescents, those with character disorders and a history of suicidal behavior, alcohol and drug abusers, physical abusers.

NURSING ASSESSMENT: In addition to the general psychiatric admission assessment, the following information is especially important. Assess and document acting-out behavior patterns as described above.

A. *Decreases acting out behavior*

INTERVENTION:
1. Intervene promptly in response to patient's acting-out behavior by setting clear, consistent, and firm limits. Methods may involve:
    a. Verbal instruction in calm, direct nondefensive manner
    b. Removal to a quiet area
    c. Restraints
2. Avoid punitive or judgmental attitude.
3. Reinforce appropriate behavior.
4. Initiate interactions with patient at times when limit-setting is not an issue.

B. *Recognizes needs being met through behavior*

5. Observe pattern of acting-out behavior and note precipitating circumstances.
6. Explore with patient how he sees his own behavior.
7. Share with patient your observation of his behavior in an attempt to raise his awareness of patterns and underlying feelings.
8. Assist patient to realize that acting out hehavior:
    a. Provides immediate relief but does not resolve underlying conflicts
    b. Creates new problems

C. *Exhibits appropriate behavior in getting needs met*

9. Encourage and assist patient to explore alternative means of dealing with conflicts.
    a. Guide patient in choosing appropriate alternative behaviors.
    b. Elicit from patient his fantasies of responses to new behaviors and feelings concerning these responses.
    c. Provide recreational and occupational activities which allow channeling and discharging of energy levels.
10. Evaluate with the patient and the rest of treatment team the ability to apply interactional skills after a home visit or therapeutic leave of absence.

D. *Participates in discharge planning*

11. Establish discharge plan with patient.
    a. Identify current support systems. Assess whether or not they are functioning.
        • Work with functional support systems to increase their effectiveness and assist patient to identify and develop new support systems as they are needed, such as family, church, community groups, mental health resources, and other significant people.
    b. Discuss with patient realistic plan following discharge.
        • Help patient define short and long-term goals, *e.g.,* career, living situation, diversions. Consider time beyond the next six months.
    c. Review follow-up health care plans.
        • Inform patient whom to call in crisis.
        • Instruct patient about prescribed medications, frequency, amount, effects, side effects, and synergistic action.

Patient Outcome	Process

The patient is able to participate in treatment plan and benefit from therapeutic environment. This includes:

DESCRIPTION: The patient's chief problem in the following categories of behavior is anxiety which stems from an underlying conflict. This anxiety may be felt directly and expressed or may be unconscious and automatically controlled by various psychological defense mechanisms. These individuals often have difficulty knowing what they want and don't want and, therefore, have difficulty making decisions. They often feel inferior and worthless. Their attempts to relieve or alleviate anxiety result in specific patterns of behavior, some of which may be described as follows:

- *Depressive:* Characterized by self-depreciating behavior and depressive affect; usually follows a loss. Guilt may result because of unacceptable anger felt toward the lost relationship and be introjected.
- *Anxiety reaction:* Patient is unable to identify source of anxiety; free-floating.
- *Obsessive-compulsive reaction:* Anxiety controlled by repetitive thoughts and performance of acts. The patient recognizes the unreasonableness of the thoughts and acts but is unable to control them.
- *Conversion reaction:* The reaction to a conflict which results in anxiety being converted into symptoms of a sensory-motor disability, *e.g.,* blindness, paralysis
- *Phobic:* Characterized by specific fear which is out of proportion to the feared object or situation
- *Dissociative reaction:* Characterized by disorganization within the individual, disturbances of conscious memory, *e.g.,* amnesia, fugue states, multiple personalities
- *Hypochondriac:* Characterized by persistent preoccupation with physical or emotional health, somatic symptoms which have no demonstrated organic basis

NURSING ASSESSMENT: In addition to the general psychiatric admission assessment, the following information is especially important.

1. Assess and document mental status.
   a. Orientation to:
      - Time, place, person, self
   b. Affect and feelings while acting out behaviors
2. Assess and document extent, degree, and kind of symptoms. Examples:
   a. Sleep disturbance, appetite disturbance
   b. Tachycardia, frequent urination, diarrhea, constipation, diaphoresis
   c. Pain, discomfort: backache, headache
   d. Tenseness, restlessness, agitation
   e. Apprehension
   f. Selective inattention
3. Determine if symptoms interfere with physiological well-being or daily functioning including relationships with others. Symptoms may include activity disturbances, neglect of appearance, or behaviors that suggest need for protective precautions, *e.g.,* potential for harming self or others.
4. Assess patient's understanding of symptoms and causes of behaviors (Do not interpret causation to patient).
   - Determine nature of past, current, and impending life changes.

A. *Exhibits decreased anxiety*

INTERVENTION:

1. Establish trust relationship. To do this:
   a. Accept behavior.
   b. Give information, answer questions.
   c. Reassure patient that (s) he will be cared for.
   d. Allow patient to be dependent as long as necessary.
   e. Provide consistency in terms of scheduling activities, nursing approach.
   f. Refrain from interpretive statements.
   g. Discuss neutral "here and now" topics.
2. Evaluate effects of medication on behavior.
   a. Desired goal: decrease anxiety to a functional level
   b. When patient requests p.r.n. medication, give medication and later discuss possible causes for request.
3. Evaluate degree to which patient's anxiety producing symptoms change.
   Adjust care plan as necessary if symptoms do not decrease.

Patient Outcome	Process

B. *Identifies causes of anxieties*	4. Help patient to recognize anxiety:
	   a. Encourage description of feeling state, including body sensations.
	   b. Explore basis for ''here and now'' feelings.
	5. Aid patient to formulate possible rationale for current state.
	   a. Explore events preceding anxious behavior and patterns occurring over time in an effort to establish a cause and effect relationship.
	   b. Continue to explore anxiety producing situations in an attempt to aid patient to gain insight, realizing that this may be threatening.
	6. Encourage and assist patient to explore alternative means for dealing with behaviors.
	   a. Guide patient in choosing appropriate alternative behaviors.
	   b. Elicit from patient his fantasies of responses to new behaviors and his feelings concerning these responses.
	   c. Give opportunities to practice alternative behaviors.
	   d. Give positive feedback to patient for efforts toward wellness and appropriate new behavior.
	     • Evaluate with patient the effectiveness of new behaviors and possible modifications.
	7. Evaluate with the patient and the treatment team patient's ability to apply interactional skills after a home visit or therapeutic leave of absence.

C. *Participates in discharge planning*	8. Establish discharge plan with the patient.
	   a. Identify current support systems. Assess whether or not they are functioning.
	     • Work with functional support systems to increase their effectiveness and assist patient to identify and develop new support systems as they are needed such as family, church, community groups, mental health resources, and other significant people.
	   b. Discuss with the patient realistic plan following discharge.
	     • Help patient define short and long-term goals, *e.g.*, career, living situation, diversions. Consider time beyond the next six months.
	   c. Review follow-up health care plans.
	     • Inform patient whom to call in crisis.
	     • Instruct patient about prescribed medications, frequency, amount, effects, side effects, and synergistic action.

Patient Outcome

*The patient is able
to participate in
treatment plan and
benefit from thera-
peutic environment
This includes:*

Process

DESCRIPTION: Any patient whose behavior is characterized by hallucinations, looseness of association, disorganization, confusion, delusions, ambivalence, and autism has a disturbance of reality orientation. Diagnosis of schizophrenia, drug toxicity, organicity, psychotic depression, and manic states are disturbances of reality orientation. If the diagnosis is schizophrenia, it may be categorized as simple, hebephrenic, catatonic, or paranoid. Progress should be measured by positive movement toward reaching outcomes and less than 100 per cent achievement is realistic.

NURSING ASSESSMENT: In addition to the general psychiatric admission assessment, the following information is especially important.
1. Assess and document mental status.
   a. Content of conversations for evidence of thought disorders such as
      • Hallucinations
      • Delusions
      • Paranoid thoughts
      • Misperceptions/misinterpretations
   b. Appropriateness of verbal communication
      • Understandable content, logical sequence
      • Facts are accurate, this may not be possible to verify.
   c. Nonverbal behavior
      • Affect appropriate to verbal communication
      • Gestures, posture, actions appropriate
   d. Orientation to:
      • Person
      • Place
      • Time
      • Situation
   e. Usual level of functioning including past history of this type of behavior.
   f. General appearance.
2. Assess and document physical ability to care for own needs such as
   a. Activities of daily living
   b. Nutritional needs

INTERVENTION:
1. Interview family to verify information given by patient and to help identify approaches that have been helpful in dealing with patient in the past.
2. Establish plan to meet physical care needs.
   a. Identify areas of physical care in which patient needs assistance, *e.g.,* nutrition, bathing, dressing, elimination, sleep, activity.
   b. Incorporate in care plan how needs will be met; who will be involved. Evaluate and revise plan as needs change.
3. Establish trust relationship. To do this:
   a. Recognize that the patient generally has fear of interpersonal relationships and that his overt verbal behavior may not convey his true underlying feelings.
   b. Reorient to reality as needed.
   c. Attempt to limit the number of staff members interacting with patient in order to provide consistency.
   d. Establish limits and content of relationship and adhere to these.
   e. Be regular in seeing patient and faithful in meeting appointments. Explain any absences.
   f. Be consistent in conveying a caring attitude. Exhibit patience and remember that the patient may be testing your interest in him.
   g. Be conscious of the patient's awareness of surroundings and conversation regardless of his level of response, *i.e.,* explain everything to be done, particularly that which involves physical contact.
   h. Search constantly for alternate ways to reach the patient, *e.g.,* objects and activities. Notice patient's response and adjust approach accordingly.
4. Identify the patient's strengths including interactional skills and interests and utilize them in forming care plan. Incorporate information family has offered.
5. Discuss with patient situations of difficulty and consider new behaviors.
   a. Consider with patient how he expects other people to respond to his new behaviors.
   b. Give positive feedback to patient for efforts toward wellness and appropriate new behavior.

A. *Maintains physical
well being*

B. *Improves ability
to communicate*
C. *Identifies potential
stress situations and
methods of coping*

Patient Outcome

Process

c. Help patient to recognize behaviors which do not get the desired response and discuss possible modifications.

6. Evaluate patient's ability to assume increasing responsibility for self by:
   a. Verbalizing one or more new learned behavior(s) and exhibiting same within the hospital
   b. Identifying pre-existing personal and interpersonal problems and verbalizing realistic application of new learned behaviors
   c. Identifying potential problems which may arise in response to new behaviors and ways to deal with them.

7. Monitor patient's ability to use leisure time effectively and consult with recreational therapist as needed.

8. Be aware that the patient may regress in behavior in response to different stresses, *e.g.*, changes in care people, changes in environment, patient population, schedule.

9. Take steps to prepare patient for potential stress such as explaining new procedures and discuss approaching changes in environment.

D. *Participates in discharge planning*

10. Establish discharge plan with patient.
   a. Identify current support systems. Assess whether or not they are functioning.
      • Work with functional support systems to increase their effectiveness and assist patient to identify and develop new support systems as they are needed such as family, community groups, church, mental health resources, and other significant people.
   b. Discuss with patient realistic plan following discharge.
      • Help patient define short and long-term goals, *e.g.*, career, living situation, partner status, economic, diversions. Consider time beyond the next six months.
   c. Review follow-up health care plans.
      • Inform patient whom to call in crises.
      • Instruct patient about prescribed medications: frequency, amount, effects, side effects.

Patient Outcome	Process

The patient is able to participate in treatment plan and benefit from therapeutic environment. This includes:

DESCRIPTION: These guidelines are applicable to the patient who has made an overt suicide attempt or has verbalized intent to perform a self-destructive act. The patient is hospitalized for psychiatric treatment.

NURSING ASSESSMENT: In addition to the general psychiatric admission assessment, the following information is especially important.

1. Assess and document the degree of potential for suicide.
   b. Verbalization of attempt with or without specific plan
   c. History of suicide attempt and recency
   d. Other historical data which categorizes patient with high potential for suicide:
      • Transition
      • Recent loss
      • Recent depression
      • Within three months of emotional crisis.
   e. Failure to make positive reference to the future

2. Assess and document physical status including:
   a. Weight
   b. Eating pattern
   c. Condition of skin, mouth, hair, etc.
   d. Sleep pattern

A. *Maintains life*

INTERVENTION:

1. Provide a safe environment.
   a. Maintain room free from self-destructive devices.
   b. Provide appropriate staff-patient ratio for surveillance (1:1 for actively suicidal or potentially impulsive).
   c. Observe people interacting with patient for passage of dangerous objects.
   d. Use chemical and/or physical restraints and seclusion appropriately. Justify use with rationale in chart.

2. Provide for maintenance of physical status.
   a. Nutrition
   b. Elimination
   c. Personal hygiene
   d. Sleep

B. *Exhibits no self-destructive behavior*

3. Identify personal behavioral patterns, situations, and/or issues which for this individual may trigger a self-destructive act.

4. Employ a variety of techniques which have the effect of reducing suicidal behavior such as
   a. Drug therapy
   b. "No-suicide" contract
   c. Insight session
   d. Group and community peer pressure

5. Assist patient to identify personal behavioral patterns, situations, and issues and take his or her own preventive measures.

6. Assist patient to reduce own suicidal behavior through:
   a. Avoiding a precipitating situation
   b. Seeking appropriate help
   c. Building on strengths
   d. Identifying and utilizing support systems

C. *Recognizes and expresses feelings*

7. Assess through verbal and nonverbal cues the behaviors the patient is exhibiting.

8. Reflect, clarify, summarize, and interpret level and kind of feelings, *e.g.*, anger.

9. Facilitate patient's expressions of feelings.
   a. Encourage patient to express and deal with feelings as they arise.
   b. Assist family or significant others to provide support for patient in his efforts to be more expressive of feelings.

Patient Outcome	Process
D. *Develops and maintains individual support systems*	10. Identify current support systems. Assess whether or not they are functioning. a. Work with functional support systems to increase their effectiveness. b. Assist patient to identify and develop new support systems as they are needed such as family, community groups, church, mental health resources, and other significant people.
E. *Relates to future with realistic plan*	11. Establish discharge plan with patient. a. Discuss with patient realistic plans following discharge. • Help patient define short and long-term goals, *e.g.,* career, living situation, economic, diversions. Consider time beyond the next six months. b. Review follow-up health care plans. • Inform patient whom to call in crisis. • Instruct patient about prescribed drugs to include amount, frequency, effects, and side effects. Discuss precautions.

Patient Outcome	Process

The patient is able to participate in treatment plan and benefit from therapeutic environment. This includes:

DESCRIPTION: The patient may exhibit behaviors such as: stays in own room, excludes self from interpersonal interchange, exhibits unrealistic fears of other people or things, or displays a lack of interest in self and other things. This does not include psychotic behavior such as delusions, hallucinations, etc.

NURSING ASSESSMENT: In addition to the general psychiatric admission assessment, the following information is especially important.
1. Assess and document usual patterns of behavior.
   a. Sleep
   b. Eating
   c. Interaction
   d. Activities—how patient typically spends time
   e. Affect
2. Assess patient's current ability to care for own physical and environmental needs.

A. *Takes part in interpersonal relationships*

INTERVENTION:
1. Establish trust relationship. To do this:
   a. Recognize that the patient generally has low self-esteem and a fear of interpersonal relationships.
   b. Provide an accepting, nonthreatening friendly environment.
   c. Attempt to limit the number of staff members interacting with patient in order to provide consistency.
   d. Establish limits and content of relationship and adhere to these.
   e. Be regular in seeing patient and faithful in meeting appointments. Explain any absences.
   f. Be consistent in attitude and sense of caring. Exhibit patience; remember that the patient may be testing your interest in him.
   g. Be conscious of the patient's awareness of surroundings and conversation regardless of his level of response, *i.e.,* explain everything that will be done before it is done, particularly that which will involve physical contact.
   h. Search constantly for alternate ways to reach the patient, *e.g.,* objects and activities. Notice patient's response and adjust your approach on its basis.
2. Identify the patient's strengths including interactional skills and utilize them in forming care plan.
3. Keep initial conversations nonthreatening and gradually proceed to more insight related as patient is able to tolerate.
4. Assess patient for general level of functioning in interpersonal relationships and apply information in selecting interventions.
   Work with patient to integrate strengths into more satisfying relationships and evaluate degree of success with patient.
5. Observe patient's behavior which indicates a greater degree of comfort in the environment and an interest in involvement with other people.
6. Plan with patient a schedule of activities which foster personal achievement and restore self-esteem.
   Give assistance to patients who need help with activities of daily living.

B. *Demonstrates active involvement with environment*

7. Determine involvement in environment through assessment of behavior which includes:
   a. Amount of time in room and how occupied. Describe, *e.g.,* sleeping, reading.
   b. Amount of time outside of room and behavior in relation to others
   c. Interaction: (Consider tone of voice, rate of speaking, subject matter, content.)
      • No response
      • Responds to questions
      • Initiates interaction in, or within a 1:1 basis only, with a small group, large group
   d. Eating pattern:
      • Requires feeding
      • Other-initiated
      • Self-initiated
   e. Sleeping pattern:
      • Amount of sleep and when
      • Describe difficulties such as falling asleep, remaining asleep, or nightmares

Patient Outcome	Process
	f. Activities:
	• Does not attend to personal physical needs (consider bathing, shaving, elimination, appearance, etc.)
	• Attends to own physical needs
	• Participates in individual diversionary activities
	• Participates in small group activities
	• Participates in large group activities
	• Initiates activities with others (describe)
	g. Affect, body posture:
	• Body posture indicative of withdrawal, *e.g.*, fetal position, tensed arms and legs, head down, little or no eye contact, staring, intent, fearful gaze, tears, wringing hands, sweaty palms
	• More relaxed body posture, more purposeful body movement, muscles more relaxed, facial expression less tense
	• Posture appropriate to improved feeling state and level of functioning in walk, seated position, facial expression, hands, etc.
C. *Demonstrates interactional skills necessary to living at home and in the community*	8. Evaluate with the patient and the others in treatment team patients' ability to apply interactional skills after a home visit or therapeutic leave of absence.
	9. Identify areas of need and incorporate these into the discharge plans. Components of plan should include:
	a. Discuss resources that person will utilize for further psychiatric treatment and crisis intervention.
	b. Discuss realistic plan after discharge, *e.g.*, career family, recreation.
	• Day-to-day plan
	• Anticipating problems and how they will be managed
	c. Review follow-up health care plan.
	• Inform patient whom to call in crisis.
	• Instruct patient about prescribed medications including amount, frequency, effects, side effects, and synergistic actions.

CHAPTER VII
Guidelines For The Obstetric Patient

INTRODUCTION: Patient care outcomes are identified along with related nursing process in this section for the mother during labor, delivery and the postpartum phases. Guidelines for the care of the normal newborn are described. The highly skilled nursing interventions facilitate the desired patient outcomes necessary for the physiological and psychological well-being of the child-bearing woman.

The guidelines are written in the context of the family unit. Therefore, reference is often made to care of the infant when planning care with the mother and to normal obstetric care when pertinent to more complex situations or patient problems that require specific nursing interventions.

Patient Outcome	Process

The patient experiences informed, safe, and comfortable evaluation for possible admission for delivery. This includes:

DESCRIPTION: These guidelines are applicable for any patient with a pregnancy of greater than 20 weeks who presents in the emergency room or clinic with symptoms requiring further evaluation.

NURSING ASSESSMENT: One nurse is designated to interview, assess, and assist with evaluation to determine need for diagnostic studies, and/or admission to the hospital or discharge. In addition to the general admission assessment, the following information is especially important.
1. Assess and document presenting symptoms.
   a. Ask patient "What problems are you having?"
   b. Review symptoms including:
      • Ruptured membranes
      • Mucus plug
      • Bleeding
      • Pain and location, quality
      • Frequency and duration of contractions
      • Time of initiation of regular contractions
      • Voiding difficulties
      • Dizziness, fainting, headaches, blurred vision, abdominal pain unrelated to contractions
      • Increased blood pressure
      • Vomiting
      • Swelling
2. Assess and document general information.
   a. Parity and calculated date of confinement
   b. Problems related to previous labor and delivery
   c. Drug allergies
   d. Admission vital signs (TPR, BP, fetal heart rate, height, weight)
      • If fetal heart rate less than or equal to 120 or greater than or equal to 160, notify physician.
      • If blood pressure greater than or equal to 140/90, notify physician.

A. *Is aware of need for evaluation and evaluation process*

INTERVENTION:
1. Orient to immediate environment.
2. Institute preparation for examination and provide care.
   a. Assist in getting ready for physical examination.
   b. Obtain urine specimen and test for protein, glucose, and ketones.
   c. Explain to patient that physician will perform pelvic and physical examination and discuss care.
   d. Notify physician of patient status, any significant observations, and readiness to be examined.
   e. Remain with patient during examination and
      • Provide emotional support.
      • Observe body hygiene.
      • Assess response to examination indicating need for further nursing support.
      • Assist physician.
      • Interpret physician's findings to patient, as needed.
   f. Document findings of examination in nurses' notes and need for:
      • Diagnostic studies such as sterile urine specimen, ultra sound, speculum examination, amniocentesis, oxytocin challenge test
      • Preparation for labor and delivery (skin preparation and enema)
   g. Transfer to appropriate room for diagnostic study or admission to hospital.

B. *Is maintaining physiological function of the maternal/fetal unit*

C. *Is achieving relative comfort*

3. Provide continuing care which may include:
   a. Monitor maternal and fetal vital signs as necessary for specific procedures and according to patient status.
   b. Institute physical and emotional comfort measures.
      • Calm, controlled, uncluttered environment
      • Continuous emotional support; answer questions.
      • Privacy
      • Positioning on side, semi-Fowler's position, or with one hip slightly elevated on pillow, for comfort, ventilation, and to avoid maternal hypotension and fetal bradycardia
      • Back rubs
      • Clean, dry underpads

Patient Outcome	Process

D. *Is prepared for admission/or discharge and self-care*	c. Be aware of physician's decision about admission/discharge. Be present during physician's explanation to patient to answer questions and clarify information.
	d. Prepare patient for admission according to established protocol and appropriate guidelines.
	    • Perineal preparation
	    • Enema
	    • Electronic fetal monitoring
	    • Antacid, if ordered
	e. Instruct patient for discharge:
	    • Care to be performed at home
	    • Symptoms to be reported immediately to physician such as increased contractions, bleeding, rupture of membranes
	    • Anticipate return to hospital with presenting symptoms.

Patient Outcome

The mother and newborn experience safe labor and delivery. This includes:

A. *Is prepared for labor and delivery*

B. *Is achieving relative state of comfort*

C. *Is maintaining stable maternal/fetal unit physiological function during labor and delivery*

Process

DESCRIPTION: These guidelines are to be used in conjunction with guidelines for Obstetric patients for evaluation/possible admission p. 257 and apply to any patient who is 36 weeks pregnant and/or who has rhythmic uterine contractions, cervical dilation, and effacement.

NURSING ASSESSMENT: In addition to the general admission assessment, the following information is especially important.
1. Assess and document progression of labor.
   a. Frequency, duration, strength of contractions, manual or electronic means
   b. Quality and progress of labor
   c. Presence of hyperstimulation
   d. Behavior indicating change in labor status:
      • Increase in concentration
      • Irritability
      • Vomiting
      • Loss of emotional control
      • Bearing down
      • Feeling of increasing pressure, need to move bowels
   e. Status of membranes; presence of meconium or blood in amniotic fluid or foul odor.
2. Assess and document fetal status.
   a. Quality and rate of fetal heart tone
   b. Fetal position

INTERVENTION:
1. Explain visiting policy. Identify who patient's significant other will be and restrict other visitors.
2. Teach patient/significant other about the following:
   a. Analgesia and anesthesia
   b. Nothing by mouth status
   c. Reason of IV
   d. Admistration of medications, *e.g.,* mylanta
   e. Fetal monitoring
   f. Breathing techniques and muscular relaxation
      • Slow, deep breathing
      • Panting
      • Pushing
      • Total body relaxation
   g. Process of labor, *i.e.,* dilation, effacement
   h. Process of delivery, including episiotomy
3. Caution patient whose membranes have ruptured or who has internal monitoring devices not to get out of bed. Others may be allowed to go the bathroom to void.
4. Provide physical and emotional comfort measures to aid in labor and reduce chance of infection.
   a. Evaluate patients with poor body hygiene and, if labor status permits, assist patient to bathe.
   b. Provide calm, controlled, uncluttered environment.
   c. Give continuous emotional support; answer questions.
   d. Allow as much privacy as possible.
   e. Position on side, semi-Fowler's position, or with one hip slightly elevated on pillow, for comfort, ventilation, and to avoid maternal hypotension and fetal bradycardia.
   f. Give back rubs.
   g. Encourage patient to void at least every 1 to 3 hours. Observe for bladder distention.
   h. Provide clean, dry underpads.
   i. Provide frequent perineal care at least q 3 to 4 hours, after voiding and as needed.
5. Monitor and maintain fluid/electrolyte balance:
   a. Provide strict intake and output.
   b. Maintain IV fluids.
   c. Be aware of result of electrolyte determinations.
6. Monitor maternal/fetal status throughout labor:
   a. Take vital signs (BP, P, fetal heart rate) according to stage of labor and stability of patient's condition; for example:

Patient Outcome

Process

- First stage of labor
  Latent phase when cervix dilated 0 to 4 to 5 cm, take vital signs q 1 hour.
  Active phase when cervix dilated 4 to 5 to 8 cm, take vital signs q 30 minutes.
  Transition phase when cervix dilated 8 to 10 cm, take vital signs q 15 minutes.
- Second stage of labor
  Take vital signs q 15 minutes.

  b. Monitor patients receiving epidural anesthesia or requiring special surveillance according to their needs.
  c. Observe for signs of fetal distress such as:
  - Lack of beat to beat variability (Fig. 7-1.)
  - Deceleration of fetal heart rate (Fig. 7-2. and 7-3.)
  - Prolonged tachycardia
  - Prolonged bradycardia
  d. In the event of getal distress: Give mother oxygen (6 to 8 liters per minute) and turn to left side. Notify physician.
7. Assist with amniotomy (artificial rupture of membranes) if indicated and placement of internal fetal scalp electrode and intrauterine pressure monitoring device (IUPMD).

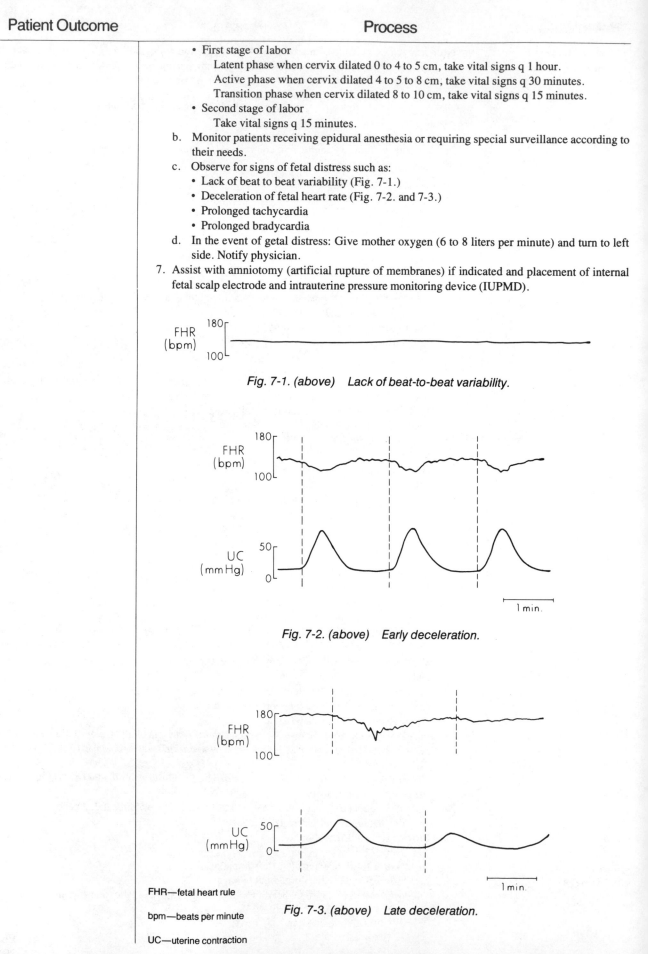

Fig. 7-1. (above)   Lack of beat-to-beat variability.

Fig. 7-2. (above)   Early deceleration.

FHR—fetal heart rule

bpm—beats per minute

Fig. 7-3. (above)   Late deceleration.

UC—uterine contraction

Patient Outcome	Process

	8. Prepare patient/significant other for actual transfer to Delivery Room.
	   a. Check for proper identification of mother and predelivery information in nurses labor and delivery notes.
	   b. Instruct significant other to dress in scrub clothes and wash hands.
	9. Remain with patient to give information, explain progress, and provide support and encouragement.
	   a. Teach about sterile field and patient's responsibility.
	   b. Evaluate need for wrist restraints.
	   c. Adjust mirror for patient's/significant other's visualization.
	   d. Identify people present in delivery room and their function.
	   e. Coach patient in appropriate breathing techniques, *e.g.*, panting versus pushing.
	10. Provide physical preparation:
	   a. Place patient in lithotomy position:
	     • Raise legs simultaneously into stirrups.
	     • Adjust stirrups for comfort.
	   b. Intervene for patient's comfort such as
	     • Massage leg cramps.
	     • Provide extra covers.
	     • Moisten lips.
	     • Position hand grips to aid patient in bearing down.
	   c. Provide oxygen per face mask, if indicated.
	11. Monitor:
	   a. Fetal heart tone after each contraction if manual or continually if electronic monitor used
	   b. Maternal blood pressure, pulse and respirations, q 5 to 10 minutes
	   c. IV infusion
	12. Inform mother of baby's sex and keep her informed of baby's condition.
	13. Provide immediate care of newborn:
	   a. Maintain patent airway.
	   b. Dry infant and allow him to remain uncovered under heater.
	   c. Observe for anomalies.
	   d. Assign Apgar scores per hospital policy.
	   e. Weigh infant.
	   f. Identify infant with ID bracelet, foot print, or according to hospital policy.
	   g. Complete written labor and delivery forms per hospital policy.
	14. Initiate maternal-fetal bonding (include significant other).
	   a. Move baby warmer (Krieslmann) to mother's side and encourage mother (and/or significant other) to touch and hold infant.
	   b. Cover infant to ensure warmth during holding.
	   c. Stand next to mother to assure baby's safety.
	   d. Assist mother who wishes to begin breast feeding immediately. Reassure her not to be discouraged since breast feeding is difficult in this position and another opportunity will be provided in Recovery Room.
	15. Prepare for transfer to Recovery Room:
	   a. Remove legs from stirrups simultaneously.
	   b. Assist patient to clean bed and raise side rails.
	   c. Place baby in mother's arms.

D. *Is maintaining stable status during immediate post-partum period (First two hours)*	16. Provide immediate postpartum care. Explain to patient rationale for care. This includes:
	   a. Monitor BP, P, R and height, position and firmness of fundus q 15 minutes for 1 hour, then q 1 hour for 6 hours.
	     • Be alert to patient who is more likely to have postpartum bleeding due to problems such as:
	        Grand multiparity
	        Large doses of oxytocin (Pitocin)
	        Multiple gestations
	        Polyhydramnios
	        Precipitous labor (less than two hours)
	        Delivery of large baby
	        Retained placenta requiring manual removal or curettage
	   b. Institute measures for excessive bleeding.
	     • Observe for signs of shock.

Patient Outcome	Process

- Increase frequency of vital signs, fundal checks, and fundal massage.
- Treat for shock as indicated:
  Trendelenburg position
  Blankets for warmth
- Provide supportive measures to minimize anxiety.
- Anticipate physician's orders for:
  Increasing rate of IV
  Oxytocic drugs
  Methylergonovine (Methergine) (p.o. or IM)
  Possible curettage

c. Check temperature on admission to Recovery Room, then q 4 hours unless elevated or otherwise indicated.

d. Check episiotomy q 15 minutes for 1 hour.

e. Provide pad count with peri-pad change and cleaning of perineum.

f. Apply ice pack to perineum as ordered.

g. Monitor postanesthesia recovery:
- For patients who received analgesics, *e.g.*, meperidine (Demerol), promethazine (Phenergan), small amounts of nitrous oxide:
  Monitor alertness, responsiveness, and quality of respirations while monitoring vital signs.
- For patients who received epidural, spinal (saddle-block) anesthesia:
  Check mobility of lower extremities and alertness.
  Instruct to lie flat for 12 hours if patient had spinal.
  Do not transfer patient to postpartum unit until sensory and motor control of lower extremities return and epidural catheter is removed.
- For patients who received general anesthesia:
  Check alertness and responsiveness.
  Administer O_2 by mask, 6 to 8 liters per minute.
  Suction as needed.
  Position for optimal ventilation.
  Monitor breath sounds and vital signs per routine.

h. Provide comfort measures:
- Administer medication for relief of pain, discomfort, nausea.
- Consider amount of medication ordered and check with anesthesiologist and/or attending physician if indicated.
- Institute care for postpartum "shaking":
  Provide warmed blanket, especially to feet.
  Reassure patient that this is a normal and temporary response.

i. Provide fluids and monitor amounts and kind:
- Maintain IV fluids and/or encourage p.o. intake as ordered.
- Accurate intake and output record

j. Take measures to prevent bladder distention:
- Observe for bladder distention, q 15 minutes for 1 hour and then q 1 hour for 6 hours.
- Encourage patient to void within 6 hours.
- Use measures to assist patient to initiate voiding, *e.g.*, offer bedpan frequently, assure privacy, assist patient to a sitting position in bed or on chair, turn on water faucet, ambulate to bathroom unless contraindicated.

17. Promote maternal/significant other-infant bonding:
a. Allow mother to hold infant as desired during time infant remains in Recovery Room.
b. Assist mother in breast feeding as she desires.
c. Encourage interaction between mother/significant other and baby. Examples:
- Allow to hold; show how to if necessary.
- Briefly unwrap baby and allow to touch.
- Decrease light in room and hold baby so that (s)he is able to open eyes.
- Explain newborn's appearance and behavior, *e.g.*, crying, sleeping, movements, color.
d. Explain reason for brief stay of baby in Recovery Room and placement of baby in Nursery.

18. Facilitate infant's transfer to Nursery.
a. Call Nursery to transport baby. Obtain baby bed.
b. Send cord blood samples with infant per hospital policy.

Patient Outcome	Process

c. Send all documentation with infant. Report significant information of maternal-infant status.

19. Facilitate mother's transfer to postpartum unit.
    a. Obtain room assignment and alert postpartum nurse of impending transfer and needed equipment.
    b. Provide perineal care.
    c. Write transfer note to include:
       • Summary of admission and labor process.
       • Delivery data and infant condition: time, kind of delivery, episiotomy, infant's sex, weight, Apgar score
       • Maternal condition during immediate postpartum period:
          Vital sign stability and range, fundal height and firmness, description of lochia, activity status, voiding status, diet toleration, emotional response to labor/delivery of baby
       • Breast or bottle feeding
       • Where prenatal care given and cause if high risk
       • Summary of available data, *e.g.*, blood type, gonococcal culture, venereal disease research laboratories (VDRL), Pap smear, rubella titer, sickle cell prep
       • Medications received and time administered during immediate postpartum period, and if medications sent with patient
    d. Transfer according to activity status. Make sure personal possessions are transferred also.
    e. Assist patient to bed in postpartum unit.
    f. Verbally report significant information of maternal-infant status to assigned nurse in postpartum unit.

Patient Outcome	Process

DESCRIPTION: These guidelines are applicable to the patient who has had a normal, spontaneous vaginal delivery of a viable infant. The guidelines may be used in conjunction with the Normal Labor and Delivery and Normal Newborn Guidelines; pp. 259–263; 273–281.

A. *The patient knows about hospital environment and therapeutic routine care*

1. Orient the patient to room, unit, and care routines.
   a. Activity within ward but not outside
   b. Visitor restrictions
   c. Location of supplies (peri-pads, underpads, etc.)
   d. How to call Nursery to contact personnel or to see baby
   e. Daily routines (sitz baths, lamps, pericare, vital signs)
   f. Use of bathroom trash can to dispose of peri-pads

B. *The patient/baby are safe in the environment*

2. Provide safe environment.
   a. Explain mother's responsibility.
   b. Emphasize importance of having nursing assistance especially during the first time out of bed.
   c. Take special precautions for mother holding baby.
      • Provide footstools while sitting on edge of bed, as needed.
      • No walking with baby outside of room
      • Do not leave baby unattended. When not being held, place baby in crib.
   d. Teach hand-washing techniques to mother and handwashing and gowning to allowed visitors.
   e. Inform mother of visitor restrictions and reasons for this.
   f. Enforce visitor restrictions as needed.

C. *The patient has progressive involution of uterus and controlled bleeding*

3. Provide and teach care related to progressive uterine involution and control of bleeding.
   a. Facilitate uterine involution:
      • Assess and document level of fundus. Massage fundus to stimulate firmness and express clots or pooled blood. The frequency depends upon the amount and kind of lochia, kind of delivery, and length of time following delivery. Usual frequency of massage is:
         Every 15 to 30 minutes for 1 hour postpartum and upon arrival in postpartum unit; q 1 hour for 2 hours, 4 hours for first 24 hours, then q 8 hours.
   b. Assess amount of lochia.
      • Keep accurate pad count.
      • Instruct mother to report immediately if lochia seems excessive.
   c. Provide explanation to mother that contractions, although uncomfortable, are normal and will gradually decrease in severity and frequency.
   d. Teach patient with "boggy" fundus to massage own fundus with firm but gentle pressure. Observe return demonstration.
   e. Give oxytocic medications as ordered:
      • Methergine p.o. or IM 0.2 mgm. q.i.d. (dependent upon bleeding and blood pressure). Give after measuring blood pressure. Diastolic pressure should be less than 90.
      • Oxytocin (Pitocin:) IV 10 to 30 units per liter or IM (dependent upon bleeding)
   f. Provide care for patient who is bleeding excessively.
      • Monitor pulse and blood pressure q 15 to 30 minutes.
      • Notify physician.
      • Keep strict pad count.
      • Massage fundus frequently.
      • Give medications as ordered.

D. *The patient has minimal breast engorgement (nonbreast-feeding mother) or is able to breast feed adequately and with minimal discomfort (breast-feeding mother)*

4. Assist mother to adapt to chosen method of infant feeding.
   a. Interview patient to determine whether breast or bottle feeding.
   b. Provide care for mother who bottle feeds baby.
      • Remind to wear tight support bra all of the time (day and night).
      • Use binders as substitute for bra if desired.
      • Apply ice packs to reduce congestion and swelling.
      • Check breasts twice a day for discomfort.
      • Inform patient analgesics are available if breasts become painful.
      • An estrogen compound may be prescribed to suppress lactation. If mother then decides to breast feed, physician will discuss with patient the possibility of maternal side effects such as blood clots, thrombophlebitis.

265

Patient Outcome	Process

c. Provide care for mother who breast feeds baby.
- Assess for potential problems with breast feeding such as inverted nipples, flat nipples, sensitive skin.
  - Use nipple shield for inverted nipples.
  - Use heat lamp for 15 minutes after each feeding and prior to application of nipple cream for cracked nipples. Be careful not to burn tender breast skin.
- Check breasts once each 8 hours for soreness, cracked nipples, skin blisters, bleeding.
- Teach mother to inspect breasts and report signs of problems.

d. Teach and/or assess mother's knowledge and skills related to feeding. This includes:
- Wash hands; wash and rinse areola (start at center and wash toward periphery) before and after each feeding.
- Position self and baby.
- Place nipple in baby's mouth.
- Feed every 3 to 4 hours depending on needs of baby per physician's order:
  - First 24 hours: 5 minutes on each breast
  - Second 24 hours: 10 minutes on each breast
  - Third 24 hours: up to 15 minutes on each breast—never more than 30 minutes total nursing time
- Reassure mother that baby does not need to nurse for longer periods and that nipples may be injured if nursing is prolonged. Teach mother how to break suction before removing nipple from baby's mouth.
- Wash nipple, pat dry, and apply breast cream as needed.

e. Consider methods to promote milk "let-down".
- Syntocinon nasal spray may be prescribed to be administered 15 minutes before feeding to stimulate "let-down" of milk.
- Shower
- Warm, moist towel application

f. Assist with use of breast pump or manual expression of milk as indicated to relieve discomfort or for baby not able to come to the breast.

g. Observe for signs of severe engorgement which may lead to mastitis, *e.g.*, redness, tenderness, fever, pain.
- Notify physician.
- Anticipate use of ice packs, tight binder, analgesic.

h. Remain aware of situations which may temporarily interfere with mother's ability to breast feed such as:
- Fever of mother higher than 38°C
- Isolation of mother
- Certain medications, *e.g.*, sulfonamides, phenobarbital, other sedatives
- Inadequate milk supply (baby may need supplementary feedings temporarily)

i. Determine reasons if mother has poor milk supply.

5. Assist mother to maintain personal hygiene.

a. Encourage daily shower with soap. May use deodorant and shampoo hair if desired.

b. Provide and teach perineal care to include:
- Check for allergy to iodine.
- Explain/demonstrate perineal cleansing with povidone-iodine after each use of the toilet. If patient allergic to iodine, may use prepackaged medicated towelettes.
- Do not touch stitches: air dry.
- Replace fresh pad after each use of toilet.
- Caution not to powder perineum.
- Apply heat lamp to perineum b.i.d.
  - Place 15 to 20 inches away from body.
  - Instruct to call nurse if uncomfortable.
- Check perineum and episiotomy daily for redness, swelling, stitch breakdown, hematoma, hemorrhoids. Report abnormalities.
- Provide sitz bath as ordered to relieve perineal and rectal discomfort.

E. *The patient is comfortable and adequately rested*

6. Promote adequate rest and comfort.

a. Assess the patient's rest/comfort needs considering:
- Experience in labor and delivery
  - Length of labor and difficulties

Patient Outcome	Process

Type of delivery
Sensory stimulation (number of other patients in recovery room, noise level)
Anesthesia and medications
- General physical status of mother, including hunger and thirst.
- Anxiety of mother including concerns for self, baby, family and home situation.

b. Plan with patient to meet comfort/rest needs.
- Encourage patient to try to rest even though elated feelings may make this difficult.
- Consider mother's need to have physical contact with baby and conversation with family members before she can relax.
- Offer food, fluids, medications as ordered.
- Explain availability of pain medications and sedative.
- Check with patient periodically to determine level of comfort.
  Before rest periods patient may need to void or have analgesic.
- Plan time for nap periods; early afternoon is often a good time.
- Provide for a quiet, darkened environment.
- Plan care to provide undisturbed rest periods.
- Provide comfort measures as needed such as back rubs, repositioning, and cushion.
- Give sitz bath as ordered to relieve perineal and rectal discomforts.
- Restrict visitors, per unit policy, in terms of time and number to allow rest periods. Explain rationale to mother and visitors.
  Place sign on door to remind staff/visitors that patient is resting.
- Evaluate with patient to determine whether rest/comfort needs are being met effectively. Revise plan as needed.

7. Facilitate return to normal bowel and bladder function and nutritional status.
  a. Assess for potential problems in voiding considering:
  - Kind of anesthesia: epidural; spinal; saddle-block will interrupt sensation and ability to void.
  - Type of delivery; difficult delivery may cause excessive periurethral edema, tissue damage.
  - Full bladder during delivery may allow bladder to be slightly damaged and hematuria may result.
  b. Assure adequate urinary output.
  - Use techniques to induce voiding, *e.g.*, give analgesic, upright position, running water, warm towels, apply warm water over perineum, shower, rubbing ice cubes over bladder.
  - Catheterize after six hours unless otherwise ordered. Check with physician if still unable to void within six hours after catheterization.
  - Check for symptoms of overdistention of bladder.
    Small frequent amounts of urine
    Displaced uterus
    Increased lochia
    Abdominal discomfort
  - Encourage fluid intake (2000 to 3000 cc daily) unless on fluid restrictions.
  - Record intake-output for at least first 24 hours. Continue if there are voiding problems or need for controlled intake.
  - Check for sign of dehydration:
    Output considerably less than intake
    Elevated temperature
    Elevated urine specific gravity
    Unusual thirst
  - Collect and send urine specimens for urinalysis and culture as ordered.
  - Provide care related to indwelling catheter.
    Provide routine perineal care and catheter care.
    Collect urine specimen for culture prior to removal of catheter.
  c. Promote adequate nutritional intake.
  - Assess special dietary needs through observing amount of food and fluids ingested and asking about patient satisfaction with food.
    Make special diet requests due to medical condition, patient preference, and religion.
    Obtain dietary consult as needed.

Patient Outcome	Process

	• Consider special needs of breast-feeding mothers:
	    Encourage ample fluid intake including milk or substitutes such as cheese or puddings.
	    Encourage well-balanced diet.
	    Teach awareness of any foods that seem to affect the baby, *e.g.*, cabbage, orange juice, and onions.
	  d. Promote return of optimal bowel function. Refer to Chapter 2 Bowel Care Guidelines when there is Deviation from Normal Bowel Function, p. 25.
	    • Assess for potential bowel function problems such as constipation. Consider:
	        Bowel status prior to labor
	        Enema or laxative given prior to or during labor.
	        Medications, *e.g.*, iron supplement
	        Anesthesia
	        Episiotomy
	        Hemorrhoids
	    • Begin bowel care program within 24 hours postdelivery. Discontinue after first normal stool.
	        Sodium sulfosuccinate (Colace) 100 mg p.o., b.i.d. as ordered
	        Milk of magnesia 30 cc p.o., b.i.d. as ordered.
	    • Collaborate with physician for suppository or lubricating enema if necessary.
	    • Keep bowel record.
	    • Reassure patient that having a bowel movement will not tear perineum.
	    • Consult with physician for medications to relieve hemorrhoids.

G. *The patient is free of thrombophlebitis*	8. Provide measures to prevent/minimize occurrence of thrombophlebitis.
	  a. Assess for predisposing factors of thrombophlebitis:
	    • Increase in blood volume, slowing of venous return, increase in clotting ability during pregnancy.
	    • Presence of varicosities, edema
	    • Prolonged periods of bed rest before or after delivery
	    • Past history of thrombophlebitis
	    • Age factor (over 40)
	    • Postsurgery, *e.g.*, cesearean section
	    • Systemic infection
	    • Direct injury to vein, *e.g.,* prolonged period in stirrups, IV site
	  b. Observe for signs and symptoms of thrombophlebitis:
	    • Redness, swelling of vein
	    • Pain, tenderness in lower extremity
	    • Positive Homan's sign
	    • High fever unresponsive to antibiotics (pelvic thrombophlebitis)
	  c. Provide preventive care. Instruct patient and explain importance of the following care measures.
	    • Early ambulation and exercise to maintain circulation
	    • Proper position of legs, *e.g.*, do not cross legs at knees, no prolonged dangling of legs (use footstool)
	    • Ankle and leg exercises for bed patients q 4 hours
	    • Support hose, as ordered
	    • Avoidance of restrictive wearing apparel, *e.g.*, knee high hose, garters
	    • Adequate fluid intake
	    • Early recognition of symptoms of thrombophlebitis
	  d. Provide therapeutic care, initiated by nurse and/or ordered by physician.
	    • Apply antiembolic hose as ordered.
	    • Encourage bed rest.
	    • Instruct patient not to massage affected leg.
	    • Elevate legs 20° by raising foot of bed: no acute angle at hips.
	    • Apply heating pad to area as ordered.
	    • Maintain hydration.
	    • Check temperature frequently.
	    • Give medications as ordered, *e.g.*, heparin, analgesics.

H. *The patient achieves a realistic level of emotional stability*	9. Assist the patient to achieve emotional stability. a. Assess verbal and nonverbal behaviors that indicate adjustment to childbirth experience.

Patient Outcome	Process

b. Consider factors that may influence adjustment. Identify and document current or potential problems.
- Previous and current labor and delivery experience, *e.g.*, sleep deprivation
- Health of mother and baby
- Past history of emotional stability
- Effects, side effects of drugs
- Present feelings about baby
- Age of patient
- Number and ages of other children
- Personal responsibilities, *e.g.*, career, extended family
- Financial status
- Support system and how available to patient (under- or overavailability)
- Cultural influences including communication

c. Be aware that emotions may be affected by lack of sleep, lack of privacy, hormonal changes, and pain.

d. Help mother and family understand rationale for care being given. Examples are:
- Intravenous infusions
- Medications
- Urine samples
- Treatments, examinations
- Schedules, *e.g.*, nursery
- Separation from infant as it occurs

e. Help mother/family understand care being given to baby. Make special arrangements if baby is not normal newborn to have pediatrician and/or nursery staff talk with mother/family.

f. Help patient to express feelings openly.
- Spend time talking and listening, especially with patients who have been identified as having current or potential problems.
- Problem-solve with patient about immediate concerns, *e.g.*, contact with baby.

g. Consider other resources that may be helpful, *e.g.*, social worker, psychologist, public health nurse.

h. Encourage patient to participate in diversional activities, *e.g.*, games, conversations with other patients.

i. Provide for contact with other patients who may share common concerns.

j. Be aware of behaviors or circumstances which might indicate emotional instability and/or potential for child abuse. Document behaviors.
- Indifference towards baby:
  Holds baby away from body
  Impersonal references to baby
  Lack of interest in seeing, touching
  Attitude change from interest to disinterest when visitors leave
- Lack of interest in mothering role:
  Jealousy of baby or attention received
  Unwillingness to be responsible for a person other than self
- Denial or rejection of pregnancy that persists throughout pregnancy
- Unfavorable circumstances associated with pregnancy, *e.g.*, dislike of father, pregnancy resulting from rape
- Excessive fatigue, many questions
- Relationship with patient's mother

k. Consult resource people who can assist in helping patient who may have emotional problems.
- Psychiatric consult as ordered by physician
- Psychiatric social worker (who may interview patient/family and may arrange to have social worker visit home)
- Psychiatric nurse (who may confer with staff regarding specific patient problems)
- Public health nurse (who may visit patient/family for supervision at home and may refer patient to a mental health outpatient facility)

Patient Outcome	Process

I. *The patient and family have knowledge and skills related to mother and baby care*	10. Plan home care with patient and family.
	
	  a. Assess patient knowledge regarding care of self and baby as early as possible in hospitalization. Consider:
	    • Patient's prior knowledge:
	      Previous experience with postpartum and baby care
	      Previous education: TV, reading, classes
	    • Interest in learning may be modified by:
	      Family situation, environment
	      Age
	      Anxiety
	    • Ability to learn
	    • Degree of comfort
	    • Communication between nurse/patient
	
	  b. Identify patient whose financial situation may prevent family from providing adequate home care.
	    • Contact social services immediately to initiate assistance.
	    • Alert Nursery personnel to special needs.
	    • Discuss acceptable but less expensive alternatives with patient.
	    • Obtain free samples of products when available from Nursery or physician's office.
	    • Notify public health nurse of mother/baby needs. Nursery personnel will help write referral.
	
	  c. Plan for individual and/or group teaching.
	  d. Use every opportunity to teach patient while performing care.
	    • Explain treatments and other care.
	    • Include appropriate family member who will share care responsibilities.

• *Activity/exercise*	e. Teach regarding resumption of activity.
	    • Coordinate mother's and baby's rest period.
	    • Resume shower and shampoo as desired.
	    • Suggest limitations:
	      First week: Mother's activities should be limited to own and baby's care needs. Limit stair climbing to twice daily.
	      Second week: Increase activities to include cooking and light house work. Limit demanding activities, *e.g.*, lifting heavy loads.
	      Third week: Mother may resume driving.
	      Fourth to Sixth week: According to physician's orders, mother may resume tub bath, douching, use of tampons, and sexual activity.
	      Sixth week: Mother may resume all normal activities.
	
	  f. Teach exercises to regain normal muscle tone. Watch return demonstration.
	    • Initial exercises in hospital (mild)
	      Breathing exercises
	      Buttock tightening
	      Head lift
	    • Predischarge exercises (more strenuous)
	      Pelvic tilt
	      Abdominal strengthening
	    • Ambulation

• *Hygiene*	g. Teach regarding hygiene measures to include:
	    • No tub baths for first four weeks unless ordered by physician. Daily shower or body sponge baths advised.
	    • Review principles of wiping/washing perineal area from front to back.
	    • Change perineal pad frequently, or at every use of bathroom even though not very soiled until soreness of episiotomy is gone.
	    • Special care of breasts and perineum.

• *Nutrition/Bowel*	h. Counsel regarding well-balanced diet:
	    • Encourage intake of meat, vegetables, fruit, and bread daily. Consider cultural influences.
	    • Drink ample fluids.
	    • Exercise as tolerated to avoid constipation.
	    • Help patient identify foods that are not constipating or will promote bowel function.

Patient Outcome	Process

- *Family planning*

- Use laxative such as 30 ml milk of magnesia if needed: breast feeding mother should avoid laxative.
  i. Teach about family planning.
  - Review patient history for contraindications to certain methods of birth control such as oral contraceptive.
    Oral contraceptive: heavy menstrual periods or unusual bleeding, uterine fibroids, cesarean section, pelvic inflammatory disease, breast feeding
  - Interview patient for preferred method of birth control (Previous method may be preferred).
    Oral
    Intrauterine device (IUD)
    Diaphragm
    Condom
    Spermicidal jelly
    Rhythm
    Abstinence
    Coitus interruptus
    Tubal ligation
    Hysterectomy
    Vasectomy
  - Provide basic written information as needed to include sexual function and discuss alternative methods of birth control.
  - Use demonstration kits/models and audiovisual aids for teaching.
  - Encourage discussion with partner so that it will be a mutually agreed upon decision.
  - Teach patient about selected method of birth control and give written information. Emphasize signs/symptoms of problems that should be reported to physician.
    Check for correct information through verbal feedback.
    If patient selects diaphragm or IUD, this will probably be fitted after six week check-up and further instructions given.
    Patients who select a surgical procedure such as tubal ligation, hysterectomy, (or if husband selects vasectomy) should discuss choice with physician.
  - Discuss of return of menses following delivery.

- *Emotional needs*

  j. Counsel mother about normal emotional needs.
  - Consider that:
    Hormone change may cause patient to experience feelings of "depression" or moodiness.
    The patient may be disappointed with body appearance and need reassurance and encouragement regarding gradual return toward prepregnant appearance.
  - Encourage patient to plan a time for meeting her own important personal needs, *e.g.*, rest and relaxation.
  - Discuss the need for re-establishing relationships with husband and children to include redistributing time and attention.

- *Illness*

  k. Teach patient signs and symptoms of illness to report to physician:
  - Bleeding between periods or very heavy bleeding
  - Severe headaches, nausea, vomiting, dizziness
  - Pain, more severe and/or in a different location than experienced in hospital
  - Swelling, discharge, increased tenderness around episiotomy
  - Fever and/or chills
  - Frequency, burning on urination

- *Baby care*

  l. Teach and/or share teaching of baby care with Nursery staff. Refer to Normal Newborn Guidelines, p. 273 for specific teaching related to:
  - Breast feeding techniques
  - Bottle feeding
  - Burping
  - Cord care
  - Circumcision care
  - Effect of hormones on baby's breasts, vaginal discharge
  - Bathing and skin care
  - Diapering and cleansing diaper area

Patient Outcome	Process
	• Positioning and holding baby
	• Clipping finger nails
	• Appropriate clothing
	• Sleeping accommodations
	• Stimulation of infant
	• Normal activity, sleeping pattern
	• Safety of baby, *e.g.*, do not leave baby on bed or unattended; protect from young children
	• Importance of regular medical care
	• Care of sick baby:
	Taking temperature (axillary for neonate)
	Signs and symptoms to report to physician: fever, abnormal color or consistency of stools, loss of appetite, loss of weight, respiratory distress, irritability, vomiting, poor skin color, lethargy
	m. Give return appointment for six week evaluation.

Patient Outcome	Process

A. *The infant maintains physiological functions*	1. Assess and document general physical status on admission or transfer to Nursery.
	   a. Obtain baseline data:
	     • Temperature, pulse, respirations
	     • Blood pressure
	     • Head and chest circumference
	     • Length
	     • Weight
	     • Gestational age
	   b. Observe for normal and abnormal physiological functions, physical deformities.
	   c. Check for proper identification.
	   d. Check for medications given such as silver nitrate, vitamin K.
	   e. Check for blood studies such as tests for syphilis, phenylketonuria, Coombs' test, blood type.
	   f. Determine if there was previous contact with parents.

• *Temperature regulation*	2. Facilitate temperature regulation.
	   a. Check axillary temperature on admission. If less than 36.5°, place in warming crib. If greater than 36.5° × 2 and in no distress, baby may be bathed.
	   b. Check temperature 30 minutes after bathing. If greater than 36.5°, may be warmly wrapped and placed in open crib.
	   c. Check temperature frequently:
	     • q 1 hour until stable
	     • q 4 hours × 12 hours
	     • q 8 hours unless irregular temperature which requires more frequent checking
	   d. Use heat lamp to increase baby's temperature as needed (60 watt bulb, at least 16 inches above crib). If temperature does not rise, baby may be returned to warming crib or Isolette. Temperature probe must not be placed over bony prominence.

• *Respiratory*	3. Assist infant to maintain respiratory function.
	   a. Assess for signs of respiratory abnormality and distress:
	     • Cyanosis
	     • Retractions
	     • Flaring of nares
	     • Audible grunting
	     • Tachypnea
	     • Excess secretions
	     • Choking
	     • Seesaw respirations
	     • Abnormal breath sounds/or heard in unusual place, *e.g.*, pneumothorax may be present.
	     • Barrel chest
	   b. Maintain open airway:
	     • Position on side or stomach to drain secretions.
	     • Suction as needed with nasogastric or bulb suction. Position on right side.
	     • Lower head and chest and pat firmly on back for choking.
	   c. Provide adequate ventilation:
	     • Give free O_2 via cannula with humidity at 4 liters per minute. May be given without physician's order per hospital policy.
	     • Request respiratory therapist to set proper mist and percentage of continuous O_2 if prescribed.

• *Cardiovascular*	4. Assist infant to maintain cardiovascular function.
	   a. Assess for signs of abnormal cardiovascular function:
	     • Rate, rhythm, strength of apical pulse
	     • Abnormal heart sounds or sounds heard in unusual position
	     • Color change; especially note when baby unclothed or during activities such as feeding
	     • Signs of shock (low blood pressure, diaphoresis, cold clammy skin)
	   b. Begin cardiopulmonary resuscitation as indicated according to hospital policy.

• *Gastrointestinal*	5. Assist infant to maintain gastrointestinal function.
	   a. Assess for normal function and signs of abnormalities.
	     • Initial bowel movement within 24 hours (meconium plug)
	     • Consistency, size, color, odor, and frequency of stools indicating normal stages of bowel evacuation

Patient Outcome	Process

- Signs of abnormalities
  Mouth: thrush, cleft palate, gum cysts
  Imperforate anus
  Vomiting, including meconium or green vomitus
  Abnormal stools: absence of stool, foul odor, water margin around stool
  Frequent stools
  Blood or suspected blood in stools
  b. Provide infant feeding according to hospital policy.
  - General feeding principles:
    Observe barrier technique, changing covering in front of uniform to protect against cross contamination.
    Hold infant with head elevated above level of stomach during feeding.
    Assure that neck of bottle and nipple are filled with fluid and nipple is placed on top of tongue.
    Observe for problems such as poor feeding, color change, choking, regurgitation, and incomplete closure of palate or lip.
    Burp as frequently as necessary and place on right side or stomach after feeding.
    Elevate head of bed for baby who regurgitates frequently.
  - For normal baby: (This routine varies according to institution)
    N.p.o. for 4 hours unless otherwise ordered
    First feeding: D_5W (dextrose 5 per cent in water) not to exceed 15cc
    Formula or breast q 3 to 4 hours, dependent upon demand
      Usual schedule for breast feeding first three days:
        First 24 hours—5 minutes each breast
        Second 24 hours—10 minutes each breast
        Third 24 hours—15 minutes each breast
        Following each breast feeding with D_5W for 48 hours.
      Progress formula per age not to exceed:
        First 24 hours—45 cc per feeding
        Second 24 hours—75 cc per feeding
        Third 24 hours—90 cc per feeding
        Fourth 24 hours—120 cc per feeding
  - For baby with suspected glucose problems: baby of diabetic mother, baby with birth weight greater than 4000 gm or less than 2500 gm, baby that is small for gestational age (SGA), or baby with intrauterine growth retardation (IUGR).
    N.p.o. for 3 hours or as prescribed
    First feeding: D_5W
    Formula q 3 hours for 24 hours
    Test blood for glucose using Dextrostix at admission, 1, 2, 3 hours and before feeding × 24 hours. Report results less than 45 or greater than 130 mg per 100 ml.
  - For "sick baby", *e.g.,* respiratory, cardiac or gastrointestinal problems, baby with IV. Depending upon need of baby, physician will order amount, feeding method and frequency. May include:
    Gavage feeding
    Smaller, more frequent feedings
    Special positioning after feeding
    Further orders by physician
  - For premature baby without associated problems:
    N.p.o. for 3 hours or as prescribed
    Nipple or gavage feeding, as ordered
    First feeding: D_5W
    Formula q 3 hours, until otherwise ordered
    Further orders by physician
  - For newborn with hyperbilirubinemia:
    N.p.o. 3 hours
    Formula q 3 hours or breast feed alternately with formula as ordered
    Laboratory tests as ordered
  - For baby with cleft palate:
    Observe for problems with secretions.
    Feeding routines: Chetwood syringe, gavage feeding, special nipples

Patient Outcome	Process

• *Skin and cord*	6. Promote skin integrity and cord healing.
	   a. Observe skin for normal or abnormal color (pallor, plethora, jaundice, cyanosis) birth marks, abnormalities, lacerations, probe and forceps marks, mongolian spots, petechiae, blisters, pustules.
	   b. Bathe infant and provide cord care according to hospital policy.
	   c. Provide special skin care.
	     • Lacerations:
	      Apply povidone-iodine every 8 hours. Expose to air. Physician may order antibiotic ointment.
	     • Rashes of buttocks:
	      Expose to air and lamp light.
	      Apply ointment p.r.n. as ordered.
	     • Monilial infection of perineum:
	      Apply antifungal ointment as ordered.
	     • Long finger nails:
	      Clip nails with finger nail scissors.

• *Eyes*	7. Assist infant to maintain eye function.
	   a. Observe eyes for clarity, eye and pupil position, shape, swelling, discoloration, discharge, laceration of skin around eye and cornea, broken blood vessels.
	   b. Follow Credé method for eyes once if already done in Delivery Room, twice if not done in Delivery Room, and three times if mother has positive test for venereal disease.
	   c. Protect eyes of baby under bilirubin reduction lights using eye cover. Remove during feeding. Prior to discharge, physician will check baby for corneal abrasions. If a baby is under 2000 gm. weight at birth and received O_2, eye consult will be needed to rule out retrolental fibroplasia. Before eye examination, dilate pupils per order.

• *Genitourinary*	8. Assist infant to maintain urinary function.
	   a. Observe for normal/abnormal urinary function:
	     • Check voiding within first 24 hours.
	     • Check specific gravities or collect urine samples per physician order.
	     • Observe abnormalities:
	      Unusual voiding pattern, color, concentration of urine
	      Hypospadias, epispadias
	     • Absence of normal external sexual characteristics
	     • Provide care prior to and following circumcision.

• *Neurological*	9. Assist infant to maintain neurological function.
	   a. Observe for normal/abnormal neurological development:
	     • Size and shape of head in proportion to body size and gestational age. Notify physician of abnormally large or small measurement.
	     • Fontanelle
	     • Cry (vigorous, nonshrill)
	     • Muscle tone
	     • Response to stimulation
	     • Sucking reflex
	     • Grasping reflex
	     • Note abnormalities (Consider effect of maternal medication or history of drugs or alcohol):
	      Unusual shape of head
	      Facial palsies, Erb's palsy
	      Shrill cry
	      Lack of/or poor muscle tone, or hypertonia
	      Lethargy
	      Abnormal response to stimulation
	      Bulging, sunken fontaneles; overriding or closed sutures
	      Poor temperature control
	      Down's syndrome: low set ears, simian crease, loose skin covering back of neck, protruding tongue, epicanthal folds causing oriental appearance to eyes, muscular hypotonia

• *Musculoskeletal*	10. Assist infant to maintain musculoskeletal function.
	   a. Observe for normal/abnormal musculoskeletal development:
	     • Note presence of all extremities and digits.

Patient Outcome	Process
	• Note if trunk and extremities are aligned normally and move through normal range of motion.
	• Note abnormalities:
	Appearance indicating congenital abnormality or birth injury, *e.g.,* absence of extremity or digits; presence of extra digit; "lobster claw"; drooping shoulder (fractured clavicle); clubbing; dislocation; spinal curvature; meningocele
	Abnormal range of motion: "clicking sounds", hyperextension of knee joint
	b. Provide care for baby with musculoskeletal problem per physician orders.
	• Extra digits
	Physician obtains permit to ligate digit.
	Keep area covered and taped as necessary.
	• Absence of part of extremity:
	Provide range of motion to extremity.
	• Hip dislocation:
	Use double diapering.
	Use Frejka pillow splint.
	• Disorders of the leg and foot, *e.g.,* clubbed foot
	Provide cast care.
	• Meningocele:
	Apply sterile dressing moistened with saline.
	• Fractured clavicle
	Keep off affected side.
	Use open front T-shirt.
• *Endocrine*	11. Assist infant to maintain endocrine function.
	a. Observe for signs of normal/abnormal endocrine function:
	• For baby with suspected glucose problems
	Check blood for glucose using Dextrostix at admission, 1,2,3 hours and before feeding × 24 hours.
	Notify physician if less than 45 mg per 100 ml or greater than 130 mg per 100 ml.
	b. For baby with tremors
	• Check blood with Dextrostix; notify physician who may order calcium determination.
	c. For baby with hypocalcemia:
	• Remind physician to regularly obtain calcium level.
	d. For baby of mother with hypo- or hyperthyroidism:
	• Observe for bulging eyes, irritability, temperature control instability, poor feeding.
B. *The infant is in a safe environment*	12. Provide a safe environment.
	a. Identify baby properly in Delivery Room. Check baby's armband with mother's armband. Have mother verbally spell name.
	b. Transport infant from Delivery Room to Nursery in crib; include bulb syringe.
	c. Do not leave baby unattended for first 12 hours in or out of crib; after 12 hours, never leave unattended outside of crib.
	d. Restrict visitors according to hospital policy.
	e. Adhere to strict cleaning routines:
	• Equipment: Clean counters, scales, heated cribs, circumcision board, measuring tray between babies.
	• When baby is in bed more than seven days, clean bed or Isolette.
	• Personnel, visitors:
	Initial wash in nursery: scrub with povidone-iodine or other antimicrobial solution to elbows (two minutes), wear gown over clothing.
	f. Assist mother to maintain safety precautions.
	• Check physical readiness of mother to receive baby (consider medications, strength, alertness, disabilities).
	• Check for safety hazards in room (electric cords, other obstructions).
	• Make sure bulb syringe is available and mother knows how to use it.
	• Instruct mother and designated visitors in hand-washing and gowning before handling baby.
	• Instruct in proper feeding technique, burping and positioning baby after feeding.
	• Discuss visiting policies and importance of them.

Patient Outcome	Process

Process content:

- Caution mother against:
  - Placing baby in mother's bed
  - Leaving baby alone in room
  - Visiting with baby in another room
- g. Transportation of baby to other areas:
  - Attend baby at all times by Nursery personnel.
  - Transport in baby's crib; bulb syringe included.
13. Use special isolation techniques to prevent cross contamination.
  - a. Indications:
    - Suspected infections of mother, *e.g.,* herpes simplex, hepatitis, rubella, scabies
    - Exposure of mother prior to delivery to diseases such as chickenpox, rubella, mumps
    - Suspected infections of baby: Klebsiella, Salmonella, Staphlococcus, Streptococcus, Escherichia coli
  - b. Isolation techniques include:
    - Isolation corner in unit (whenever possible)
    - Isolette as ordered by physician
    - Regular bed with special precautions
    - Rooming in with mother (private room)
    - Precautions as ordered, which may include: gown, glove, linen, trash, needle, stool

C. *The baby is free of or has minimal complications following special therapies*
• Circumcision

14. Intervene for infant requiring circumcision.
  - a. Explain circumcision to parents to include:
    - *Purpose:* To remove foreskin for purposes of cleanliness, or as a religious ritual.
    - *Procedure:* The procedure varies depending on type of equipment. The baby is strapped to a circumcision board using gauze strips with velcro closures. He is draped and the penis is prepped with antiseptic solution. A probe is inserted between foreskin and penis to free any adhesions. The foreskin is clamped and a small cut is made to allow placement of bell part of the Gomco clamp. After the bell is placed over the meatus, the foreskin is pulled up around the outside of the bell and pinned. The clamp is tightened for hemostasis and the skin is cut and removed. The clamp is then removed and the area is observed for excessive bleeding. Vaseline gauze is applied and baby removed from the board. He may be fed immediately.
  - b. Institute preparation for procedure:
    - Be aware of these considerations:
      - Baby must be at least 12 hours old.
      - Baby must have a physical examination to rule out any contraindications to procedure such as questionable sexual determination or hypospadias.
      - Procedure is contraindicated in families with history of hemophilia (Check bleeding, clotting time).
      - Must not be receiving fluorescent light therapy or blood checks for glucose.
    - Check for permit signed by mother (Jewish parents may prefer to have ritual circumcision performed by a rabbi).
    - Keep n.p.o. at least three hours or as ordered.
  - c. Provide post-procedure care.
    - Observe for excessive bleeding; apply pressure dressing; notify physician for adrenalin order or sutures.
    - Check initial voiding.
    - Redress and teach mother to redress with vaseline gauze every diaper change for three days.

• Photatherapy

15. Provide care for baby receiving photatherapy.
  - a. Reinforce physician's explanation of need for therapy.
    - *Purpose:* To break down bilirubin through chemical decomposition which changes into nontoxic particles
    - *Procedure:* Clothing is removed, eyes are covered, and baby is positioned on either side or stomach under light. The baby is removed only for routine care and feeding until the bilirubin level is within normal limits.
  - b. Provide care during therapy.
    - Increase frequency of feedings to q 3 hours because of loss of fluid through bowel and skin.
    - Keep penis taped to prevent urination on heat lamp light bulb which might cause bulb to shatter.

Patient Outcome	Process

• *Isolette*	16. Provide care for baby in Isolette.
	  a. Reinforce physician's explanation to mother.
	    • *Purpose:* To maintain body temperature for babies with temperature instability due to being small for gestational age, and/or intrauterine growth retardation or for protective isolation
	  b. Provide routine care in Isolette rather than outside with removal for weighing only.
	  c. Maintain Isolette temperature level 90°F, unless otherwise ordered.
	  d. Check baby's temperature as frequently as needed.
	  e. Allow parents to visit in Nursery. The mother must not have a fever.

• *Intravenous therapy*	17. Provide care for baby receiving intravenous therapy.
	  a. Reinforce physician's explanation of therapy.
	    • *Purpose:* Adequate nutrition, fluid and electrolyte balance, giving medications
	  b. Assist in starting infusion.
	    • Maintain proper position of baby.
	    • Protect infusion site.
	  c. Observe and maintain proper equipment and infusion.
	  d. Observe for signs of complications.
	    • Swelling around IV site
	    • Lack of blood return
	    • Nonfunctioning IV
	  e. Change tubing q 24 hours.
	  f. Assure IV site change q 48 hours or as needed for special circumstances. Document exceptions.
	  g. Use infusion pump for safety.

• *Lumbar puncture*	18. Provide care for baby requiring lumbar puncture.
	  a. Reinforce physician's explanation to parent.
	  b. Assist with procedure as needed.
	    • Maintain proper position: sitting, side-lying.
	  c. Observe for abnormal irritability, apnea, bradycardia, and leakage from puncture site during postprocedure period.

• *Suprapubic bladder tap*	19. Provide care for baby having suprapubic bladder tap.
	  a. Reinforce physician's explanation to parent.
	  b. Assist with tap; properly position baby.
	  c. Observe for bloody urine during postprocedure period.

D. *The parents attain knowledge and skills related to home care*	20. Provide teaching about normal newborn care.
	  a. Share teaching of baby care with obstetric nursing staff; hold conferences as needed to assess
	    • Mother's attitude regarding baby and learning
	    • Current level of knowledge
	    • General condition of baby, any abnormalities
	    • Condition of mother that might affect care or learning about care
	    • Socioeconomic factors that might affect baby care
	    • What role each nursing staff will take regarding teaching of baby care
	  b. Give daily instructions to mother (include father and/or other family members when appropriate); continually assess learning; reinforce information as necessary.
	  c. Explain normal characteristics of baby:
	    • Head molding
	    • Milia
	    • Reaction of eyes to silver nitrate (swelling, drainage)
	    • Fontanelles, overriding sutures
	    • "Newborn rash", peeling skin
	    • Abrasions resulting from fetal monitor
	    • Complexion
	    • Breast engorgement, discharge
	    • Condition of cord, dye
	    • Genitalia, vaginal discharge, circumcision
	    • Color and consistency of bowels
	    • Mongolian spots, birth marks
	    • Abrasions or lacerations due to delivery
	    • Remaining lanugo

Patient Outcome	Process

    d. Give bath demonstration.
- Head/hair, skin, umbilical cord, genitalia
- Special emphasis on crevices, fontanelles.

    e. Discuss feeding and formula preparation.
- Breast feeding: Follow usual schedule.
- Breast care, pumping, shields, freezing of milk, breast pads, supplementary bottle, vitamins.
- Bottle feeding:
    - Sterilization of formula and bottles
    - Types of formulas, amount per age
    - Holding bottle properly
    - Holding baby during feeding/no propping
- General feeding measures:
    - Frequency ("on-demand", about every 3 to 4 hours)
    - Positioning during feeding
    - Burping
    - Positioning after feeding
    - Sterile water between feedings

    f. Teach skin care
- Apply lotion to dry skin; avoid powder and petroleum jelly.
- Observe for allergic reactions.
- Trim nails.

    g. Teach observation of stools to include:
- Color, consistency, odor, frequency, amount of stool dependent upon baby's age, feeding, and health.

    h. Discuss sensory stimulation.
- Consider mobiles, colors, change in light, music boxes, and textured toys.
- Instruct about holding, changing position, talking, providing for sucking needs, gentle touch.

    i. Discuss safety measures.
- Discourage parents from sleeping with baby.
- Stress proper hand washing.
- Keep out of crowds and away from those with infections.
- Provide proper clothing.
- Don't leave unattended in potentially dangerous situation, *e.g.*, with other young children or alone in house.
- Encourage parents to use car seat for baby whenever operating a moving vehicle.

21. Teach special feeding techniques for babies with feeding problems which may include: cleft palate, prematures, babies with respiratory or cardiac problems, poor sucking response, facial palsy.
    a. Use of special feeding devices for cleft palate or prematures:
- Chetwood syringe
- Premature nipple

    b. Positioning after feedings (at least one half hour)
- Raise head of bed, lay on right side or stomach, never on back.
- Infant-seat position, attended by adult.

    c. Baby should not be left on back except when attended by adult.

22. Teach care of baby with orthopedic problem/nerve damage.
    a. Fractured clavicle:
- Position on unaffected side only.
- Use open front T-shirts.
- Provide passive range of motion after first week.
- Avoid movement of extremity but allow baby freedom of movement.

    b. "Hip click" (socket problem):
- Double or triple diapering with cloth diapers
- Return orthopaedic appointment

    c. Club foot/feet:
- If casted, teach cast care.
- Return orthopaedic appointment

Patient Outcome	Process

      d.   Extra digits or skin tags:
- Keep covered with bandage if necessary.
- Watch for separation.
- Be aware if bone involved, may require later surgery. Return orthopaedic appointment.

      e.   Erb's palsy (brachial nerve 5, 6, 7):
- Teach passive range of motion.
- Should resolve gradually

23. Teach proper administration of medications. Assess skills and knowledge related to medications—purpose, frequency, course, side effects.

      a.   Antifungal, antibiotic for thrush
- Place medication on tongue to retain in mouth as long as possible.

      b.   Saline nose drops for stuffy nose
- Teach to make at home.
- Suction after drops administered.

      c.   Eye medication: drops or ointment

24. Teach wound care for probe, forcep, and scalpel lacerations.

25. Teach special skin care for rashes, extremely dry skin, fungus infection.

      a.   Expose buttocks to air as much as possible.

      b.   Use ointment or lotion prescribed.

      c.   Keep rubber pants off.

      d.   Wash buttocks after each stool.

      e.   Rinse diapers thoroughly after washing to remove any detergent.

      f.   Do not irritate rashes or milia because of increased possibility of infection.

26. Teach about illness.

      a.   Signs and symptoms of illness and when to notify physician:
- Fever (37.5°C or above) in conjunction with other symptoms
- Regurgitating large amounts, vomiting
- Coughing, chest congestion
- Runny noses, especially yellow nasal discharge
- Refusal to eat a number of feedings
- Irritable
- Flushed
- Unable to arouse
- Diarrhea
- Red, swollen, foul-smelling, warm, umbilical cord area.

      b.   Caution parents *not to*:
- Administer medications without specific instruction from physician.
- Feed baby when vomiting.
- Overfeed baby having diarrhea.
- Expose to people with infections.

      c.   Give suggestions for care of baby who becomes ill:
- Call physician for fever; may then sponge baby with cool water.
- Use cool-mist vaporizer for congestion.
- Give medications as prescribed for entire course of therapy.
- Give extra attention to ill baby.

E. *The parents are coping with events during post-partum period*

27. Assist parents to cope with events during postpartum period.

      a.   Observe verbal and nonverbal reactions to baby and baby care instructions.
- Interest or reluctance in providing care
- Signs of anxiety, apprehension, hostility

      b.   Explore parents' interests and concerns.

      c.   Encourage parents to have as much physical contact with baby as possible.

      d.   Reassure parents that they should not feel guilty about having baby with defect or abnormality. Use appropriate interventions as needed.

      e.   Give appropriate written information in addition to direct teaching.

      f.   Consider special needs of parents with multiple births.
- Watch for verbal and nonverbal behavior of parents which may indicate problems in caring for more than one baby.
- Assess home situation, *e.g.,* other children to care for, facilities ready for babies' care, whether mother will have help in caring for babies.

Patient Outcome	Process
	• Encourage contact with babies in Nursery (feeding, holding, learning care) if births are premature. Help to dispel fears, promote closeness.
	• Send public health nursing referral to any anticipated problems.
	g. Provide special help for parents learning to care for baby with a physical problem.
	• Consider situations/conditions as:
	Physical defects such as cleft palate, meningomyelocele, absence or deformity of an extremity, abnormal genitalia, blindness, hydrocephalus, Down's syndrome
	Birth injuries such as fractured clavicle, nerve damage, skull injury
	Illness such as respiratory problems, kidney problems
	h. Provide supportive care while teaching about the baby.
	• Stay with parents while they become familiar with baby but do not promote dependency on the nurse.
	• Determine if the doctor has discussed the problem sufficiently to insure parents' understanding.
	i. Consider special needs when baby must remain in hospital.
	• Allow parents to express feelings about leaving baby.
	• Encourage parents to return to hospital to visit baby as frequently as they can and/or to phone. Signature is necessary prior to mother's discharge for identification purposes.
	• Encourage physical contact with baby. Teach feeding techniques and other care that parent can provide.
	• Explain care needs of baby and answer questions.
	• Record and inform physician of parental visitors and progress.
	28. Consider special discharge planning for parents who may need assistance in accepting child care responsibilities.
	a. Respond to needs related to:
	• Mother who demonstrates difficulty in learning about child care responsibilities
	• Retarded mother
	• Very young mother
	• Problems identified in home situation
	• High-risk situations for child abuse
	b. Initiate interagency referral.
	c. Contact social service agency.
F. *The parents are knowledgeable about resources for continuity of care at home*	29. Inform parents of other community agencies which may provide assistance in continuity of care, especially in long-term hospital care/special home care.
	a. Financial aid
	b. Equipment and supplies
	c. Food
	d. Clothing

Patient Outcome	Process

The mother and new-born experience safe cesarean delivery. This includes:

DESCRIPTION: Patients who have had cesarean section(s) or uterine surgery, *e.g.,* myomectomy, hysterotomy, or with known cephalopelvic disproportion are usually delivered by cesarean section after fetal maturity has been determined by ultrasound and/or amniocentesis. Other indications for cesarean section include significant maternal or fetal distress (with or without labor).

NURSING ASSESSMENT: Follow suggested assessment in guidelines for Obstetric Patients for Evaluation/Possible Admission, p. 257. If the patient is in labor, follow suggested assessment in guidelines for Normal Labor and Delivery, p. 259. In addition, assess and document patient's/significant other's understanding of need for delivery by cesarean section.

INTERVENTION:

A. *Is prepared for operative procedure and delivery*

1. Provide physical care of mother. Refer to Normal Labor and Delivery guidelines, p. 259.
2. Reinforce physician's explanation of need for surgery and method of anesthesia.
   a. Clarify information.
   b. Correct misconceptions.
3. Summarize usual preoperative preparation and provide care per hospital routine and physician's orders.
   a. Assure skin preparation of abdominal/perineal areas.
   b. Insert indwelling catheter.
   c. Keep n.p.o.
   d. Remove prostheses, valuables.
   e. Check for operative permit.
   f. Place identification bracelet on patient per hospital policy.
   g. Document availability of blood for transfusion.
   h. Give medication as ordered.
   i. Alert pediatric and anesthesia staff per hospital policy.
   j. Transport mother to OR with appropriately documented records including newborn identification.
4. Provide assistance to significant other. Physician will decide if significant other can be present during surgery.
   a. If significant other will be present:
      • Provide proper attire and instruct in hand-washing routine.
      • Explain procedure for cesarean delivery.
      • Describe methods of maintaining sterile environment and take to area for observation.
      • Explain what to do if individual has difficulty coping with the experience.
   b. If significant other is not present during delivery:
      • Explain and show him to waiting area.
      • Keep informed of patient's progress and arrange for individual to see baby after delivery and before baby goes to Nursery.
   c. Request significant other who holds baby to wash hands and wear gown.
5. Verify that the resuscitation unit is available for delivery. This includes:
   a. O_2
   b. Suction
   c. Resuscitation equipment
6. Assist physician who initiates newborn assessment and care.
7. Take baby after status is stabilized to mother (if awake) and allow her to touch.
   a. Permit significant other, if present, to hold baby.
8. Provide routine newborn care per hospital policy such as
   a. Record foot prints and apply identification bands.
   b. Weigh baby.
   c. Position baby on side under warmer.
   d. Document passage of meconium and/or urine.
   e. Obtain and label three tubes of cord blood.
   f. Weigh placenta.
   g. Call Nursery to receive baby (from Operating Room if maternal span in OR is greater than one hour; otherwise baby may go to Recovery Room with mother).
      • Obtain baby bed.
      • Include appropriate documentation of labor and delivery, footprint record, and cord blood samples.
      • Verbally report to nurse significant information of maternal-infant status.

Patient Outcome	Process

B. *Is free of or has minimal discomfort or complications*	9. Provide immediate postpartum care and explain rationale for care to mother.
	  a. Prepare for transfer to Recovery Room.
	    • Cleanse patient of all blood, amniotic fluid, surgical scrub solution, and apply perineal pad. Change patient's gown.
	    • Check patency of indwelling catheter.
	    • Assist patient to transfer from operating room table to bed. Raise side rails.
	    • Transfer according to judgment of anesthesiologist. Send personal possessions with patient.
	  b. Observe for postpartum bleeding.
	    • Monitor BP, P, R, height, position and firmness of fundus q 15 minutes for 1 hour, then q 1 hour for 6 hours.
	    • Be alert to patient who is more likely to have postpartum bleeding due to problems such as
	        Grand multiparity
	        Large doses of oxytocin (Pitocin)
	        Multiple gestations
	        Polyhydramnious
	        Delivery of large baby
	    • Intervene for excessive bleeding.
	        Notify physician.
	        Observe for signs of shock.
	        Increase frequency of vital signs, fundal checks and fundal massage.
	        Treat for shock as indicated:
	          Trendelenburg position
	          Blankets for warmth
	        Provide supportive measures to minimize anxiety.
	    • Anticipate physician's orders for:
	        Increasing rate of IV
	        Oxytocic drugs
	        Methylergonovine (Methergine) p.o. or IM
	  c. Check temperature on admission to Recovery Room, then q 4 hours unless elevated or otherwise indicated.
	  d. Check abdominal dressing q 15 minutes. Expect small amount of serous drainage. Report any bleeding.
	  e. Provide pad count with peri-pad change and cleaning of perineum.
	  f. Monitor postanesthesia recovery:
	    • For patients who received epidural, spinal (saddle-block) anesthesia:
	        Check mobility of lower extremities and alertness.
	        Instruct to lie flat for 12 hours if patient had spinal.
	        Do not transfer patient to postpartum unit until sensory and motor control of lower extremities return and epidural catheter is removed.
	    • For patients who received general anesthesia:
	        Check alertness and responsiveness.
	        Suction as needed.
	        Position for optimal ventilation.
	        Monitor breath sounds and vital signs per routine.
	  g. Provide comfort measures.
	    • Administer medication for relief of pain, discomfort, and nausea.
	    • Consider amount of medication ordered and check with anesthesiologist and/or attending physician, if indicated.
	    • Give care for postpartum "shaking":
	        Provide warmed blanket, especially to feet.
	        Reassure patient that this is a normal and temporary response.
	    • Offer ice chips, sips of water as ordered. If n.p.o., explain rationale to patient.
	  h. Provide fluids and monitor amount and kind.
	    • Maintain IV fluids as ordered and/or encourage p.o. intake.
	    • Accurate intake–output. Measure indwelling catheter drainage q 1 hour and determine specific gravity.

Patient Outcome	Process

10. Promote maternal/significant other-infant bonding if baby remains with mother in Recovery Room.
    a. Allow mother to hold infant as desired during time infant remains with mother in Recovery Room. Provide warmed blankets.
    b. Assist mother in breast feeding as she desires.
    c. Encourage interaction between mother/significant other and baby. Examples:
       • Allow to hold; show how to hold if necessary.
       • Briefly unwrap baby and allow to touch.
       • Decrease light in room and hold baby so that (s)he is able to open eyes.
       • Explain newborn's appearance and behavior, *e.g.*, crying, sleeping, movements, color.
    d. Explain reason for brief stay of baby in Recovery Room and placement of baby in Nursery.
11. Facilitate infant's transfer to Nursery.
    a. Call Nursery to transport baby. Obtain baby bed.
    b. Send cord blood samples with infant per hospital policy.
    c. Send all documentation with infant. Report significant information of maternal-infant status.
12. Facilitate mother's transfer to postpartum unit.
    a. Write transfer note to include:
       • Patient care summary
       • Delivery data and infant condition: time, kind and reason for cesarean section, infant's sex, weight, and Apgar scores
       • Maternal condition during immediate postpartum period
       • Vital sign stability and range, fundal height and firmness, description of lochia, activity status, intake-output record, emotional response to delivery, status of dressing
       • Breast or bottle feeding
       • Where prenatal care given and cause if high risk.
       • Summary of available data, *e.g.*, blood type, gonococcal culture, veneral disease research laboratories (VDRL), Pap smear, rubella titer, sickle cell prep.
       • Medications received through out delivery and immediate postpartum period
    b. Obtain room assignment and alert postpartum nurse of impending transfer and needed equipment.
    c. Assist patient to bed in postpartum unit.
    d. Verbally report significant information of maternal-infant status to assigned nurse in postpartum unit.

Patient Outcome	Process

The mother and new born experience safe induced labor and delivery. This includes:

DESCRIPTION: Patients are selected for this treatment on the basis of physiological status, *e.g.*, diabetes mellitus, postdatism, ruptured membranes with potential or documented infection. If it has been determined that patient has adequate pelvis for vaginal delivery and, if elected, that fetal maturity has been verified by amniocentesis and ultrasound. The guidelines for Normal Labor and Delivery p. 259 should be used for patients having oxytocin-induced labor with the following additions and/or exceptions.

NURSING ASSESSMENT: Follow suggested assessment in guideline Obstetric Patient For Evaluation/Possible Admission, p. 257.

INTERVENTION

A. *Is prepared for induction procedure*

1. Explain induction of labor versus spontaneous labor. Include information such as
   a. May take several hours to establish effectual contraction pattern
   b. Induction may require more than one day depending upon progress of the cervix for labor.
   c. Oxytocin used 8 to 12 hours only unless significant cervical change indicates impending delivery.
   d. If no significant cervical change after 8 to 12 hours, patient will rest until next morning and may have a regular diet.
   e. Intensity of induced contractions will differ from spontaneous contractions; they may peak more rapidly and last longer.
2. Explain necessity for constant nursing observation and equipment.
   a. IV and infusion pump
   b. Continuous electronic monitoring of fetal heart tone patterns and uterine contraction pattern
   c. Frequent vital signs
3. Provide diversional activities during latent phase of labor. May have TV, radio, reading materials, etc.
4. Reassure frequently of progress and explain possibility of prolonged latent phase.

B. *Is maintaining stable maternal/fetal unit physiological function*

5. Follow guidelines for Normal Labor and Delivery p. with additional elements of care.
   a. Recognize signs of adverse maternal/fetal physiological response to oxytocin:
      • Observe for hyperstimulation and/or tetany.
      • Observe for variations in fetal heart tone.
   b. Discontinue oxytocin, administer O_2 per mask at 6 to 8 liters per minute and notify physician if adverse response occurs.
   c. Have medication at bedside to counteract hyperstimulation, *e.g.*, amyl nitrite, epinephrine.

Patient Outcome	Process

The patient experiences informed, comfortable, and safe maintenance of maternal/fetal unit. This includes:

DESCRIPTION: These guidelines are applicable to any patient in labor who is less than 36 weeks pregnant. Medical management for patients with intact or ruptured membranes may include: administration of vasodilators to arrest uterine activity and steroids to enhance fetal lung maturity. In case of clinical signs of infection, the patient is supported to continue labor and delivery while receiving treatment for the infection.

NURSING ASSESSMENT: In addition to nursing assessment described in Obstetric Patient for Evaluation/Possible Admission guidelines, p. 257, the following information is especially important.

1. Assess and document fetal heart tone and uterine activity via electronic monitor.

INTERVENTION:

A. *Is aware of need for evaluation and plan of care*

1. Explain rationale for:
   a. Monitoring equipment
   b. Vaginal examinations
   c. Process of labor
   d. Ultrasound study
   e. Blood test
   f. Intravenous fluids
   g. Catheterized urine specimen
   h. Close observation by a number of personnel
2. Reinforce and clarify explanation of physician regarding plan of care.
   a. Patient should understand that at least 48 hours hospitalization is involved.
   b. Depending upon physical examination and laboratory findings, one of the following regimens will be instituted:
      • Continue labor and eventual delivery
         If no spontaneous labor and indications of infection, labor will be induced. Refer to Oxytocin Induced Labor guidelines, p. 287.
      • Attempt to arrest uterine activity with fluid load and/or vasodilators.

B. *Is maintaining stable maternal/fetal unit physiological function*

3. Provide care if patient is to continue to labor and delivery. Refer to guidelines for Normal Labor and Delivery, p. 259. Include additional elements of care as:
   a. Keep patient/significant other informed of current plan of care.
   b. Provide additional emotional support because of likelihood of small baby.
   c. Assure that fetal monitor is used.
   d. Check laboratory values carefully:
      • Coagulation studies
      • CBC
   e. Initiate contact with neonatal nurse to discuss aspects of premature care.
   f. Observe for signs/symptoms of infection.
      • Monitor temperature q 1 hour.
      • Check WBC results b.i.d.
   g. Carry out prophylactic measures to prevent infection:
      • Avoid vaginal examination unless absolutely necessary.
      • Assist with sterile speculum examinations to obtain appropriate cultures.
   h. Anticipate that labor will progress faster than for full-term baby.
   i. Collect heparinized cord blood after delivery.
4. Provide general nursing care measures. Include:
   a. Monitor vital signs q 2 hours or as indicated by physician's orders.
   b. Record daily weight.
   c. Maintain strict intake and output record.
   d. Turn q 2 hours.
   e. Maintain bed rest in lateral position and/or Trendelenburg position as ordered.
   f. Apply antiembolic hose.
5. Plan diversional activities for patients on prolonged treatment.
   a. Consider use of TV, radio, books, and crafts.
   b. Incorporate support people as appropriate.

C. *Is knowledgeable about self-care and resources for continuity of care*

6. Plan with undelivered patient for discharge.
   a. Assess patient's home environment and responsibilities in order to plan with patient and family for self-care related to environment/situation. Consider:
      • Child care and household duties
      • Employment

Patient Outcome	Process
	• Sexual activity • Family relationships and availability of support people • Activity limitations related to condition as ordered by physician b. Reinforce physician's discharge plan of care and evaluate understanding by patient/ significant other. c. Review prescribed medications to include dosage, effects, signs and symptoms to report to physician. d. Initiate interagency referral. e. Consider sending nursing care summary to nursing unit of home hospital designated by patient.

CHAPTER VIII
Guidelines for the pediatric patient

INTRODUCTION: Consideration should be given to the Pediatric General Care Guidelines for the hospitalized child regardless of age, illness, or therapy. Key nursing intervention is identified to meet the child's needs for safety, rest, comfort, nutrition, personal identity and acceptance, maintenance of body functions, and health knowledge related to self-care. There is emphasis on the child as an individual as well as part of the family unit.

Guidelines are presented which describe patient care outcomes and associated nursing process for the child with specific conditions and illnesses. Nursing interventions are identified which promote the ability of the child and family to function at an optimal level within limitations due to illness and therapy.

Frequent reference is made to guidelines based on the common features of nursing care needed during the preoperative and predischarge phases of hospitalization.

Patient Outcome	Process

A. *The child is in a safe environment*	1. Provide a safe environment.
	   a. Identify child and records accurately including special information as indicated. This includes:
	   • Addressograph plate
	   • Arm band with name, history number, patient unit
	   • Door card
	   • Bed card
	   • Chart cover marked with special precautions and allergies
	   • Special precautions regarding questionable infection or recent exposure to communicable diseases
	   b. Inform child and parent or guardian about room and unit as they will need to use it.
	   c. Maintain surveillance of room and unit to eliminate preventable hazards. Consider cleanliness, operative condition, physical arrangement. These include:
	   • Floor
	   • Furniture
	   • Equipment
	   • Electrical connections including unused wall outlets
	   • Lighting
	   • Necessary items (bellcord, side rails, personal belongings, toys, thermometers)
	   • Materials that may be contaminated or are unnecessary
	   • Dangerous supplies, drugs, potentially hazardous objects, *e.g.*, oxygen suction, window blinds and cords, open safety pins
	   • Smoking (allowed only in designated areas)
	   d. Plan child's bed environment to eliminate hazards.
	   • Demonstrate and explain to child and parent/guardian needed safety precautions.
	   • Use siderails, plastic crib tops, bumper guards when indicated.
	   • Maintain proper height of child's bed ("low" position when unattended).
	   • Use restraints when indicated. Record justification in patient's chart. Provide close observation.
	   e. Evaluate child's capacity for safeguarding self.
	   • Assess need for supervision of activities via conference with parent and observation of child.
	   • Provide for supervision and nursing assistance.
	   f. Plan child's physical care considering the following:
	   • Developmental level
	   • Body alignment and positioning
	   • Transfer between bed and stretcher/chair
	   • Ambulation
	   • Bathing
	   • Elimination (maintenance of previously established bowel and bladder habits)
	   • Personal hygiene (skin, mouth care, hair, nails)
	   • Eating
	   • Medications
	   • Diagnostic studies
	   • Treatments and special procedures
	   g. Initiate and maintain isolation when necessary for child/family/staff protection.
	   • Wound and skin precautions
	   • Enteric precautions
	   • Needle precautions
	   • Respiratory isolation
	   • Protective isolation
	   • Strict isolation
	   h. Maintain alertness and ability to protect child and family in the event of a fire or disaster.

B. *The child has optimal rest*	2. Assure adequate rest.
	   a. Evaluate sleep patterns.
	   b. Encourage appropriate bedtime according to age or age group.
	   c. Assure that child has afternoon rest period.
	   d. Attempt to place child in appropriate bed space according to developmental level, sex, condition.

Patient Outcome	Process
	e. Coordinate activities of health personnel providing services to allow for periods of rest. • Plan giving of medications, treatments, etc. • Avoid "hurtful" procedures during rest periods. f. Attempt to restrict visitors to approved times and numbers. g. Exercise control over unnecessary noise and lights. h. Encourage rest periods and breaks for parents/guardians.
C. *The child maintains optimal nutritional status*	3. Provide for maintenance of nutritional status. a. Check for proper diet order, meal distribution, and nourishment between meals. b. Inform child and/or family regarding dietary routine and specific diet to include: • Dietary and fluid restrictions • Food should not be left in the child's room. c. Carry out and record feedings (nipple, gavage, gastrostomy, duodenal tube, syringe, trays) per physician's orders with regard to amount, frequency, and nutritional needs. d. Maintain hourly checks of IV fluids and special tube feedings. e. Observe child's total nutritional intake including ingestion and retention of feedings and administration of IV fluids. f. Assess changing nutritional needs and modify diet accordingly. g. Assist with food selection with consideration of cultural dietary habits. h. Request dietary consultation as needed. i. Reinforce importance of proper nutrition as a part of child's health status.
D. *The child functions within physiological capacity* • *Sensory*	4. Assist the patient to maintain sensory perception. a. Determine presence of any sensory impairment. Consider stage of growth and development as it relates to hearing, vision, touch, smell, taste. b. Provide for development of sensory perception and adequate stimulation. Examples are: • Mobiles, washable toys, radios • Playroom activities c. Maintain awareness of amount and kinds of sensory stimulation and attempt to modify according to child's current needs. These stimuli may include: • Verbal and nonverbal communication; need for reorientation • Noise, light, odors in environment • Sleep, rest, and activity patterns • Effects of medications • Need for physical contact, *e.g.,* importance of touch and closeness with other children. d. Provide child/parent with assistance as necessary; request physician to order appropriate services, *e.g.,* physical therapy or supportive aids when indicated. e. Assist child/parent in protection from loss and care of supportive aids and articles from home.
• *Motor*	5. Assist the patient to maintain motor ability. a. Assess present status and pertinent past history that may affect motor ability of child. Considerations include: • Orthopaedic and neurological disabilities • Cardiovascular and respiratory status • Visual problems • Pain • Psychosocial factors • Prostheses b. Consult with child/parent/physician regarding desirable child activities and establish activity program. Re-evaluate and adjust according to child's needs. c. Provide assistance as necessary. • Consider physical therapy services or supportive aids as appropriate.
• *Circulatory*	6. Assist patient to maintain cardiovascular function. a. Assess present cardiovascular status and pertinent past history. • Congenital defects • Chronic states as rheumatic heart disease, hypertension • Drugs • Dietary habits b. Assess and record on admission and throughout hospitalization: • Heart rate, rhythm, and strength • Blood pressure

Patient Outcome	Process
	• Height and weight

- Height and weight
- Peripheral circulation; skin—color, condition
- Respiratory rate and character—note stridor, retractions
- Dyspnea (with or without increased activity)
- Lethargy

c. Support normal circulation by:
- Appropriate exercise and activity
- Change of body position and skin care
- Maintenance of proper body temperature

d. Support normal fluid balance by:
- Monitor intake and output.
- Check for signs of fluid overload or dehydration, *e.g.,* weight gain or loss.

e. Administer drugs carefully and observe for desired effects and side effects.

• *Skin*

7. Maintain integrity of skin.
   a. Assess present status and pertinent past history considering:
   - Bruises, lacerations, abrasions, rashes, excoriated areas, allergies, birthmarks, decubiti
   - Description of skin; dry, oily, turgor
   - Open wound or stoma
   - Poor skin hygiene
   - Edema
   - Diarrhea—excoriated perineum
   - Obesity or emaciation

   b. Plan generalized skin care program.
   - Bathe patient every day unless otherwise indicated.
   - General skin care considerations:
       Dry skin: mild soap, oil in bath water, lotion
       Oily skin: frequent washing
       Dry, scaly feet: soak in warm, soapy water; apply emollient.
   - Hair and scalp care: Shampoo as needed.
   - Buttocks care: Bathe with soap and water; apply ointments and/or lotion; use heat lamp; frequent diaper changes or leave diaper off.
   - Decubiti care: prevention, turn frequently—keep off pressure area, clean area and apply medication as ordered.

• *Respiratory*

8. Assist patient to maintain respiratory function.
   a. Assess present status and pertinent past history. Consider:
   - Rate, depth and character of respirations
       Cyanosis, pallor
       Dyspnea, orthopnea
       Stridor
       Coughing
       Wheezing
       Production of sputum
   - Child's posture, *e.g.,* squatting

   b. History of respiratory problems from parent and/or patient such as
   - Obstruction
   - Infection

   c. Support respiratory function.
   - Position patient for comfort and ease of respirations.
   - Turn, cough, deep breathe patients confined to bed; frequency determined by patient needs.
   - Use assistive devices as ordered:
       Blow bottles
       IPPB
       Humidifier
       Oxygen
       Croup tents
       Play activities—blowing pingpong balls, soap bubbles, balloons

Patient Outcome	Process

• *Urinary*	9. Assist the patient to maintain urinary function.
	  a. Interview child and/or parent to determine:
	    • Pre-existing bladder problems
	    • Usual habits, words used, stage of toilet training, level of control
	  b. Assure adequate fluid intake (100 to 150 cc per kg body weight per day up to 1000 to 2000 cc per day unless contraindicated). Encourage active participation by child and/or parent.
	  c. Assess child's urinary output in relation to:
	    • Fluid intake
	    • Time since last voiding
	    • Bladder distention, discomfort
	    • Pain inhibiting voluntary response to void
	    • Normal voiding habit
	    • Provision of privacy
	    • Position (restrictive devices, etc.)
	  d. Record fluid intake (time and amount) and output (time and amount) as ordered by nurse or physician.
	  e. Assure good periurethral hygiene once daily with bath and more often if indicated.
	  f. Initiate measures to stimulate voiding as needed, *e.g.,* pour warm water over perineum.
	  g. Catheterize child if indicated.
	    • Provide adequate explanation to child and parent.
	    • Follow sterile techniques in catheterization, collecting specimens, and irrigation.
	    • Use strict catheter management techniques in routine care.
	    • Avoid catheterizing children unless absolutely necessary and all other measures fail.
	  h. Assist physician as necessary in suprapubic tap.

• *Bowel*	10. Assist the patient to maintain bowel function.
	  a. Interview child and/or parent to determine:
	    • Pre-existing bowel problems, *e.g.,* constipation, diarrhea, impaction, constipation, misuse of bowel stimulants
	    • Usual habits, words used, stage of toilet training, level of control
	  b. Keep record of time, amount, consistency, and color of stools. Check for signs and symptoms of bowel complications such as distention, diarrhea, presence of blood, intestinal parasites.
	  c. Consider factors influencing child's normal bowel evacuation such as
	    • Immobility, decreased activity
	    • Stress
	    • Medications
	    • Fluid and food intake
	    • Lack of privacy
	    • Hospitalization

E. *The child has minimal pain and/or discomfort*	11. Intervene to minimize child's physical discomfort.
	  a. Evaluate child's discomfort.
	    • Objective:
	      Covert and overt behavior, *e.g.,* body language, facial expression, guarding or splinting, decrease in play activity or play interests, irritability
	      Deviation from usual behavior patterns
	      Interference in sleep patterns, *e.g.,* restlessness
	    • Subjective:
	      Description of pain or discomfort in child's own words including kind, location, degree, and intensity
	      Consider parents' assessment of child's discomfort.
	    • Psychological influences:
	      Suggestability
	      Attitude of parents and staff
	      Fear of child or parent
	  b. Report excessive, unusual, or new pain to physician. Note and report changes in vital signs and condition.

Patient Outcome	Process

	c. Provide measures to alleviate pain and/or discomfort:
	• Observe for factors that may contribute to pain or discomfort:
	  Distention (full bladder, gas)
	  Constipation
	  Constriction (tight bandages, casts, etc.)
	  Restrictive devices (restraints, isolation)
	  Obstructed drainage tubes or infiltrated intravenous infusion
	  Edema
	  Bruising
	  Changes in body temperature
	  Vomiting, diarrhea
	  Coughing
	  Itching
	• Maintain good body alignment with supportive devices such as pillows.
	• Change body position frequently.
	• Provide basic hygiene measures, *i.e.,* skin and mouth care
	• Maintain environment conducive to rest (room temperature, noise, visitors).
	• Apply heat and/or cold as indicated, tepid bath.
	• Elevate body part as indicated.
	• Maintain adequate hydration.
	• Support adequate air exchange by turning, coughing, deep breathing, suctioning, using supportive devices as respirators, nebulizers.
	• Use diversionary methods with discretion.
	• Collaborate with physician for appropriate medication orders.
	  Observe response, duration, untoward side effects.
	  Employ nursing measures to enhance effectiveness of medications.

F. *The child and parents are emotionally stable*	12. Support ability of child and parents to maintain emotional stability.
	a. Assess child's needs for emotional support through observing behaviors. Examples are:
	• Crying when no physical reason can be ascertained, *e.g.,* wet diaper, need for elimination, hunger, cold
	• Facial expression, *e.g.,* sad, wistful, lonely, avoidance of eye contact, superficial smile
	• Attitude, *e.g.,* too quiet, too "good", withdrawn, hostile, overly aggressive, angry, demanding excessive attention
	• Activity, *e.g.,* inactive, hyperactive, temper tantrums
	• Special mannerism, *e.g.,* thumbsucking, nailbiting, masturbation, hair pulling or twisting, rocking motions
	b. Provide measures to offer emotional support of child.
	• Provide consistent relationship.
	• Maintain awareness of special needs of various age groups and recognize normal regression during illness. Encourage parents to exhibit acceptance.
	  Infant, *e.g.,* cuddling, rocking, pacifier p.r.n.
	  Toddler, *e.g.,* cuddling, holding, allowing some independence, favorite toy, security blanket, night light
	  Preschooler, *e.g.,* allow to ask questions, bedtime rituals, read stories, some cuddling, limit setting.
	  Schoolage, *e.g.,* participation in care, encourage peer activity and relationships, play games with child, watch appropriate TV programs with child and discuss same.
	  Adolescent, *e.g.,* allow own decision making when possible, peer activity, games, TV, opportunity to question treatments, provide for privacy, limit setting.
	• Praise any cooperation no matter how small.
	• Avoid humiliating child through shaming, etc.
	• Explain purpose of procedures, equipment, treatments, medications, in language child can understand, find out what child already knows.
	• Talk with child while caring for, feeding, bathing, etc.
	• Encourage child to ventilate by talking or "playing out" fears and worries.
	• Encourage constructive ways of dealing with tension and stress.
	• Engage child in peer, ward, and playroom activities.
	• Listen to what the child says. Observe body language, question appropriately.
	• Give honest answers to questions—geared to age group.

Patient Outcome	Process
	• Set limits on behavior; reasonable and appropriate discipline helps child to feel more secure.
	• Maintain sense of humor, encourage laughter.
	• Exhibit calm, confident, positive attitude with expectation of cooperation.
	• Make hospitalization as much of a positive experience as possible in the child's emotional growth.
	• Maintain nonjudgmental attitude.
	• Be aware of religious strengths.
	• Note which family members offer support to child and enlist their help.
	• Teach, encourage, and assist parents in providing support through visits, etc.
	• Avoid creating fearful attitude toward medical personnel and treatments in the child.
	c. Assess parents' needs for emotional support through observing behavior.
	• Fatigue
	• Guilt
	• Worry
	• Anger, hostility
	• Frustration
	• Fear
	• Need for excessive, frequent reassurance and attention
	• Frequent complaints and criticism of medical personnel
	• Frequent requests for unnecessary items
	• Lack of interest in appearance and surroundings
	• Attitude toward child, *e.g.*, overly protective
	• Attitude toward staff, *e.g.*, overly dependent, hostile
	d. Provide measures to offer emotional support to parents.
	• Establish an attitude of trust and concern for the child and parents and promote a sense of security.
	• Introduce self to parent by name, title, function.
	• Encourage discussion of problem by parent.
	• Assist with problem-solving; answer questions.
	• Recognize that anger is not necessarily personally directed.
	• Provide for parents' needs. Examples are:
	Place and time for rest
	Place to bathe and tend to personal hygiene needs
	Place and food to eat
	Time to be with child and time to be away from child
	• Provide realistic reassurance concerning care and condition of child.
	• Explain tests, treatments, medications, etc.
	• Assure that results from tests and studies will be discussed as soon as possible.
	• Encourage reasonable participation in child's care and provide positive feedback for efforts.
	• Assess parent's view of help needed.
	• Display concern, interest, and knowledge about child and his condition.
	• Share questions child has asked and the answers nurse has given with the parents.
	• Offer support and comfort by being present and available—spending time with parent. Help parents to identify their support systems.
G. *The child and parents have sense of value and personal identity*	13. Assist the patient and parents to maintain sense of personal identity and values.
	a. Convey a sense of concern and warmth and clearly identify self on initial contact with child and parent.
	b. Assist child and parent to become familiar with environment and hospital equipment.
	c. Approach child and parent with respectful and caring attitude.
	d. Be aware that child's and parents' behaviors are indicative of inner feelings.
	• Child is very sensitive to cues picked up from parents and behavior may reflect their anxieties.
	• Explore reasons for behavior with child and parent and encourage expression of feelings and constructive means of dealing with stress.
	e. Recognize changes in physical appearance and/or functioning may affect child's and parent's behavior.
	f. Anticipate needs of child and parent and supply these before being asked such as diaper supply, formula, extra blanket, juices.

Patient Outcome	Process
	g. Respond as promptly as possible to any child or parent request and explain if a request cannot be met.
	h. Recognize that children are unique individuals with needs that vary according to their stage of growth and development.
	i. Accept child and parent as members of the health team and promote cooperation.
	• Accept their right to question, request information and their right to refuse procedures, treatments, and medications.
	j. Be considerate of child's needs for privacy and modesty and prevent undue exposure during bath, toileting, and treatments.
	k. Be aware of any special needs and comply in so far as possible such as dietary phobias, fear of the dark, fear of elevators.
	l. Avoid talking about child in his presence unless he is included.
	m. Avoid personal conversation among staff in child's or parents' presence without including them.
	n. Use parent's or child's proper name or name preference when interacting.
	o. Avoid belittling, or humiliating child for unavoidable accidents such as spilled food, or bedwetting.
H. *The child is participating in recreational activity at level of growth and development*	14. Initiate recreational activity as appropriate part of therapy.
	a. Recognize the importance of play in the child's life and in progressing through the various stages of growth and development.
	• Realize that children understand, learn, and cope through playing-out activities and imitating adults.
	b. Determine child's present stage of growth and development (mental, physical, emotional, social) and deviations from normal.
	• Be familiar with usual form of activity used by the particular age group—active and passive.
	c. Recognize limitations imposed on child by health status and find methods to overcome limitations in order to promote feeling of mastery of hospitalization.
	d. Participate in interdisciplinary conferences to plan recreational program to meet child's needs.
	e. Use play activities for relaxation, fun, recreation, learning, relief of tension, release of emotions, relief of stress, interaction with peers, mastery of hospitalization, control, and correction of misconceptions.
	• Utilize child's natural interests and curiosity to master the new frightening environment.
	f. Supervise play and prevent injuries from too boisterious activity and unsafe toys.
	• Provide appropriate materials for play.
	• Improvise as necessary and have parents bring favorite toy from home.
	g. Select activities to maximize physical potential.
	h. Be aware of individual needs for low-key activities as well as stimulating activities.
	i. Encourage participation in play room activities at child's own pace of readiness.
	j. Consult recreational therapist in planning for child's activities and recreation. Give child choice of when to come and leave playroom.
	k. Eliminate "hurtful" procedures during playroom time.
	l. Collaborate with recreational therapist in evaluating and assessing child's behavior and needs and their relationship to health status and stage of growth and development.
I. *The child and parents are knowledgeable about nature of illness, procedures, treatments, and planned program directed toward health restoration and maintenance*	15. Teach child and parents about health-illness state and plan for health restoration and maintenance.
	a. Begin at admission to assess child's and parents':
	• Level of understanding
	• Ability to comprehend and to cooperate in care
	• Response to hospitalization, level of acceptance
	• Physical, mental, and emotional limitations
	• Cultural, religious, and environmental aspects
	• Parent/child relationships
	• Familial relationships
	b. Assess child/parent perception of diagnosis, prognosis, and needs.
	c. Reinforce information given to child/parent by physician.
	d. Explain tests, procedures, and treatments to child and parent in terms that they can understand and repeat explanation as often as needed.

Patient Outcome	Process
	e. Teach and promote good health habits (hygiene, dietary, rest, exercise, etc.) during hospitalization.
	f. Use appropriate available aids in teaching.
	• Audiovisual media, *e.g.,* movies, tapes
	• Written material, *e.g.,* booklets, pamphlets
	• Toys, play therapy, hospital supplies, *e.g.,* syringes
	• Community resources
	g. Enlist child and parent participation in and continuation of health care program.
	h. Assess child's and parents' perception of current health status, limitations, and its effect on the stage of growth and development.
	i. Be aware of the effect of the child's illness on other siblings and family members and family life-style.
	j. Discuss plans for discharge with child and parents. Include:
	• Diet
	• Medication
	• Activity
	• Importance of follow-up care
	• Necessary supplies and equipment
	k. Inform child and parent of facilities available for continuity of care, *e.g.,* public health agency, school health, clinics.

Preoperative phase of hospitalization (infants–adolescents)

Patient Outcome	Process

The patient/family experience informed and comfortable preoperative phase of hospitalization. This includes:	1. Gather information about patient's condition, reason for admission, planned surgical procedure, parents' and patient's understanding of illness and the degree of anxiety/frustration.
	2. Discuss with the parents the emotional status and developmental level of child. It is important to note:
	  a. Child's concept of reason for hospitalization
	  b. Etiology of problem
	  c. Previous experiences or admissions that might contribute or be detrimental to emotional well-being
	  d. Sibling relationships
	3. Explore with parents their plans for visiting and presence on day of surgery. Place emergency telephone number of parents in chart.
	4. Discuss actual surgical procedure and include:
	  a. Location of planned surgery
	  b. Probable size of incision(s)
	  c. Function of body or limb/organ to be altered
	  d. Change in postoperative appearance or body function
	  e. Expected time of surgery
	  f. Expected length of surgery
	  g. Preanesthesia routines
	5. Alert patient and family to postoperative expectations.
	  a. Immediate postoperative location
	  b. Knowledge of equipment such as IV, drainage tubes, etc.
	  c. Provision for relief of pain when indicated and limits on use and frequency
	  d. Observation schedule of nursing staff and expected parent role
	  e. Turning, coughing, and deep breathing exercise routine
	  f. Changes in bowel or bladder function
	  g. Progressive diet changes (fluids to regular diet)
	  h. Expectations of progressive ambulation
	  i. Progression of resuming previous level of self-care

A. *Is emotionally prepared for surgery*	6. Be aware of patient's and parents' feelings and needs.
	  a. Encourage verbalization about surgery and recognize concerns.
	  b. Listen and observe for misconceptions and signs of anxiety.
	  c. Assess support systems available to child and family.
	7. Attempt to reduce anxiety.
	  a. Determine basis of anxiety.
	  b. Consult support personnel such as social worker, chaplain, clinician.
	  c. Provide care as indicated.
	  d. Maintain an environment that meets the needs of the patient, *e.g.,* need for privacy, comfort. Include objects important to the child, *e.g.,* stuffed animal.
	  e. Be aware of parents' role in care of child during hospitalization.
	  f. Provide means based on child's development for expressing anxiety, *e.g.,* play therapy.

B. *Is physically prepared for surgery*	8. Provide immediate preoperative care.
	  a. Explain preoperative procedures to the patient and assist parents in delivery of care if they so desire.
	  b. Carry out written orders for medication and treatment.
	  c. Keep n.p.o. as ordered in relation to patient's age.
	  d. Give bowel cleansing as indicated.
	  e. Give mouth care if age appropriate and antimicrobial soap bath.
	  f. Empty bladder if bladder control has been established.
	  g. Restrict activity for safety.
	  h. Safeguard valuables and prostheses.
	  i. List allergies on record.
	  j. Assure signed consent form on chart.
	  k. Give patient gown and apply identification bracelet.
	  l. Accompany patient to Operating Room, providing support and reassurance during transfer.

Predischarge phase of hospitalization (infants–adolescents)

Patient Outcome	Process

The patient/family are knowledgeable about nature of illness, care at home, and resources for continuity of care	1. Reinforce information relating to body image changes, limitations according to patient condition, and physician orders.
	2. Consult with other health care personnel, patient, and parents in planning toward discharge.
	3. Assist family unit to gain knowledge and skills necessary for self-care after discharge. Assess patient participation when developmentally appropriate and indicated. Include:
	  a. Physical activity restrictions and progression
	  b. Wound care
	  c. Use and care of prosthesis if indicated
	  d. Where to buy equipment and supplies and resources if financial support necessary
	  e. Dietary modifications and diet instructions
	  f. Teaching regarding health-illness state
	  g. Medication therapy
	    • Type of medication
	    • Dosages and time schedule
	    • Side effects
	    • Safety factors
	    • Make certain appropriate prescriptions have been written and given to parents
	  h. Symptoms of complications and whom to call
	  i. Provisions of follow-up care
	    • Return to physician.
	    • Return to clinic(s) and appointment slips.
	4. Assess with family and patient the suitability of home for convalescence.
	  • Suggest modifications as necessary.
	5. Initiate interagency referral for patients who need help in planning for and adjusting to illness, return appointments, and/or follow-up care.
	6. Discuss specific community agencies available to assist patient and family, such as Heart Fund, Cancer Society, Colostomy clubs, rehabilitation centers, homebound teachers.
	7. Answer questions and concerns about home care. Reassure family.

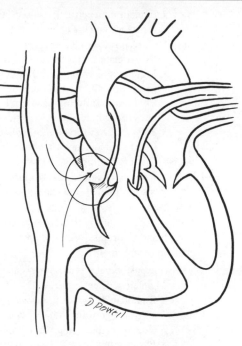

Fig. 8-1.   Atrial septal defect.

The patient/family experience informed, safe, and comfortable preoperative, post-operative, and pre-discharge phases of hospitalization. This includes:

DESCRIPTION: An atrial septal defect (ASD) is an opening between the atria that allows blood to pass from the left atrium to the lower pressured right atrium (Fig. 8-1.). Diagnosis is most often made in early childhood; it is frequently noted at a preschool physical examination. Symptoms may vary from no symptoms at all to vague complaints of fatigue on exertion and/or upper-respiratory infections.

PROCEDURE: The incision is made using a right anterolateral thoracotomy or a medium sternotomy depending on location of the defect. The heart is visualized and cardiopulmonary bypass utilized. The atrium is opened and the defect is closed using either a primary or patch (dacron, pericardium) closure. The atrial incision is then closed and bypass is discontinued.

NURSING ASSESSMENT: In the general admission assessment, the following information is especially important.
1. Assess and document physical status.
    a.   Activity level
    b.   Allergies
    c.   Vital signs
    d.   Peripheral pulses
    e.   Current medications
    f.   History of any recent illness, allergies
    g.   Physical appearance: growth; color
2. Assess and document response to information about the disease process, implications and anticipated surgery.
    a.   Apparent anxiety level of patient and family
    b.   Previous experience with surgery
3. Assess and document understanding of disease process, implications, and anticipated surgery.
    a.   Evaluate parents' perception of child's expectation.
    b.   Evaluate child's perception of what is to happen.

A. *Is prepared for surgery*

INTERVENTION:
1. Reinforce understanding of patient and family regarding disease process, implication, and anticipated surgery. Consider developmental level of patient.
    a.   Explain anatomy and possible etiology of defect.
    b.   Emphasize that surgical correction is done not for current symptoms but for prevention of lung damage.

Patient Outcome	Process
	• Explain concept of increased pulmonary blood flow contributing to pulmonary vascular resistance and the underlying danger.
	c. Discuss postoperative expectations.
	• Will remain in special care unit overnight
	• May require endotracheal tube with mechanical ventilation for several hours. Following extubation, O_2 mask is used for 4 to 6 hours.
	• Constant monitoring of arterial pressures, central venous pressures (CVP), temperature, pulse, respiration and blood pressure, and electrocardiogram EKG
	• Foley catheter for monitoring hourly urine output
	• Chest drainage tube attached to suction
	• Chest radiographs
	• Pulmonary care: deep breathing, coughing, postural drainage
	d. Reassure patient and family that explanations will be given about care, procedures, and progress.
	2. Summarize features of preoperative phase and provide care needed per hospital routine and physician's orders. See Chapter 8, Preoperative Phase of Hospitalization (Infants—Adolescents), p. 301.
B. *Is free of or has minimal discomfort or postoperative complications*	3. Provide postoperative care. Intervene in the critical elements of care.
	a. Maintain a patent airway.
• Respiratory	• If intubated, suction as necessary using saline irrigations to thin secretions.
	Note signs of respiratory distress.
	Give medication p.r.n. for splinting respirations
• Cardiovascular	• Physical therapy will be done q 2 to 4 hours as necessary after returning to ward to prevent atelectasis and pneumonia.
	b. Maintain stable cardiovascular function.
	• Monitor vital signs including central venous pressure per routine. Notify physician of any variable from normal for age.
	• Check peripheral pulses q 1 hour. Note temperature and color of extremities especially where arterial lines are located.
	• Watch closely for arrhythmias—atrial arrhythmias are common postoperatively.
	Run rhythm strip; note time and document. Run 12-lead EKG if indicated.
	• Assess carefully for bleeding.
	Measure drainage from chest tubes q 15 minutes—1 hour as indicated and replace volume as necessary.
	Check other sites for bleeding: arterial line, Foley catheter, endotracheal tube.
• Fluid/electrolyte balance	c. Provide continual and careful assessment of fluid and electrolyte balance.
	• Maintain intake and output record.
	• Measure urine on return from Operating Room then q 1 hour.
	Diuresis will occur postcardiopulmonary bypass. Observe carefully to maintain adequate potassium levels.
	Call physician if urine drops below 1 cc per kg per hour or becomes increasingly bloody.
	• Assess fluid and electrolyte status.
	Note and document amount of fluid lost through blood loss, urine, emesis.
	Notify physician of significant change in the following:
	EKG
	CVP and vital signs
	Pulmonary status
	Serum electrolytes
	Blood chemistries are extremely important in children in the immediate postoperative period. Potassium may be administered on a hourly basis as necessary. Calcium may be given q 1 hour as needed. Electrolytes will be checked q 4 hours until the following morning then once a day for 2 to 3 days.
• Gastrointestinal	d. Facilitate gastrointestinal function.
	• Watch closely for abdominal distention as this restricts respiratory effort and indicates that nausea and vomiting could occur.
	• Assess for returning function of bowel, *i.e.,* sounds.
	• Give ice chips 4 hours postextubation, then sips of clear fluids if no nausea noted. Full liquid breakfast morning following surgery. Progress to regular diet as desired.

Patient Outcome	Process
• *Neurological*	e. Assess patient for symptoms indicating neurological deficit.
	• Assess level of consciousness and mental status and compare with baseline.
• *Comfort*	f. Anticipate and evaluate patient's needs for pain control. Provide necessary relief measures.
	• Administer medication to relieve discomfort, anxiety, and coughing and facilitate movement.
	• Position child comfortably to relieve discomfort.
• *Wound healing*	g. Assess incision for healing daily. Notify physician and document any drainage, redness, etc.
	• Initial dressing done in recovery area then changed p.r.n. until removed by physician.
	• Closure of skin stitches is subcuticular which does not require removal.
C. *Is knowledgeable about nature of illness, care, and resources for continuity of care*	4. See Chapter 8, Predischarge Phase of Hospitalization (Infants—Adolescents), p. 303. Include additional essential elements of preparation for discharge.
	a. Instruct patient/family regarding resumption of activities.
	• Provide short rest periods.
	• Avoid ''organized'' games in extreme weather for two weeks.
	• May return to normal level of activity in one month unless otherwise indicated.
	• May return to school in seven days unless otherwise indicated.
	b. Discuss with parents the possible behavioral changes that may occur after major surgery in children.
	• Increased dependency
	• Nightmares
	• Bedwetting
	• Eating or sleeping problems
	c. Discuss need for pain medication and type.
	• Younger children (3 to 7) may take acetaminophen (Tylenol) for fever or pain.
	• Older children may be given prescriptions per physician for pain medication.
	• Instruct parents in the proper way of giving medication and how to dispose of medication after it is no longer required for relief of discomfort.
	d. Provide written instructions about:
	• Activity
	• Bathing
	• Medications
	• Return to school/church
	• Emergency phone number for physician contact to report chest pain, fever for several days or night, productive cough that does not improve, and complaint of ''feeling bad''.
	• Clinic return appointment
	e. Discuss community agencies which may assist in continuity of care, *e.g.*, school health office.
	f. Initiate interagency referral as needed.

Patient Outcome	Process

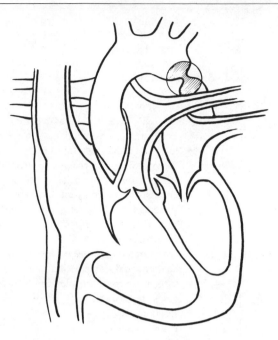

Fig. 8-2. Coarctation of the aorta.

The patient/family experience informed, safe, and comfortable pre-operative, post-operative, and pre-discharge, phases of hospitalization. This includes:

DESCRIPTION: Coarctation is a narrowing of the lumen of the aorta, usually at the site of insertion of the ductus (Fig. 8-2.). The blood flow to the lower body is thus obstructed.

PROCEDURE: The patient is in a lateral position with left side up. An incision is made from the anterior axillary line to midway between the vertebral column and scapula. The chest is entered through the fourth intercostal space. The area of coarctation is excised and anastomosis is performed either primarily, utilizing a portion of the subclavian, or when necessary, a dacron patch. Care is taken to watch for bleeding from multiple collateral vessels. The chest is closed and a chest drainage tube is left in place for 24 hours.

NURSING ASSESSMENT: In addition to the general admission assessment, the following information is especially important.
1. Assess and document physical status.
   a. Level of activity, symptoms on exertion
   b. Quality of peripheral pulses, especially comparison of upper and lower extremities and femoral pulses
   c. Current medication
   d. History of recent febrile illness, allergies, family history of congenital heart disease
   e. Blood pressure in all extremities
2. Assess and document response to information about the disease process, implications, and anticipated surgery.
   a. Apparent anxiety level of patient and family
   b. Previous experience with surgery
3. Assess and document understanding of the disease process, implications, and anticipated surgery.
   a. Evaluate parents' perception of child's expectation.
   b. Evaluate child's perception of what is to happen.

A. *Is prepared for surgery*

INTERVENTION:
1. Reinforce understanding of patient and family regarding the disease process, implications, and anticipated surgery.
   • Emphasize postoperative expectations:
     • Will remain in special care unit for 24 to 48 hours
     • Will be extubated following repair of defect and have a mist O_2 mask for several hours
     • Constant monitoring of the arterial pressure, vital signs, and EKG

Patient Outcome	Process
	• Foley catheter for monitoring urine output for several hours
	• Chest drainage tube attached to suction
	• Chest radiographs
	• Pulmonary care: deep breathing, coughing, postural drainage
	2. Summarize features of preoperative phase and provide care needed per hospital routine and physician's orders. See Chapter 8, Preoperative Phase of Hospitalization (Infants—Adolescents), p. 301.
B. *Is free of or has minimal discomfort or postoperative complications*	3. Provide postoperative care. Intervene in the critical elements of care.
	a. Maintain adequate ventilation.
• Respiratory	• Note signs and symptoms of respiratory distress.
	• Observe for sudden changes in arterial blood gas values.
	• Medicate to prevent inadequate respirations due to splinting.
	• Chest physical therapy may be done q 4 hours until 5 to 6 days postoperatively if needed.
	• Encourage coughing, deep breathing q 2 hours in immediate postoperative period.
	• Prevent abdominal distension in small children using nasogastric tube or burping.
	• Listen to breath sounds.
• Cardiovascular	b. Maintain stable cardiovascular function.
	• Monitor and document vital signs. Notify physician of any changes from normal for age.
	• Remain aware of accepted limits of blood pressure and heart rate when antihypertensive agents are required.
	• Observe EKG for arrhythmias.
	• Measure drainage from chest tubes and replace volume as indicated.
• Fluid/electrolyte balance	c. Provide continual and accurate observation of fluid and electrolyte balance.
	• Maintain intake-output record.
	• Measure urine output q 1 hour. Notify physician of any decrease.
	• Assess fluid and electrolyte status.
	Document fluids lost through blood loss, urine, and emesis. Document time of loss and replacement if indicated.
	Notify physician of significant changes in the following:
	EKG
	Vital signs, especially blood pressure
	Pulmonary status
	Arterial blood gases
	Blood chemistries
	Watch electrolytes carefully in the immediate postoperative period. Potassium may be replaced hourly according to need.
• Gastrointestinal	d. Facilitate gastrointestinal function.
	• Observe closely for abdominal distention, nausea, and vomiting in the immediate and late postoperative period.
	• Assess and document the return of bowel sounds.
	• Offer ice chips in small amounts 4 to 6 hours postextubation. If the abdomen remains flat and bowel sounds return, progress to clear liquids by late evening.
• Neurological	e. Assess patient for symptoms indicating neurological deficit.
	• Observe for movement of lower limbs on command to rule out paraplegia as postoperative complication.
	• Assess level of consciousness and mental status and compare with baseline data.
• Comfort	f. Anticipate and evaluate patient's needs for pain control. Provide necessary relief measures.
	• Administer medication to relieve discomfort, anxiety, coughing, and facilitate movement.
	• Change position of patient as needed to relieve discomfort.
• Wound healing	g. Assess wound for redness, drainage, or inflammation daily.
	• Initial dressing change will be done in recovery area and then dressed as necessary with dry, sterile dressings.
	• Skin sutures will be removed on the seventh postoperative day.
	h. Provide family with periods of time to visit and offer emotional support.
	• Accompany parents on first visit to answer questions, explain equipment and treatment.
C. *Is knowledgeable about nature of illness, care, and resources for continuity of care*	4. See Chapter 8, Predischarge Phase of Hospitalization (Infants—Adolescents), p. 303. Include additional essential elements of preparation for discharge.
	a. Instruct patient and family regarding resumption of activities.
	• Provide periods of rest for 7 to 10 days.
	• Avoid excessive activity in extreme weather.

Patient Outcome	Process
	• Resume normal level of activity in one month unless otherwise indicated.
	• Return to school/day care in 7 to 10 days after discharge unless otherwise indicated.
	b. Discuss medication dosages, schedule, precautions and length of time to continue taking.
	c. Instruct family in follow-up care.
	• Provide written guidelines to explain:
	Activity
	Bathing
	Medications
	Emergency phone numbers for physician contact to report:
	Chest pain
	Dizziness/fainting
	Elevated temperature over several days
	Productive cough that doesn't improve
	Complaints of malaise or fatigue
	d. Discuss community agencies which may assist in continuity of care, *e.g.,* school health office.
	e. Initiate interagency referral as needed.

Patient Outcome	Process
The patient functions comfortably within limitations due to an immunologic deficiency state. This includes:	**DESCRIPTION:** Inherited immunologic deficiency states in children may be characterized by agammaglobulinemia, hypogammaglobulinemia, defect in cellular immunity, or a combination of deficits. Children may be diagnosed as newborns or later in life depending upon the severity of the deficiency. These deficiencies result in increased susceptibility to infection and decreased ability to ward off infection.

NURSING ASSESSMENT: In addition to the general admission assessment, the following information is especially important.

1. Assess and document physical status.
    a. Skin condition, abscesses, bruises, mouth infection
    b. Nutritional status
    c. Bowel function
    d. Level of activity
    e. History of or current infection
    f. History of allergies
    g. Other congenital abnormalities
    h. Current medications
2. Assess and document emotional status.
    a. Mother-child relationships
    b. Current coping strategy of child/parent
3. Assess and document patient's/family's understanding of the disease process, implications, and treatment.

INTERVENTION:

A. Is prepared for diagnostic studies

1. Explain/answer questions about diagnostic studies. Refer to Chapter 3 Guidelines on The Patient Undergoing Diagnostic Studies, p. 33. Studies may include:
    a. Numerous blood studies requiring large volumes of blood
    b. Skin tests

B. Is benefiting from protective environment

2. Collaborate with physician to extablish appropriate environment to minimize infection.
    a. Complete isolation (laminar flow room)
       • Use for patients with severe immune defects.
       • Maintain entirely sterile environment: wear sterile gowns, gloves, mask, hood, and shoe covers. Check that everything entering room is sterile.
    b. Protective isolation
       • Use if laminar flow room unavailable for patients with agammaglobulinemia or other deficiency.
       • Wear clean gowns, and mask.
       • Use good hand-washing technique.
       • Give patient mask to wear if taken out of room.
       • Minimize patient's time out of room.
       • Limit traffic in and out of room, including family members.
    c. Teach family procedure to protect child when visiting.
3. Provide for and teach health maintenance measures.
    a. Skin/hair/nail care:
       • Bathe daily with frequent hair shampooing.
       • Use lotions only as prescribed.
       • Observe for skin breaks, irritations, rashes.
       • Give special care to buttocks if diarrhea is present.
    b. Mouth:
       • Establish routine mouth care appropriate to age.
       • Observe for sores and infection, *e.g.*, monilia.
       • Refer dental problems to physician.
    c. Respiratory system:
       • Observe for signs and symptoms of respiratory infection. Report to physician.
       • Avoid exposure to infected others.
    d. Gastrointestinal system:
       • Evaluate tolerance to oral intake.
       • Observe stools for consistency, amount, and frequency. Report any abnormalities to physician.

Patient Outcome	Process

C. *Is free of or has minimal discomfort or complications from therapy*	4. Intervene for the patient undergoing specific therapies. These may include:
	  a. Fetal liver transplant, thymus transplant, bone marrow transplant
	     • Observe for and report signs and symptoms of graft versus host reaction.
	       Fever
	       Rash
	       Anorexia
	       Diarrhea
	  b. Irradiated blood transfusion
	     • Observe for and report signs and symptoms of blood transfusion reaction.
	       Fever
	       Chills
	       Rash
	       Back pain
	       Hypotension
	       Tachycardia
	  c. Other therapies: plasma transfusion, gamma globulin (IM or IV)
	     • Observe for signs and symptoms of blood transfusion reaction.
	     • Observe for reactions to large amounts of solution in intramuscular injections of gamma globulin, *e.g.*, pain, induration at injection sites.
	  d. Monitor vital signs frequently.
	  e. Maintain strict intake-output record.
	  f. Record daily weight.
	  g. Administer antibiotic as ordered.
	  h. Provide opportunity for expression of concerns, fears, and questions.
	  i. Explain care of patient and involve family in daily care as appropriate.

D. *Is knowledgeable about nature of illness, self-care, and resources for continuity of care*	5. Plan for discharge with patient/family.
	  a. Evaluate teaching/understanding to include:
	     • Health maintenance measures
	     • Preventive measures
	     • Medications
	     • Diet
	  b. Discuss importance of follow-up care.
	  c. Inform patient/family of community agencies which may assist in continuity of care.
	  d. Initiate public health referral as needed.
	  e. Inform parents of available genetic counseling.

Patent ductus arteriosus (first year of life excluding infants with respiratory distress syndrome)

Patient Outcome	Process

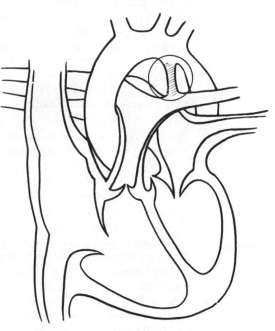

Fig. 8-3. Patent ductus arteriosus.

The patient/family experience informed, safe, and comfortable preoperative, postoperative, and predischarge phases of hospitalization. This includes:

DESCRIPTION: Patent ductus arteriosus is the fetal arterial pathway between the pulmonary artery and aorta that normally closes soon after birth (Fig. 8-3.)

PROCEDURE: The left chest is entered through a left posterolateral incision in the third intercostal space. After the lung is retracted, the ductus is exposed and ligated.

NURSING ASSESSMENT: In addition to the general admission assessment, the following information is especially important.
1. Assess and document physical status.
   a. Activity level
   b. Vital signs
   c. Peripheral pulses
   d. Current medications
   e. History of recent illness
2. Assess and document parents' response to information about the disease process, implications, and anticipated surgery.
   a. Apparent anxiety level of parents
   b. Previous experience with surgery
3. Assess and document parents' understanding of the disease process, implications, and anticipated surgery.

INTERVENTION:

A. *Is prepared for surgery*

1. Reinforce parents' understanding regarding the disease process, implications, and anticipated surgery.
   • Emphasize postoperative expectations.
      • Will remain in recovery area from 4 to 24 hours
      • Will receive O_2 via mask until fully awake
      • Continuous monitoring of arterial pressure, pulse, and possibly central venous pressure
      • Will receive IV fluids through central and peripheral veins until next day
      • Chest drainage tube attached to suction until lung is fully expanded
      • Bed rest for 24 hours, then out of bed
      • Pain control by medication as needed
2. Summarize features of preoperative phase and provide care needed per hospital routine and physician's orders. See Chapter 8 Preoperative Phase of Hospitalization (Infants—Adolescents), p. 301.

Patient Outcome	Process

B. *Is free of or has minimal discomfort or postoperative complications*	3. Provide postoperative care. Intervene in the critical elements of care.
	   a. Maintain adequate ventilation.
	     • Maintain patent airway and note signs of respiratory distress.
	     • Give O_2 and humidity by mask for 4 to 8 hours.
	     • Turn frequently.
	     • Chest physical therapy for 24 hours and longer if necessary
	     • Give pain relief medications.
	     • Position for comfort and adequate respirations.

• *Cardiovascular*	b. Maintain stable and cardiovascular function.
	     • Monitor vital signs and report deviations from normal for age.
	     • Check peripheral pulse.
	     • Observe for bleeding.
	     • Assess and document location and amount of bleeding. Provide replacement as ordered to maintain homeostasis.

• *Fluid/electrolyte balance*	c. Provide continual and careful assessment of fluid and electrolyte status.
	     • Maintain intake and output record.
	     • Measure urinary output by Foley catheter, diaper weight, or urine collection bags.
	     • Call physician if no output for six hours or less than 1 cc per kg hourly with Foley catheter in place.
	     • Assess fluid and electrolyte status.
	        Note amount of blood loss and fluid replacement during surgery.
	        Notify physician of changes in:
	           EKG
	           Blood chemistries and blood gases
	           Vital signs
	           Skin turgor
	           Pulmonary congestion.

• *Gastrointestinal*	d. Facilitate gastrointestinal function.
	     • Observe closely for abdominal distention.
	     • Assess for return of bowel sounds.
	     • Keep n.p.o. for six hours; then give sips of fluid and progress diet as tolerated.

• *Neurological*	e. Assess for symptoms indicating neurologic deficit. • Assess level of consciousness and check with baseline data.
• *Comfort*	f. Anticipate and evaluate patient's need for pain control. Provide necessary relief measures. • Assist movement to position which seems comfortable. Turn from side to side to prevent atelectasis.

• *Wound healing*	g. Provide wound care.
	     • Observe for signs of infection.
	     • Change dry dressings as necessary.

C. *Is knowledgeable about nature of illness, care, and resources for continuity of care*	4. See Chapter 8 Predischarge Phase of Hospitalization (Infants—Adolescents), p. 303. Include additional essential elements of preparation for discharge.
	   a. Instruct family concerning return to normal level of activity.
	     • Periodic naps will be necessary for about 5 to 6 days after discharge or per normal home routine.
	     • May return to day care or nursery care approximately one week after discharge.
	   b. Instruct that there are no routine discharge medications.
	     • Acetaminophen (Tylenol) may be given for pain and/or temperature control in appropriate dose.
	   c. Instruct family to notify physician of signs and symptoms such as
	     • Fever • Congestion
	     • Incisional tenderness and inflammation • General malaise
	   d. Provide written guidelines about specifics of care as needed.
	   e. Give return appointment.
	   f. Inform family of community agencies which may assist in continuity of care.
	   g. Initiate interagency referral as needed.

Patient Outcome	Process

The child and family function at optimal level within limitations due to illness and therapy. This includes:

DESCRIPTION: Pediatric cancer nursing concerns children, from birth through adolescence, who have cancer; it also incorporates their families. Nursing care is based on the philosophy that each child with cancer and his family have the right to quality nursing care based on current standards which guide the nurse in providing that care. The philosophy further includes communication between the multi-disciplinary staff and family/child unit. Nursing is directed toward supporting a day-to-day outlook for the child and family with a continuity of physical and psychological care. The purpose in stating general guidelines is to enable the nurse to determine basic parameters for assessing the child and family and thereby increasing her skill to direct nursing intervention and evaluation.

NURSING ASSESSMENT: In the general admission assessment, the following information is especially important.

1. Assess and document physical and mental status.
   a. Cardiovascular
      - Blood pressure
      - Pulse
   b. Respiratory
      - Dyspnea
      - Increased coughing
      - Increased secretions
      - Hemoptysis
   c. Temperature (axillary if oral or rectal lesions present)
   d. Skin
      - Color: pale, flushed
      - Temperature: cool, clammy, warm
      - Areas of breakdown due to friable tissue
      - Increases in petechiae and/or bruises, especially over chest, back, and abdomen
      - Abscesses: perianal, other body sores
      - Edema
      - Dehydration: poor skin turgor, dry skin and mucous membranes, "sunken eyes"
   e. Mucous membranes (vaginal, oral, rectal, nasopharyngeal)
      - Color
      - Integrity
      - Bleeding, exudate
      - Lesions: circumoral, buccal, rectal
   f. Changes in bowel/bladder function
      - Bladder: pyuria, hematuria, polyuria, dysuria, oliguria
      - Bowel: diarrhea, constipation, "bloody" or "tarry" stools
   g. Changes in appetite, weight loss, vomiting, anorexia
   h. Deviations from usual height and weight at current developmental level
   i. Changes in activity tolerance: fatigue
   j. Pain: increases or decreases
   k. Neurological and/or sensory deficits or alterations: Bell's palsy, unequal hand grasp, changes in level of consciousness, ptosis, changes in gait
   l. Personality changes
   m. Alterations in CBC, platelet and reticulocyte count
   n. Complete immunization history and history of past contagious disease of child and other siblings: chicken pox, measles, mumps

2. Assess hematologic laboratory data in relation to normal findings in appropriate age group.

A. *Is achieving maximum protection from infectious organisms*

INTERVENTION:
1. Establish protective precautions based on assessment findings.
   a. Observe nursing measures to minimize infectious organisms:
      - Strict hand washing
      - Preparation of skin with povidone-iodine prior to any invasive procedure, *e.g.,* IV
      - Evaluation of the need for IM or subcutaneous injections
      - Awareness of symptoms which indicate alteration of the mucosal linings
        Anus: occurrence of bleeding, fissures, hemorrhoids
        Gingiva: inflammation, exudate breakdown, lesions
        Urethra: changes in urine flow, color, consistency
        Vagina: unusual bleeding, drainage

Patient Outcome	Process
	<ul><li>No oral manipulation. Instead of toothbrushes, use toothettes, oral irrigation device, mouth washes such as peroxide, commercial mouthwash.</li><li>No rectal medicines, temperature or manipulation</li><li>Restrict visitors to parents and immediate family; screen visitors for infections.</li><li>Do not permit contact with airborne viral disease: Chickenpox (varicella; herpes zoster), mumps Rubella (three-day measles), rubeola (ten-day measles) Mononucleosis, toxoplasmosis, histoplasmosis, tuberculosis Cytomegalovirus (CMV), influenze B.</li><li>Record and report temperatures greater than 38.5°C orally, or greater than 38°C axillary.</li></ul>b. Provide care if patient requires white cell transfusion to include:<ul><li>Preparation of patient/family with information regarding rationale and procedure.</li><li>Monitoring patient during administration</li></ul>c. Use precautionary measures to administering IV therapy with antibiotics d. Assist patient and family to comply with precautionary measures.
B. *Is modifying activity according to degree of anemia*	2. Intervene if there is evidence of profound anemia. a. Strict bed rest b. Check pulse and respiration q 2 hours; blood pressure and temperature q 4 hours. c. Observe the following routine for patients receiving transfusions:<ul><li>Blood should be administered over a 2 to 6 hour period.</li><li>Obtain baseline, T, P, R, BP</li><li>Have an alternate IV solution and epinephrine 1:1000 available. Usual ordered dosage: 1</li><li>ml of epinephrine mixed with 9 ml of normal saline, given gradually IV.</li><li>Observe (particularly first 10 to 15 minutes) for sign of an immediate reaction. Continue observation throughout administration every 30 minutes. Itching Rash, urticaria Wheezing and/or persistent cough Temperature elevation Diaphoresis Nausea and vomiting Headache, dizziness Changes in pulse or respiration, hypotension Back pain (late symptom)</li><li>If signs and symptoms occur, discontinue administration of blood and replace with alternate IV fluids.</li><li>With an anaphylactic reaction, observe for oliguria for a minimum of 24 hours.</li></ul>
C. *Is free of or has minimal bleeding episodes*	3. Prevent and/or minimize bleeding complications. a. Observe for vulnerable areas and protect child from injury.<ul><li>No rectal medicine, temperature or manipulation</li><li>Evaluate the need for IM or subcutaneous injections.</li><li>Be aware of symptoms which indicate alteration of mucosal linings, *e.g.*, rectal, gingival.</li></ul>b. Be aware that increased time is needed to allow clot formation, *i.e.*, after a finger stick, IV, bone marrow aspiration, or biopsy.<ul><li>Use elastoplast or other pressure dressing as necessary.</li><li>Apply manual pressure for at least five minutes or until bleeding stops.</li></ul>c. Avoid trauma or irritants to mucosal linings, *i.e.*, nasogastric tube, suctioning tube.<ul><li>Record intake and output, especially stools. Check stools for presence of blood.</li><li>Be aware that constipation can predispose to fissures and bleeding.</li></ul>d. Warn against shaving with a razor blade. e. Avoid tourniquets and constricting dressings which may cause bruising, and/or decreased circulation. f. Evaluate the need for aspirin because of its interference with platelet aggregation.
D. *Is achieving adequate nutritional status*	4. Maintain adequate nutritional status. a. Provide adequate hydration and record all intake and output. The following may be used as a rough guide for hydration:<ul><li>1500 to 1800 ml per m² per day</li><li>Alternate intake schedules by weight: 0 to 10 kg—100 ml per kg 10 to 20 kg—an additional 50 ml per kg Greater than 20 kg—an additional 20 ml per kg</li></ul>

Patient Outcome	Process

- Encourage twice the maintenance intake with nephrotoxic drugs: 3000 to 3600 ml per m^2 per day

b. Rough estimate of expected urine output: 400 to 1000 ml per m^2 per day with maintenance intake

c. Encourage a high protein, nutritious diet for those who have decreased protein intake. Avoid "junk" foods when possible.
  - Consider likes and dislikes of patient.

d. Observe sodium restriction guidelines for patients receiving steroid therapy.
  - Salt should not be added in food preparation, although a small amount may be used in baking.
  - No added salt, except some "lite-salt" or salt substitute at the table.
  - No potato chips or other similarly prepared snacks unless salt-free.
  - Limited sweets, *i.e.,* hard candy, chocolate
  - Limited pork products, *i.e.,* sausage, bacon
  - Order "low sodium" diet, *i.e.,* 3 to 4 gm.

e. Consider a "dental soft" diet if child receives therapy which has or will alter oral intake.
  - Small frequent meals
  - High calorie snacks such as milkshakes

E. *Is adapting to physical alterations and implications of illness*

5. Assist patient/family to cope with illness.

a. Evaluate present psychosocial development and mechanisms for coping with stress.

b. Be aware that each patient/family does not necessarily pass through every stage of grieving to reach acceptance.

c. Gather assessment data in a nonthreatening manner.
  - Family relationships
  - Previous experience with serious illness, death
  - Previous coping mechanisms/behaviors with stress, *i.e.,* past major losses such as family member, job, home.
  - Inherent support systems such as family members, significant others, faith.
  - Available resources, *e.g.,* health team members, hospital chaplain, personal minister

d. Recognize mechanisms patient and family are using to cope with illness and select appropriate interventions.
  - ***Denial***
    (1) Behavioral assessment:
       Rejection of diagnosis
       Unwillingness to talk about present health status
       Euphoric behavior
       Restless, unspoken anxiety, e.g., fidgeting, hyperactivity
    (2) Nursing intervention:
       Support coping mechanisms that are constructive to patient, *e.g.,* respect patient/family's use of terminology regarding disease such as "lump" instead of "cancer".
       Establish reality of recent past: Relate to and discuss illness leading up to diagnosis.
       Have parent/child express what has been done during present hospitalization, establishing further reality of present.
       Clarify feelings of parents: "I know you must feel tired and worn out . . ."
       With "shock" or bewilderment, encourage activities, particularly those that have been a part of the family's routine prior to admission.
  - ***Anger***
    (1) Behavioral assessment:
       Overt anger:
         Abusive language directed toward health care team
         Incessant derogatory comments with regard to hospital or home
         Physical display of anger: slamming objects, abrupt movements
       Covert anger:
         Complaint, ingratiating, overly-generous behavior
         Smiling or denial regarding obviously painful or unpleasant procedures
         Repeated verbal expression of pleasure with present circumstances
    (2) Nursing intervention:
       For overt anger:
         Have family and patient go over events to this point.
         Determine what is the family's impression of those serving patient.

Patient Outcome	Process
	Help family identify source of their anger. What do they think about treatments? Why?

Supply consistent truthful information.

Observe for anger directed toward a specific person: self, staff member, family member.

Recognize anger and channel away from individuals and redirect energies to the present, *i.e.,* constructive participation in the child's treatment.

Reassure that the onset of disease was not anyone's "fault".

Encourage verbalization of feelings.

Offer opportunity of interaction with other parents of children with cancer who have accepted disease and treatment.

Give family decision-making opportunities.

For covert anger:

For persons unable to identify their own anger, help to recognize own feelings through use of words other than "anger" such as "upset," "irritated," "disappointed," "frustrated."

Help family identify sources of feelings; then continue as in intervention for overt anger.

- *Bargaining:*
  (1) Behavioral assessment:

  Wanting to bargain, barter for child's cure

  Feeling that rigid compliance with health measures will guarantee improvement in health and movement towards a cure.

  May overcompensate in terms of interpreting suggestions for care as inflexible rules

  (2) Nursing intervention:

  Repeat the facts as family/patient begin to bargain, *i.e.,* parents offering their "kidneys," "brains"; "I will do such if you can promise me my child will live."

  Be aware of signs of guilt, "if only."

  Provide additional information that will draw the parents/child back to reality; may begin teaching about the disease. Recognize and protect defenses.

  Encourage intrafamily support; evaluate financial and emotional resources.

- *Depression:*
  (1) Behavioral assessment:

  Decreased interest in environment, self, normal activities, *e.g.,* school work

  May be more demanding of health care givers

  May have alterations in normal patterns of daily activities, *e.g.,* food intake, sleep patterns

  May develop vague, nondescript, or acute pain unrelieved by conventional means. Pain may dissipate with increased attention.

  (2) Nursing intervention:

  Encourage consistency of people staying with child. Limit visitors which can be taxing to child and family.

  Provide scheduled times to relieve family and allow patient to rest or relax and not feel compelled to "entertain".

  Encourage routine self-care activities on part of family and child and permit them to feel productive and worthwhile.

  Offer praise for efforts expended.

  Encourage patient to progress slowly beyond activities of daily living, *e.g.,* school, play.

- *Acceptance:*
  (1) Behavioral assessment:

  Patient/family are able to discuss condition, treatment openly with health care givers and persons not associated with care of child.

  Patient/family can recognize that there will be instances in which they will be depressed, angry, denying, and bargaining.

  (2) Nursing intervention:

  Continue to provide consistent information to the parents and child, promoting trust.

Patient Outcome	Process

Ask the family to help other parents as this can keep the family at a level of acceptance/coping with their own child's disease.

Continue with positive reinforcement and realistic hope.

e. Accept patient's responses and recognize his feelings. Allow ample time for verbalization.

f. Demonstrate acceptance through active listening.

g. Encourage maintenance of normal family life.

F. *Is experiencing optimal physical comfort and freedom from pain, thus maximizing capacity for meaningful daily living*

6. Intervene to promote optimum physical comfort.

a. Assess in detail the experience of pain by the patient/family.

b. Evaluate for signs and symptoms of pain.
   • Restlessness
   • Sleeplessness
   • Decreased appetite
   • Irritability—may manifest differently with each age group
   • Tachycardia—evaluate in light of related causative factors, *e.g.,* anemia.
   • Altered respirations
   • Increase in blood pressure
   • Change in affective behavior
   • Tears

c. Consider nonpharmacologic nursing interventions.
   • Relief of tension and anxiety which precipitate and accentuate perception of pain.
      Reassure and prepare patient before painful, invasive treatments, or procedures.
      Suggest availability of means to alleviate pain.
   • General comfort measures:
      Turning, positioning, good body alignment
      Elevation of painful edematous limbs
      Skin care, mouth care
      Hot or cold application, *e.g.,* heating pad, bath
      Security object
      Adequate hydration
   • Control noxious environment stimuli:
      Loud noises
      Bright lights
      Rooming situation in the ward
      Visitors
   • Prevent fatigue by adequate rest periods.
   • Alleviate ancillary problems contributing to pain or discomfort, *i.e.,* coughing, vomiting, constipation.
   • Establish goals for the patient in accordance with his developmental level which provide purpose and meaning to daily living. Frustration and helplessness increase perception of pain.
   • Utilize relaxation techniques to decrease perception of pain:
      Lamaze breathing
      Conscious relaxation and contraction of various muscle groups
   • "Gate control theory" which states that it is possible to block or alter patient perception of painful sensations.
      (WIA) Waking Imagined Anesthesia
         Encourage patient to consciously think about or imagine pleasant experiences.
      Utilize fantasy to "block out" pain, *e.g.,*
         Story telling,
         Recall family experiences,
         Use of dolls, puppets to play out fantasies
      Provide distraction and diversional activities as any activity requiring concentration, can help block painful perceptions, *e.g.,*
         Word games, puzzles, needlework, model construction, music
      Utilize sensory and tactile stimulation
         Massage, vibration, rocking music
   • Encourage family to use their creativity and intimate knowledge of the child to help in planning interventions in the hospital and at home.

Patient Outcome	Process

	d. Consider drug therapy to provide pain relief yet keep patient as alert as possible.
	  • Consider the amount of medicine needed for a particular type of activity such as turning, sitting, activities of daily living.
	  • Administer the appropriate analgesics ordered after careful assessment of patient.
	  • Utilize nonpharmacologic measures to enhance effectiveness of medication.
	  • Continuously evaluate effectiveness of medication and/or possible need for changing medicine or dosage; consider the effects of undertreatment or overtreatment of pain.
	e. When started on a medicine and prior to discharge if patient is to receive it at home, teach the patient/family about the pain medication, its actions, side effects, etc.

G. *Is knowledgeable about nature of illness, self-care and resources for continuity of care*	7. Teach patient and family knowledge and skills related to care.
	a. Explain major facts about disease as it relates to patient:
	  • Patient/family should know the name of the disease and basic defect, *e.g.,* ''My child has leukemia which means some of the white blood cells are abnormal.''
	b. Teach regarding medications and plan for administration:
	  • Establish with the patient/family:
	    Purpose of each medication, *e.g.,* ''Vincristine helps kill tumor cells,'' ''Codeine is the pain medication.''
	    Proper administration of medication and adherence to schedule
	  • If patient is receiving analgesic medications, establish parameters for administration with family, child.
	c. Establish a plan of care to deal with problems related to treatment.
	  • *Alopecia*—Suggest a wig, cap, hat, scarf or remaining ''bald'', *e.g.,* ''Kojak.''
	  • *Mouth sores and decreased gum integrity*—Suggest mouthwash, one part peroxide one part mouthwash, every 4 hours or so while awake; toothettes, especially after eating; oral irrigating device, use of viscous lidocaine if sores are severe; soft diet.
	  • *Jaw pain, sore throat, abdominal pain*—For pain in general suggest acetaminophen (Tylenol); if not relieved in 24 hours, contact physician.
	  • *Nausea and vomiting*—Suggest small frequent meals, progressing from liquids to a soft diet to a regular diet; use of antiemetic suppositories; if vomiting persists longer than 4 to 8 hours, contact physician.
	  • *Constipation*—Suggest modifications in diet such as increase in fruits and juices and a decrease in starches; may suggest milk of magnesia: if symptoms are unrelieved in 2 to 3 days, call physician.
	  • *Weight gain/hypertension*—With steroid therapy, suggest low sodium diet.
	  • *Renal damage*—For those drugs specifically nephrotoxic such as cyclophosphamide, suggest specific amounts of fluids necessary.
	  • *Bleeding*—If a cut or bloody nose continues to bleed longer than 15 minutes, with constant pressure, contact physician; for petechiae and bruises over chest, back and abdomen, contact physician.
	  • *Infections*—
	    If temperature is elevated, contact physician.
	    Especially important: Limit exposure to communicable disease, especially chickenpox or shingles, particularly if the child has not had chickenpox. Notify physician or pediatric oncology nurse clinician immediately if exposed to chickenpox and child has not had chickenpox.
	    Counsel regarding immunizations—the child should not receive a live virus vaccine such as oral polio, measles, mumps, rubella.
	
	d. Help family identify community/personal resources.
	  • Leukemia Society of America
	  • American Cancer Society—local county chapter
	  • Candlelighters—national parents group
	  • Vocational Rehabilitation
	  • Social Services through Public Health Department
	  • Crippled Children's Funding (for those who qualify financially and geographically)
	  • Local parent support group
	e. Assist family to help school personnel to gain understanding of child and his condition when he returns to school.

Patient Outcome   Process

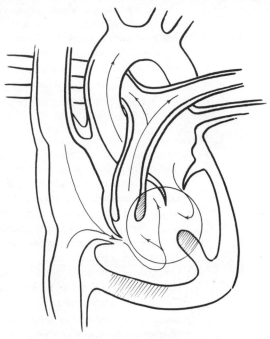

Fig. 8-4. Tetralogy of Fallot.

The patient/family experience informed, safe, and comfortable preoperative, postoperative, and pre-discharge phases of hospitalization. This includes:

DESCRIPTION: Tetralogy of Fallot describes a combination of four defects which includes (1) a ventricular septal defect, (2) infundibular and/or valvular pulmonary stenosis, (3) overriding of the aorta and, (4) hypertrophy of the right ventricle secondary to pulmonary stenosis (Fig. 8-4). It is a common congenital heart disease presenting most often in the first year of life and often necessitating palliative measures.

PROCEDURE: A median sternotomy incision is made and cardiopulmonary bypass is used during the repair of the intracardiac defects. The pulmonary artery is incised to relieve the obstruction. Infundibular hypertrophied muscle is excised and the valve cusps are excised if necessary. If the pulmonary annulus is narrowed, a pericardial patch is utilized to widen it. The ventricular septal defect is closed by fashioning a patch from percardium or dacron. The incisions are closed leaving appropriate drains, monitoring devices, and pacing wires in place.

NURSING ASSESSMENT: In addition to the general admission assessment, the following information is especially important.
1. Assess and document physical status.
   a. Level of activity
   b. Vital signs
   c. Peripheral pulses
   d. Current medications
   e. History of recent febrile illness, allergies, family history of congenital heart disease
2. Assess and document patient's/parents' response to information about the disease process, implications, and anticipated surgery.
   • Apparent anxiety level of patient/parents.
3. Assess and document patient's/parents' understanding of the disease process, implications, and anticipated surgery.
   • Evaluate parents' perception of child's expectations.

INTERVENTION:

A. Is prepared for surgery

1. Reinforce understanding of patient/parents regarding the disease and anticipated surgery.
   • Emphasize pre- and postoperative expectations:
     • Preoperative laboratory and radiograph studies
     • Antimicrobial body bath evening prior to surgery
     • Antibiotic and sedative administration p.o. and IM
     • Will remain in special care area 24 to 48 hours
     • Intubation and respiratory support will vary from a few hours to overnight.
     • Following extubation O_2 and humidity will be given for 12 to 18 hours.

Patient Outcome	Process
	• Frequent monitoring of vital signs, central venous pressure, cardiac output • Continuous monitoring of EKG and arterial pressure • Foley catheter for monitoring urine output • Chest drainage tubes (1 to 3) until adequate lung expansion • Temporary pacing wires connected to demand pacer
B. *Is free of or has minimal discomfort or post operative complications*	2. Summarize features of preoperative phase and provide care needed per hospital routine and physician's orders. See Chapter 8 Preoperative Phase of Hospitalization (Infants — Adolescents). p. 301.
	3. Provide postoperative care. Intervene in the critical elements of care.

• Respiratory	a. Maintain adequate ventilation and patent airway.
	     • Suction frequently with instillation of normal saline to thin secretion.
	     • Note signs and symptoms of respiratory distress according to age group.
	     • Observe for changes in the arterial blood gases.
	     • Medicate, if indicated, to prevent inadequate respirations due to splinting.
	     • Begin chest physical therapy on evening of surgery to prevent atelectasis.
	     • Continue physical therapy q 2 to 4 hours as needed on transfer to ward until chest is clear to percussion and auscultation.
	     • Observe for abdominal distention that will make respirations inefficient, especially in infants and small children. Insert nasogastric tube or ''burp'' as indicated.
	     • Turn, cough, deep breathe.

• Cardiovascular	b. Maintain stable cardiovascular function.
	     • Monitor and document vital signs. Notify physician of any changes from normal for age.
	     • Observe baseline cardiac output on admission to unit.
	     • Check peripheral pulses hourly.
	     • Remain aware of acceptable limits of blood pressure and heart rate when vasopressors are required. Follow hospital policy for regulating IV therapy.
	     • Document any arrhythmias, noting time and character.
	       If pacing wires are in place, they must be connected to pacer set on demand.
	         After critical period, they will be wrapped in plastic and taped to the chest ready for use.
	     • Measure drainage from chest tubes and other sites. Replace volume q 15 minutes if necessary.
	     • Observe carefully for possible tamponade.

• Fluid/electrolyte balance	c. Provide continual and accurate observation of fluid and electrolyte balance.
	     • Maintain intake and output record.
	     • Measure urine output q 1 hour on the hour.
	       Be aware diuresis will occur postcardiopulmonary bypass. Observe carefully to maintain adequate potassium with brisk diuresis.
	     • Call physician if urine drops below 1 cc per kg per hour or becomes bloody. Diuretics intravenously may be required at intervals until excess fluid is removed. Occasionally diuretics by mouth will be required for several days/weeks.
	     • Assess fluid and electrolyte status.
	       Document fluid loss through blood loss, urine, and emesis. Document time of loss and replacement fluid.
	       Notify physician of significant change in the following:
	         EKG
	         Vital signs (TPR, BP, and CVP)
	         Pulmonary status
	         Arterial blood gases
	         Blood chemistries
	       Watch electrolytes carefully in the immediate postoperative period. Potassium will be administered on an hourly basis according to need. Calcium may be given q 1 hour according to body weight. Electrolytes will be checked q 4 hours for 12 to 24 hours, then daily for 3 days.

• Gastrointestinal	d. Facilitate gastrointestinal function.
	     • Observe closely for abdominal distention, nausea, and vomiting. Insure patency of nasogastric tube.
	     • Assess and document the return of bowel sounds.

Patient Outcome	Process
	• Give ice chips in small amounts to child (three years and above) 4 to 6 hours following extubation. If no nausea and bowel sounds are present, progress to sips and full liquids within 24 hours. Progress to diet for age.
• *Neurological*	e. Assess patient for symptoms indicating neurological deficit.
	• Level of consciousness and mental status; compare with baseline.
	• Response to stimuli according to age: voice, touch, pain
• *Comfort*	f. Anticipate and evaluate needs for pain control. Provide necessary relief measures.
	• Administer medication to relieve discomfort, anxiety and coughing, facilitate movement.
	• Change position of patient to relieve discomfort.
	g. Provide family with periods of time to visit and emotional support.
	• Explain equipment.
	• Answer questions and respond to concerns.
• *Wound*	h. Assess wound for redness, drainage or inflammation, daily.
	• Initial dressing change is in recovery area then dressed p.r.n. with dry sterile dressing.
	• Skin sutures will be removed on the seventh postoperative day.
	• Keep groin incision in infant free of stool, urine.
C. *Is knowledgeable about nature of illness, care at home, and resources for continuity of care*	4. See Chapter 8 Predischarge Phase of Hospitalization (Infants—Adolescents), p. 303. Include additonal essential elements of preparation for discharge.
	a. Instruct patient/family regarding resumption of activities.
	• Provide short rest periods for two weeks.
	• Avoid activity in extreme weather.
	• Return to normal level of activity in one month unless otherwise indicated.
	• Return to school in 10 to 14 days unless otherwise indicated.
	b. Discuss medications dosages, time schedules, precautions, and length of time to take.
	c. Instruct family in follow-up care.
	• Give written guidelines to explain:
	Activity
	Bathing
	Medications
	School/church activities
	Emergency phone numbers for physician contact to report:
	Chest pain
	Elevated temperature
	Productive cough that does not improve
	Complaints of malaise and fatigue
	Shortness of breath
	Edema of periorbital area, legs, feet
	Incisional redness or drainage.
	d. Discuss community agencies which may assist in continuity of care, *e.g.,* school health office.
	e. Initiate interagency referral as needed.

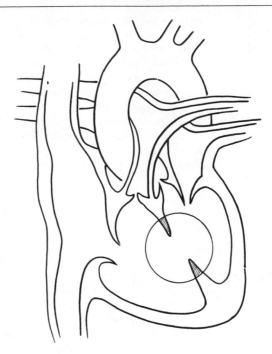

Fig. 8-5.   Ventricular septal defect.

The patient/family experience informed, safe, and comfortable preoperative, postoperative, and predischarge phases of hospitalization. This includes:

DESCRIPTION: A ventricular septal defect (VSD) is a hole or holes which allow the blood to communicate from the higher pressure left ventricle to the lower pressured right ventricle (Fig. 8-5). In turn the flow to the lungs is increased depending on the pulmonary resistance and size of defect. The severity of VSD is greatly dependent upon the degree of shunting and the amount of increased pulmonary flow and increased pulmonary hypertension. A VSD is often not suspected until a murmur is first heard at well-baby check at six weeks.

PROCEDURE: A median sternotomy incision is used to expose the heart. Cardiopulmonary bypass is utilized during repair of intracardiac defect. The heart may be opened using a right atrial or ventricular incision depending on location of VSD. The VSD is visualized and repaired using suture or patch material out of dacron or pericardium. Care is taken to prevent damage to the conduction system. The heart is closed and cardiopulmonary bypass is discontinued.

NURSING ASSESSMENT: In addition to the general admission assessment, the following information is especially important.
1. Assess and document physical status.
   a. Level of activity
   b. Vital signs
   c. Peripheral pulses
   d. Current medications
   e. History of recent febrile illness, allergies, family history of congenital heart disease.
   f. Color
2. Assess and document patient's/parents' response to information about the disease process, implications, and anticipated surgery.
   a. Apparent anxiety level of patient/parents.
   b. Previous experience with surgery.
3. Assess and document patient's/parents' understanding of disease process, implications, and anticipated surgery.
   a. Evaluate parents' perception of child's expectation.
   b. Evaluate child's perception of what is to happen.

INTERVENTION:

A. Is prepared for surgery

1. Reinforce understanding of patient/parents regarding the disease process, implications, and anticipated surgery.

Patient Outcome	Process

	• Emphasize postoperative expectations:
	  • Will remain in special care area 24 to 48 hours.
	  • Intubation and respiratory support will vary from a few hours to overnight.
	  • Following extubation, O_2 and humidity will be given for 12 to 18 hours.
	  • Constant monitoring of vital signs, central venous pressure, arterial pressure, EKG
	  • Foley catheter for monitoring urine output
	  • Chest drainage tubes (1 to 3) attached to suction until adequate lung re-expansion.
	  • Possible use of temporary pacing of heart activity
	  • Pulmonary care: coughing, deep breathing, postural drainage
	2. Summarize features of preoperative phase and provide care needed per hospital routine and physician's orders. See Chapter 8 Preoperative Phase of Hospitalization (infants—adolescents), p. 301.

B. *Is free of or has minimal discomfort or postoperative complications*
 	
• *Respiratory*
	3. Provide postoperative care. Intervene in the critical elements of care.
	  a. Maintain adequate ventilation.
	    • Suction frequently with instillation of normal saline to thin secretions.
	    • Note signs and symptoms of respiratory distress according to age group.
	    • Observe for changes in the arterial blood gases.
	    • Medicate, if indicated, to prevent inadequate respirations due to splinting.
	    • Begin chest physical therapy on evening of surgery to prevent atelectasis.
	    • Physical therapy will be continued q 2 to 4 hours as needed on transfer to ward until chest is clear to percussion and auscultation.
	    • Observe for abdominal distention that will make respirations inefficient, especially in infants and small children. Insert nasogastric tube or "burp" as indicated.

• *Cardiovascular*	b. Maintain stable cardiovascular function.
	    • Monitor and document vital signs and intracardiac pressures. Notify physician of any changes from normal for age.
	    • Remain aware of acceptable limits of blood pressure and heart rate when vasopressors are required.
	    • Document any arrhythmias, noting time and character.
	      If pacing wires are in place, they must be connected to pacer set on demand.
	        After critical period, they will be wrapped in plastic and taped to the chest for possible later use.
	    • Measure drainage from chest tubes and other sites. Replace volume q 15 minutes if necessary.
	    • Observe carefully for possible tamponade.

• *Fluid/electrolyte balance*	c. Provide continual and accurate observation of fluid and electrolyte balance.
	    • Maintain intake and output record.
	    • Measure urine output q 1 hour on the hour.
	      Be aware diuresis will occur postcardiopulmonary bypass. Observe carefully to maintain adequate potassium with brisk diuresis.
	    • Call physician if urine drops below 1 cc per kg per hour or becomes bloody. Diuretics intravenously may be required at intervals until excess fluid is removed. Occasionally diuretics by mouth will be required for several days, weeks.
	    • Assess fluid and electrolyte status.
	      Document fluid loss through blood loss, urine and, emesis. Document time of loss and replacement fluid.
	      Observe for and report presence of facial and/or peripheral edema.
	      Notify physician of significant change in the following:
	        EKG
	        Vital signs (TPR, BP, and CVP)
	        Pulmonary status
	        Arterial blood gases
	        Serum electrolytes
	      Watch electrolytes carefully in the immediate postoperative period. Potassium may be administered on an hourly basis according to need. Calcium may be given q 1 hour according to body weight. Electrolytes will be checked q 4 hours until the following morning, then q.i.d. for three days.

• *Gastrointestinal*	d. Facilitate gastrointestinal function. • Observe closely for abdominal distention, nausea, vomiting. Insure patency of nasogastric tube.

Patient Outcome	Process
	• Assess and document the return of bowel sounds.
	• Give ice chips in small amounts to child (three years and above) following extubation. If no nausea and bowel sounds are present, progress to sips and full liquids within 24 hours.
• *Neurological*	e. Assess patient for symptoms indicating neurological deficit.
	• Level of consciousness and mental status and compare with baseline.
	• Response to stimuli according to age: voice, touch, pain
• *Comfort*	f. Anticipate and evaluate needs for pain control. Provide necessary relief measures.
	• Administer medication to relieve discomfort, coughing, and anxiety and facilitate movement.
	• Change position of patient to relieve discomfort.
	g. Provide emotional support to family and schedule adequate time for visits.
	• Explain equipment.
	• Answer questions and respond to concerns.
• *Wound healing*	h. Assess wound for redness, drainage, or inflammation daily.
	• Initial dressing change is in recovery area then dressed p.r.n. with dry sterile dressing.
	• Skin sutures will be removed on the seventh postoperative day.
C. *Is knowledgeable about nature of illness, care at home, and resources for continuity of care*	4. See Chapter 8 Predischarge Phase of Hospitalization (infants—adolescents), p. 303. Include additional essential elements of preparation for discharge.
	a. Instruct patient/family regarding resumption of activities.
	• Provide short rest periods for two weeks.
	• Avoid activity in extreme weather.
	• Return to normal level of activity in one month unless otherwise indicated.
	• Return to school in 10 to 14 days unless otherwise indicated.
	b. Discuss medications: purposes, dosages, time schedules, precautions, and length of time to take.
	c. Instruct family in follow-up care.
	• Give written guidelines to explain:
	Activity
	Bathing
	Medications
	School/church activities
	Emergency phone numbers for physician contact to report:
	Chest pain
	Elevated temperature
	Productive cough that does not improve
	Complaints of malaise and fatigue
	d. Discuss community agencies which may assist in continuity of care, *e.g.*, school health office.
	e. Initiate interagency referral as needed.

CHAPTER IX
Guidelines for the critical care patient

INTRODUCTION: These guidelines describe patient care outcomes and associated nursing process for the patient who requires critical care nursing regardless of illness and therapy. There is emphasis on nursing assessment and specific interventions and the nurse's participation in detection and treatment of life-threatening events.

Consideration is given to key nursing activities directed towards preventing or minimizing the hazards of further complications which often occur during the critical illness experience.

The guideline delineating nursing process to achieve desired psychosocial outcomes is applicable to all patients and their families throughout the critical care experience.

The focus of these guidelines is directed towards the patient in a life-threatening situation; the nurse must recognize that the complexity of the current needs of the critically ill patient influences the order of priority of the nursing measures instituted.

Patient Outcome	Process	
	ASSESSMENT	INTERVENTION

PREFACE: These guidelines are intended to be comprehensive for performing a thorough cardiovascular assessment as well as describing assessment parameters for identifying low cardiac output—the cardinal feature of cardiovascular failure. The nurse establishing priorities for care of a patient in crisis may begin by assessing cardiac output and then proceed to a more general evaluation of the patient's cardiovascular status.

The patient attains optimal cardiovascular function

1. Obtain pertinent information through patient interview and chart review.
   a. Chief complaint
   b. Sociological data
   c. Current medications
   d. Signs, symptoms
      - Chest discomfort—character, duration, frequency, method of relief
      - Shortness of breath (SOB)
      - Paroxysmal nocturnal dyspnea (PND)
      - Dyspnea on exertion (DOE)
      - Hemoptysis
      - Pedal edema
      - Orthopnea
      - Recent weight change
      - Cyanosis
      - Syncope/dizziness
      - Claudication
      - Abdominal/back pain
      - Palpitations
      - Headaches
      - Blurred vision
      - Productive cough

2. Assess general physical status.
   a. Affect/orientation (appearance of distress)
   b. Body habitus (posture/position)
   c. Overt physical signs, *e.g.*,
      - Obvious pulsations
      - Deformities of chest wall
   d. Pattern/quality of respirations
   e. Skin
      - Cyanosis
      - Rosy facies
      - Pale and clammy

3. Assess peripheral vascular system.
   a. Fingernails
   b. Color of extremity
   c. Presence of swelling (edema) and/or atrophy
   d. Presence of obvious pulsations
   e. Venous pattern
   f. Neck veins (usually diffuse and undulant).
      - Presence of jugular venous distension (JVD)
      - Variations produced with respirations
      - Estimated venous pressure using internal jugular vein
   g. Assess the following pulses: carotid, brachial, radial, ulnar, femoral, popliteal, dorsalis pedis, posterior tibial.

INTERVENTION:

- Document baseline data and significant changes.

- Anticipate need for studies and therapy for patient with chest pain.
   a. Twelve-lead EKG
   b. Bilateral blood pressure
   c. Emergency blood chemistries
   d. O_2
   e. Arterial blood gases, preferably before oxygen administration
   f. Drug therapy

- Inspect for abnormalities.

- Inspect and palpate simultaneously.
   - Compare right to left to rule out pertinent negatives.

- Use three fingers to palpate pulses. Occlude pulse completely then release gradually.

Patient Outcome

Process

ASSESSMENT	INTERVENTION

- Presence or absence
  - 0—absent
  - 1—thready   3—normal
  - 2—diminished   4—bounding
- Character or quality (often reflects elasticity of wall):
  - Bounding
  - Thready
- Rhythm:
  - Regular   Tachycardia
  - Bigeminal   Bradycardia
  - Irregular
- Presence of any special qualities, *e.g.*, thrills

  h. Presence of hepatojugular reflex

  i. Homan's sign (pain in calf on rapid ankle dorsiflexion which suggests thrombophlebitis)

4. Auscultate for bruits and radiated murmurs.
   - a. Femoral arteries
   - b. Abdominal aorta
   - c. Carotid arteries

- Palpate for hepatojugular reflex:
  - a. Place patient in supine position with head elevated 45°.
  - b. Stand at patient's left side.
  - c. Place hand on right upper quadrant of abdomen just below the ribs.
  - d. Ask patient to exhale and press downward on liver.
  - e. Ask patient to inhale and note neck veins. If neck veins remain filled, this indicates a positive response.

5. Assess precordium.
   - a. Identify important anatomical landmarks:
     - Angle of Louis
     - Second intercostal space
     - Sternal border
   - b. Locate the following in relation to the identified anatomical landmarks:
     - Point of maximal impulse (PMI)
     - Aortic area
     - Tricuspid area
     - Mitral area
     - Pulmonic area
   - c. Point of maximal impulse
     - Normal forceful increased PMI occurs in:
       - Pregnancy
       - Anemia
       - Fever
       - Increased cardiac output
       - Children
     - Abnormal forceful increased PMI occurs in left ventricular hypertrophy Cardiomegaly
   - d. Note any lifts, thrills, gallops.

- Describe findings in terms of location and timing within the cardiac cycle, abnormal cardiac movements, and obvious pulsations.

- Palpate the PMI.
  - a. If difficult to palpate, tilt the patient to left side bringing the apex into closer contact with the chest wall.
  - b. Note location, size, rhythm.

6. Assess cardiac sounds.
   - a. Normal cardiac sounds:
     - S_1—beginning of ventricular systole; represents closure of mitral and tricuspid valves. S_1 is a low pitched sound loudest at the apex. May be simultaneous with carotid impulse and QRS complex of the EKG.
     - S_2—beginning of ventricular diastole;

- Auscultate sequentially through each cardiac area beginning with the mitral area.
- Describe any extra sounds, rhythm, and timing within the cardiac cycle.

Patient Outcome	Process	
	ASSESSMENT	INTERVENTION

represents closure of aortic (A_2) and pulmonic (P_2) valves. S_2 is louder than S_1 at the cardiac base.

b. Abnormal cardiac sounds and significance.

• Gallops:

Ventricular gallop or S_3—represents the initial 80 per cent filling of ventricle which is filling into overdistended or noncompliant ventricle. Indicative of impending congestive failure or fluid overload. May be indicative of incompetent mitral or tricuspid valve. May hear this sound prior to pulmonary edema. In children, pregnancy, fever this may be heard but is physiologic.

Atrial gallop or S_4—represents atrial contraction and emptying of last 20 per cent of volume into ventricle. Often a sign of noncompliant ventricle.

• Murmurs—extra cardiac sounds caused by turbulence of blood flow. Describe in relation to timing in cardiac cycle:

Systolic (early, mid, late or holosystolic)

Diastolic

Continuous

Note:

Location

Radiation

Intensity (Grade I—VI)

Quality (high, medium, or low pitch)

• Rubs—usually indicates inflammation

Pericardial—leathery sounds coinciding with the heart beat

Pleural—scratchy sound usually localized to a region of the chest and heart with either or both inspiration or expiration.

7. Assess adequacy of cardiac output to meet metabolic demands. Cardiac output is determined by factors of stroke volume and heart rate per minute. Stroke volume is the amount of blood ejected by the left ventricle each beat and is influenced by venous return, total body volume, peripheral resistance and strength of contractibility of heart.

a. Cardiac output = stroke volume × heart beat per minute

b. Early signs of decreased cardiac output:

• Reflex mechanisms which maintain homeostasis:

Relative tachycardia

INTERVENTION column:

• For sudden development of S_3

a. Note fluid balance.

b. Notify physician.

c. Note other signs of congestive failure.

• Pulmonary edema

• Ankle edema

• Respiratory distress

• Diaphoresis

• Tachycardia

• Anxiety

• Decrease in cardiac output

• For patient who has had cardiac surgery and has rub:

a. Notify physician.

b. Anticipate steroid therapy.

Patient Outcome	Process	
	ASSESSMENT	INTERVENTION

Peripheral vasoconstriction:
   Decreased skin temperature
   Decreased amplitude of periph-
      eral pulses
   Decreased pulse pressure
   Relative tachypnea
   Respiratory alkalosis: Decreased
      PCO_2
   Urinary output unchanged at this
      stage.
c. Signs of prolonged decrease in cardiac
   output and perfusion: (Reflex mech-
   anisms not maintaining homeostasis.)
   • Decreased systolic blood pressure less
      than 80 mm Hg. Hypotension may
      occur at a higher pressure in hyperten-
      sive patient.
   • Decreased urine output
   • Metabolic acidosis:
      Decreased blood pH
   • Cold, clammy extremities
   • Cyanosis
   • Decreased level of consciousness
   • Change in central venous pressure de-
      pending on underlying cause
8. Assess underlying condition causing hypo-
   perfusion state:
   a. Hypovolemia—observe for:
      • Overt signs of bleeding
      • Covert signs of bleeding
      • Hemoconcentration, *e.g.,* altered he-
         matocrit
      • Decreased central venous pressure
      • Relative tachycardia
      • Lowered pulse pressure
      • Decreased pulmonary artery and left
         atrial pressures
      • Patient populations at risk for hy-
         povolemia. Examples are:
         Burns
         Postsurgery
         Ruptured or dissecting aneurysm
         Multiple trauma
         Orthopaedic injury
         Loss of fluid from GI tract
         Hemodialysis
         Diabetes insipidus
   b. Pump failure
      • Identify signs and symptoms:
         Relative tachycardia
         Lowered pulse pressure
         Early decrease in level of con-
            sciousness
         Increased left venticular end dia-
            stolic pressure reflected by in-
            creased pulmonary artery wedge
            pressure and/or increased pulmo-
            nary artery diastolic pressure in
            the absence of hypovolemia.

• Treat cause or condition underlying hypoper-
   fusion state:
   a. Hypovolemia: notify physician and an-
      ticipate:
      • Volume replacement with:
         Electrolyte solutions such as lactated
            Ringer's solution
         Volume expanders such as albumin,
            blood products, plasmanate

• Intervene for patients with pump failure.
   Notify physician of pertinent signs and anticipate:
   a. Continuous intravenous infusion of vaso-
      pressor, vasodilator, intropic and/or anti-
      arrhythmic drugs: levarterenol (Levophed
      Bitartrate), dopamine, (Intropin), iso-
      proterenol (Isuprel Hydrochloride), nitro-
      prusside (Nipride), lidocaine (Xylocaine),
      procainamide (Pronestyl), epinephrine
      (Adrenalin)

Patient Outcome	Process

ASSESSMENT	INTERVENTION

S$_3$ or S$_4$ gallop
Decreased O$_2$ saturation
Widened arterial-venous O$_2$ difference
Decreased cardiac output as measured by thermodilution or dye injection methods in absence of hypovolemia
Cardiac arrhythmia such as bradycardia, atrial flutter with rapid ventricular response, ventricular tachycardia
• Assess underlying conditions contributing to pump failure.
    Decreased myocardial contractibility due to:
        Myocardial infarction, ischemia electrolyte imbalance (hypocalcemia, hyperkalemia), drugs such as propranolol (Inderal), cardiomyopathy, sepsis, stress of surgical manipulation of heart and/or cardiopulmonary bypass, valvular dysfunction or anomaly
        Arrhythmia: Bradycardia, tachycardia, conduction defects, decreased PO$_2$, coronary hypoperfusion, electrolyte imbalance, effects of surgery such as severed conduction pathways
    Mechanical dysfunction:
        Constrictive processes as tamponade, pericarditis, valvular insufficiency or stenosis, outflow tract obstruction
        Systemic processes
            Pregnancy, thyrotoxicosis, anemia, cor pulmonale, renal failure
c. Sepsis
    • Identify signs and symptoms:
        Increased or decreased cardiac output as measured by thermodilution or dye injection methods
        Vasodilation
        Increased temperature or extremities
        Flushing
        Decreased circulatory volume and hypovolemia
        Electrolyte imbalance
	b. Respiratory support:
	        Supplementary oxygen
	        Endotracheal tube
	        Respirator
	c. Coronary dilators, *e.g.,* nitroglycerin, morphine, nitral paste, isosorbide (Isordil)
	d. Intra-aortic balloon pump
	
	• Be aware that any patient who has had an invasive procedure, *e.g.,* indwelling catheter, is at high risk for sepsis.
	a. Notify physician of pertinent signs and symptoms and anticipate:
	    • Continuous intravenous infusion of vasoconstrictor drugs
	    • Circulatory volume enhancement
	    • Antibiotics • Antipyretics
	    • Steroids • Hypothermia
	    • Maintenance of serum albumin greater than 3.5 per cent to protect against adult respiratory distress syndrome
	b. Measure temperature hourly.
	c. Obtain cultures as indicated, *e.g.,* wound, blood, sputum, urine, invasive line.
	d. Be alert for possible cardiopulmonary arrest.

Patient Outcome	Process	
	ASSESSMENT	INTERVENTION

The patient attains optimal endocrine function	1. Assess and document signs and symptoms of abnormal endocrine function.
	  a. Assess and document signs and symptoms of hypoglycemia—low blood sugar, less than 80 mg per 100 ml. Onset may be rapid.
	    • Diaphoresis
	    • Complains of nervousness, hunger, lightheadedness
	    • Double vision
	    • Confusion: change in level of awareness
	    • Incoherent speech
	    • Behavior change, *e.g.,* irritability
	    • Tachycardia
	    • Negative urine sugar
	    • Headache
	    • Tremors, seizure activity
	    • Hypothermia
	    • Hypotension
	    • No adverse reaction to light shown on closed eyes during sleep (negative flashlight sign)
	    • Loss of consciousness
		Be aware that although patient's admitting diagnosis may not be diabetes mellitus, the management of diabetes is a major factor in maintaining health status.
		• For patient with diabetes mellitus:
		  a. Interview patient/family for self-management of diabetes.
		  b. Monitor urine sugar, acetone, blood sugar.
		  c. Monitor caloric intake (fluids, solids).
		  d. Assess subjective feelings.
		  e. Check for appropriate insulin or oral agent orders.
		  f. Monitor vital signs (VS), intake and output.
		• For patient with hypoglycemia:
		  a. Call physician.
		  b. Check blood sugar before administering glucose.
		  c. Give glucose or intravenous (IV) as appropriate.
		    • PO: sugar (2 teaspoons), or 120 cc of orange juice
		    • IV: 50 cc of $D_{50}W$ (dextrose 50 per cent in water)—through central line, if available
		  d. Monitor vital signs; if patient does not improve clinically after 10 minutes repeat glucose administration.
		  e. After patient stabilizes, attempt to evaluate cause of hypoglycemic reaction, *e.g.,*
		    • Inappropriate type or amount of insulin
		    • Change in therapy or body response that diminishes need for insulin
		  f. Continue to monitor urine sugar, acetone, blood sugar, intake and output (I&O).
		  g. Document signs, symptoms, interventions, outcomes and timing of actions.

	b. Assess and document signs and symptoms of diabetic ketoacidosis. Insidious onset; may range from hours to days.
	    • Positive urine sugar and acetone
	    • Blood sugar above normal range
	    • (80 to 120 mg per 100 ml)
	    • Increased thirst
	    • Increased frequency or urinary output
	    • Drowsiness, stupor; complaints of fatigue
	    • Nausea, vomiting, abdominal pain
	    • Sweet, fruity breath
	    • Kussmaul's breathing
	    • Decreased reflexes
		• For diabetic ketoacidosis:
		  a. Maintain airway.
		    • Have emergency equipment available
		  b. Initiate immediate and periodic blood sugar level determinations.
		  c. Call physician.
		  d. Insure patency of IV and availability of IV solutions.
		  e. Have regular insulin U100 available with syringes.
		    • Insulin may adhere to IV bag.
		    • If insulin given via continuous IV drip, a plasma binder must be included in the bag of solution, *e.g.,* albumin.
		  f. Monitor VS for hypotension.
		  g. Consider nasogastric (NG) tube and indwelling catheter.
		  h. Monitor serum electrolytes, especially potassium.
		  i. If patient on cardiac monitor, observe for changes.
		  j. Monitor I&O closely.

Patient Outcome	Process
ASSESSMENT	INTERVENTION

	k. Document signs, symptoms, interventions outcomes and timing of above actions.
	l. Provide safety precautions dependent upon patient's level of activity.
	m. Attempt to evaluate cause of diabetic ketoacidosis, *e.g.,*
	• Inappropriate insulin type or amount
	• Excessive carbohydrate intake by tube feeding, IV, p.o., or hyperalimentation
	• Increased stress due to trauma, surgery, medications, *e.g.,* steroids, antimetabolites.
c. Assess patients who are at high risk for hyperglycemia.	• Monitor critically ill patient for hyperglycemia:
• Multiple trauma	a. Qualitative and quantitative analysis of urine q 6 hours
• Burned	b. Blood sugar values
• Receiving total parenteral nutrition	
• Receiving peritoneal dialysis	• Institute measures for patient with hyperglycemia:
• Receiving steroids	a. Ascertain that insulin orders are written.
• Family history of diabetes mellitus	b. Provide preventive measures to avoid infections, *e.g.,* urinary, respiratory.
d. Identify patients at risk for diabetes insipidus.	• For patient with diabetes insipidus
• Head trauma	a. Assure patent indwelling urinary catheter
• Hypothalamic or pituitary tumor	b. Monitor
• Renal tubule dysfunction	• I&O
	• Serum electrolytes for hypernatremia
	c. Provide information and support for patient and family who may be frightened by abrupt onset and may confuse term diabetes insipidus with diabetes mellitus.
e. Assess signs and symptoms of diabetes insipidus in high risk patients.	• Clarify fluid replacement and medication orders with physician. Management usually includes:
• Large volumes of urine with low specific gravity (less than 1.005)	a. D_5W (dextrose 5 per cent in water) (avoid saline) to match output
• Dehydration, dry skin, confusion	b. May require additional IV line for larger volumes of replacement fluids
• Extreme thirst (may or may not be present)	c. For patient with extreme thirst maximize oral intake
• Urine osmolality decreases.	d. Aqueous vasopressin (Pitressin), antidiuretic hormone (ADH), ordered IM, p.r.n. dependent upon output
• Serum osmolality increases.	• For patient requiring long-term replacement of pitressin, consider Pitressin Tannate in Oil or lypressin (Diapid) spray.
2. Assess factors affecting specific uring tests.	• Document urine testing in terms of percentages; include method when recording tests.
a. Clinitest 2 drop method:	
• Not applicable to patients on certain drugs, *i.e.,* isoniazid (INH), cephalothin (Keflin), cephazolin (Ancef), tetracyclines, methyldopa (Aldomet), sulfisoxazole (Gantrisin), sulfasalazine (Azulfidine), vitamin C, phenazopyridine (Pyridium), aspirin	
• Not applicable for patients with hematuria.	

Patient Outcome	Process

ASSESSMENT	INTERVENTION

b. Tes–tape—use when above restrictions apply to patient.
c. Acetest—use in conjunction with either of above.
3. Assess patient who may require steroid replacement therapy.
   a. Identify patient who may have altered response to stress which may be due to inadequate cortisone therapy.
     • Currently receiving scheduled doses of steroids as long-term therapy
     • Has been on steroid therapy within past year
     • Has hypopituitary or hypoadrenal function
   b. Be aware that patients who have been on long-term steroid therapy:
     • Are immunosusceptible and are extremely susceptible to nosocomial infections
     • Require continuous steroid therapy or gradual decrease.
	• For patient who may have inadequate cortisone response:
	   a. Document this information and communicate as needed.
	   b. Monitor patient for signs and symptoms of inadequate cortisone in times of stress.
	     • Hypotension
	     • Lethargy
	     • Restlessness
	     • Tachycardia
	     • Increased potassium, decreased sodium
	     • Sweating, diaphoresis
	     • Increased urine output
	   c. Check with physician for possible booster doses of steroids to cover stress requirements.
	   d. Protect patient from possible sources of infection.
	   e. Ascertain that steroid replacement orders are accurate and appropriate.

c. Be aware of patients who may need short term, large doses of steroids.
These include patients with:
   • Sepsis
   • Cerebral or spinal cord edema
   • Anaphylaxis
   • Acute respiratory problems which may lead to acute respiratory distress syndrome
   • Acute renal rejection syndrome
	• For patient receiving steroids:
	   a. Monitor drug orders closely. Clarify with physician.
	     • Type of corticosteroid
	     • Dosage
	   b. Check with physician regarding a patient who has not received steroid dose as scheduled within 24 hour period.
	   c. Administer slowly if given intravenously.
	     • Monitor for hypotension.
	   d. Monitor for side effects such as
	     • Electrolyte disturbances
	     • Fluid retention
	     • Gastrointestinal disturbances, *i.e.,* bleeding
	     • Hyperglycemia
	     • Masking of infection
	     • Rapid mood changes
	   e. Monitor blood sugar levels and quantitative and qualitative urines q 6 hours.
	   f. Guaiac stools
	   g. Collaborate with physician for measures to minimize side effects, *i.e.,* give antacids.

4. Identify patients who are hypothyroid and who are on long-term thyroid replacement, *e.g.,* levothyroxine (Synthroid).	• For patient receiving thyroid replacement:
	   a. Assess ability of GI tract to absorb oral medication, *e.g.,* vomiting, hypermotility.
	   b. Consider with physician need for parenteral thyroid replacement. If thyroid replacement given, observe safety precautions, *i.e.,* give slowly.

Patient Outcome   Process

ASSESSMENT	INTERVENTION
	c. Observe for symptoms of hyperthyroidism when drug given parenterally: • Tachycardia • Elevation of blood pressure • Sweating d. Determine if patient has received daily thyroid doses as ordered. If significant number of doses missed, be alert for the following signs: • Hypotension • Bradycardia • Lethargy • Decreased respiratory drive

5. Identify patients who are hyperthyroid and be aware of circumstances which may precipate thyroid "storm".
  a. Physiological stress, *i.e.,* infection, trauma, diabetic ketoacidosis
  b. Manipulation/direct trauma to thyroid gland
  c. Noncompliance with antithyroid regimen
  d. Rapid iodine withdrawal	

6. Assess signs and symptoms of thyroid toxicosis.
  a. Fever
  b. Tachycardia with arrhythmias, especially atrial fibrillation
  c. Hypertension
  d. High cardiac output leading to congestive heart failure
  e. Extreme agitation
	• For patient who is hyperthyroid, use supportive measures to reduce secretion and production of thyroid hormones. These may include:
	  a. Antithyroid drugs and iodine
	  b. Fluids, glucose, electrolytes, vitamin B replacement
	  c. Measures to reduce fever (avoid aspirin which may increase metabolic rate)
	  d. Measures to reduce congestive heart failure, *e.g.,* digitalis, diuretics, oxygen
	  e. Large doses of steroids
	  f. Reduction of external stimuli
	• For patient with marked exopthalmos
	  a. Protect cornea with eye drops.
	  b. Avoid harsh lighting.

Patient Outcome	Process	
	ASSESSMENT	INTERVENTION

The patient attains optimal gastrointestinal function	1. Assess signs and symptoms of gastrointestinal abnormalities. Compare with baseline gastrointestinal (GI) data.
	   a. General physical assessment:
	      • General appearance, including posturing, facial expression, movement, skin color, respiratory status
	      • Presence of drainage tubes, *e.g.,* nasogastric (NG) tube
	   b. Description of pain:
	      • Type, including other sensations such as burning, rushes (growling) abdominal tightness
	      • Location
	      • Previous experience with GI pain
	      • Possible precipitating factors
	      • Methods of relief
	   c. Factors relating to current GI function:
	      • Appetite
	      • Food tolerance
	      • Thirst
	      • Diet
	      • Difficulty in swallowing
	      • Belching
	      • Nausea
	      • Vomiting
	      • Stools
	          Consistency, character, frequency, color, presence of blood and mucus, amount, odor
	      • Flatus
	      • Weight change
		• Document baseline data and significant changes.

	2. Assess preadmission health habits related to the GI system.
	   a. Bowel habits
	   b. Current medications
	   c. Eating patterns and preferences
	   d. Alcohol consumption
	   e. Stress factors
	   f. Other medical problems
		• Document health habits.
		   a. If patient on previous bowel regimen or likely to have bowel problems consult with physician for bowel regimen.
		
		   b. Consider medication side effects of salicylates, narcotics, etc.

	3. Inspect abdomen
	   a. Size, symmetry, shape
	   b. Muscle tone, herniation of bowel through muscle, bulging under skin
	   c. Skin color, warmth, pigmentation
	   d. Scars, striae, rashes
	   e. Vascular markings
	   f. Overt peristalsis
	   g. Incisions, wounds, fistulas
	   h. Irritation, granulation, swelling, drainage
	   i. Presence of drains (If unable to remove dressing to visualize drains, check for presence and location from chart or physician.)
	   j. Presence of dressings—Assess appearance of wound and drainage: character, odor, amount, color.
		• Have patient lie in supine position with hands by side and legs in comfortable position. Assure patient's privacy for examination of abdomen.
		• If distention present or anticipated:
		   a. Measure and record abdominal girths. Be sure tape is flat, the patient is in consistent position, and abdomen marked with tape position.
		   b. Position for optimal respiratory function and comfort. Change position frequently.
		• Protect skin from irritating drainage.
		   a. Establish responsibilities for dressing change with physician.
		   b. Note characteristics of drainage in progress notes. Redress as ordered.
		   c. If drainage is purulent, may send specimen for culture and sensitivity.

Patient Outcome	Process

ASSESSMENT	INTERVENTION
	d. If dressing is not to be changed, mark outline of drainage with date and time, and reinforce, if necessary. e. If wound is contaminated, maintain wound isolation precautions, prevent cross-contamination, and continue aseptic techniques.
4. Auscultate abdomen: a. Note persence, frequency, and character of sounds. • Normal bowel sounds • Absence or hypoactive bowel sounds (listen 1 to 3 minutes before considering absent) may indicate paralytic ileus or ischemic bowel. • Hyperactive bowel sounds—present with diarrhea, infection, early obstruction, and postprandial • Rushes—may be present postprandial and with obstruction • Borborygmi—loud peristaltic sounds associated with cramping pain. May be present with obstruction. • Bruit—turbulence heard in blood vessel, *e.g.,* aneurysm, aorta-femoral bypass graft	• Perform auscultation before the rest of examination to avoid alteration of bowel sounds. Be sure stethoscope diaphragm/bell is warm. Listen to all four quadrants. • For significant change in bowel sounds: a. If bowel sounds resume, contact physician for diet order. b. If bowel sounds cease, withhold oral intake and contact physician. c. If normal bowel sounds increase, consider the time and kind of food intake, early obstruction, infection. Document and notify physician if indicated.
5. Percuss abdomen for distention. a. If present differentiate between flat, fluid, flatus: • Flat: dullness on percussion • Flatus: tympanic sounds on percussion • Fluid: shifting dullness—fluid within abdomen follows force of gravity when patient's position changes. Wave-like motion seen or felt across abdomen when percussed. b. Percuss suprapubic area for bladder distention.	• For patient with urination difficulty: a. Note time of last voiding, catheter removal, fluid intake, renal status, prostate enlargement, spinal dysfunction. b. If patient is unable to void after nursing measures, *e.g.,* raise head of bed, Credés method, obtain method for catheterization.
6. Palpate abdomen. a. Relaxation/rigidity (involuntary rigidity may indicate peritoneal inflammation) b. Distention, tightness c. Warmth d. Masses	• Have patient relax and lightly palpate rectus muscles on expiration. • Consider patient's condition, *e.g.,* presence of abdominal aneurysm or diffuse abdominal cancer, before palpating deeply. • Press on abdomen firmly and slowly and withdraw fingers quickly to determine rebound tenderness.
7. Assess mouth condition including: a. Teeth, dentures b. Gums c. Mucosa d. Tongue	• Initiate mouth care as needed, at least q 4 hours. a. Use rough-textured gauze with half strength hydrogen peroxide or mouthwash, or toothbrush with toothpaste. b. Clean lips and coat with lubricating ointment.

Patient Outcome	Process	
	ASSESSMENT	**INTERVENTION**
		c. Obtain order for medicated mouthwash for symptoms of infection. d. Note loose teeth, extensive caries. Notify physician to obtain oral surgery consult.
	8. Evaluate fluid and electrolyte balance. a. Blood chemistries b. Physical signs of imbalance: muscle weakness, tetany, numbness, arrhythmias, mental status deterioration	• When assessing fluid and electrolyte balance, consider: a. Extensive NG drainage or vomiting may result in increased loss of fluids, sodium, etc. b. Extensive diarrhea may cause increased loss of fluids and electrolytes. c. Patient with abdominal distention may lose extensive amounts of fluid into abdominal space causing hypovolemia.
	9. Assess patient with active gastrointestinal bleeding (upper or lower). a. Frequent vital signs b. Observe for signs of shock: increased pulse, decreased CVP, decreased BP, increased respirations, increased anxiety. c. Estimate amount of bleeding by direct measurement and patient appearance: color, increased anxiety. d. Observe for aspiration, respiratory distress. e. Assess laboratory values.	• For patient with overt bleeding: a. Insure that patient has patent IV or insert large bore IV or control line. b. Assess amount, color, character of bleeding. Position to prevent aspiration. Assure patent NG tube. c. Initiate steps to stop bleeding, e.g., ice lavage. d. Check that blood is typed and crossmatched. e. Accompany patient to Radiology Department, etc. f. Anticipate need for Sengstaken-Blakemore tube or use of topical thrombin • For patient who is at risk for GI bleeding: a. Consider need for antacid therapy. b. Use guaiac test for occult blood as condition indicates, *e.g.,* for patient at risk for stress ulcer.
	10. Assess nasogastric tube/drainage: a. Location of NG tube	• Check location of NG tube before irrigation, tube feeding, instillation of medication. a. Listen in left epigastric area for "bubbling" while forcing air into tube. b. Aspirate fluid and check pH to indicate gastric contents.
	b. Nasogastric drainage: • Color • Character • Amount • Presence of blood • Odor • pH	• Consider special needs of patient with NG tube. a. Do not reposition tube or irrigate for patient who has high anastomosis, *e.g.,* esophageal or upper gastric surgery. b. Check nasal area for signs of irritation, necrosis. Retape tube to relieve pressure and apply protective ointment. c. Do not give patient ice chips which can cause hypotonia in stomach, loss of electrolytes through tube.
	11. Assess wound condition. a. Skin surrounding open wound, stoma, fistula. Look for: • Redness • Burning • Irritation • Swelling. • Bleeding • Itching	• Provide wound care. a. Consider using colostomy bag for wound that drains profusely. b. Wash thoroughly around wound with water and apply stoma adhesive or Karaya blanket.

Patient Outcome	Process	
	ASSESSMENT	INTERVENTION

ASSESSMENT	INTERVENTION

b. Wound complications:
  • Bleeding
  • Dehiscence—separation of wound edges
  • Evisceration—protrusion of abdominal contents through wound
  • Drainage of body fluid
  • Infection
	• Provide care for wound complications.
	  a. For dehiscence, apply steristrips to approximate edges and notify physician. Restrict patient to bed rest.
	  b. For evisceration, apply sterile pads soaked with sterile saline. Immobilize patient and notify physician.
	  c. For infection, culture wound and dress as ordered. Notify physician.

12. Inspect rectal area.
  a. Inspect sacrococcygeal and perianal areas for:
  • Lump
  • Inflammation
  • Rashes
  • Excoriation
  • Bleeding
  • Prolapse
  • Hemorrhoids
  • Fissures
  • Fistulas
  b. Assess rectum internally for:
  • Sphincter tone
  • Tenderness
  • Irregularities, consistency of stool
  • Impaction
	• Complete rectal examination by:
	  a. Ask patient to lie on left side with right hip and knee flexed.
	  b. Put glove on index finger and lubricate.
	  c. Spread buttocks with other hand.
	  d. Explain that the examination of rectum will make the patient feel as if moving bowels.
	    • Place gloved finger over sphincter and ask patient to strain down. As patient relaxes, insert finger into rectum.
	• For hemorrhoids or other rectal problem:
	  a. Avoid rectal tubes.
	  b. Consider stool softener in preventive bowel regimen.
	  c. Clean with soothing towelette.
	  d. Avoid rectal temperatures if possible.
	  e. Check with physician for removing impaction.

13. Assess general nutritional status and signs of malnutrition.
  a. Loss of skin turgor, friable, increased capillary fragility
  b. Loss of muscle mass, generalized wasting
  c. Weight change since onset of illness
  d. Slow healing of wounds
  e. Glossitis (swollen or inflammed tongue)
  f. Easy gingival bleeding
  g. Nondependent edema
  h. Muscle weakness
  i. Lassitude
  j. Eyes—dull, periorbital edema
  k. Hair—dull, sparse, plucks out easily
  l. Low serum albumin
  m. Low hemoglobin, low hematocrit, abnormal electrolyte status
  n. Bowel status, *e.g.*, diarrhea
  o. Bowel sounds—especially hypoactive
  p. Susceptibility or inability to fight infection
	• Support normal nutritional intake:
	  a. Adjust diet to decrease discomfort associated with eating, *e.g.*, cold liquids, soft foods.
	  b. Collaborate with physician to initiate measures to treat oral infection.
	  c. Provide emotional support.
	  d. Provide measures to decrease pain, especially at mealtime.
	  e. Initiate measures to decrease nausea and vomiting such as provide foods patient is able to tolerate, eliminate odors, discontinue medications causing nausea, give antiemetic.
	  f. Work closely with family and dietician to adapt diet to maximize nutritional intake.
	  g. Consider need for daily weights.

14. Assess factors which affect nutritional status:
  a. Functional status of GI tract
  b. Contraindications to oral intake even though GI tract may be functional:
  • Inability to swallow; *e.g.*, large, aortic aneurysm
  • Depressed level of consciousness	

Patient Outcome

Process

ASSESSMENT	INTERVENTION

ASSESSMENT

- Swelling or obstruction of upper airway or esophagus
- Endotracheal tube, tracheostomy
- Neural dysfunction that affects any part of GI tract
- GI bleeding
- Fistula
- N.p.o. status

c. Factors affecting appetite:
- Mouth or throat soreness or infection
- Pain
- Nausea, anorexia, vomiting

d. Underlying disease process, *e.g.,*
- Carcinoma indicating increased need for nutritional support
- Burn
- Large wound area
- Sepsis
- Alcoholism
- Malabsorption (short gut, prolonged fasting, cystic fibrosis)
- Pancreatitis
- Trauma

e. Modifications to dietary intake
- Patient's likes/dislikes
- Cultural influences
- Treatment program
- Disease processes, *i.e.,* diabetes, cardiac disease, hiatal hernia, ulcers

15. Assess nutrient intake and need for modifications in diet.
a. Evaluate quality and quantity of intake to include oral, intravenous, tube feedings, and by hyperalimentation.
- Standard IVs without nutrient additives contain water, electrolytes, and calories but do not contain adequate nutrients. Solutions such as:
D_5W = 175 calories per liter
$D_{10}W$ = 350 calories per liter
- Inadequate nutrient/content of ordered diet such as: clear liquids, low protein
b. Consider length of stay in unit.
c. Consider factors that increase nutritional needs such as burns, stress, infection, fever, fluid loss.
d. Consider length of time patient will be unable to resume dietary intake.
e. Interview patient/family and/or review chart for diet history prior to admission to critical care unit.

INTERVENTION

- For patient progressing from IV fluids to oral intake:
a. Collaborate with physician and dietician regarding consistency and type of diet.
b. Evaluate and document tolerance to diet.
c. Consider need for vitamin, mineral additives added to IV fluid until p.o. intake adequate.
- For patient with insufficient oral intake to support good functional ability of GI tract, consult with physician to initiate nutritional program.
a. For patient with normal functioning bowel consider:
- Tube feeding via small lumen (8 to 10 french) NG tube using continuous drip.
- Tube feeding every four hours with residual checks.
- Kind and amount of solution determined by physician and dietician according to patient's condition and needs.
- Evaluate and document patient's tolerance to tube feeding, diarrhea, cramping, vomiting, etc.
b. For patient with nonfunctional bowel or with contraindication to food in gut consider total parenteral nutrition (TPN).
- Collaborate with physician for consult to TPN team.

Critical care general guidelines—life support

Patient Outcome	Process	
	ASSESSMENT	INTERVENTION

The patient attains optimal life support	1. Assess and document signs and symptoms of respiratory and/or cardiac arrest: a. Level of consciousness b. Respiratory status: • Observe for chest movement. • Listen and feel for respiration. c. Circulatory status: • Check for carotid pulse for 5 to 10 seconds.

<table>
<tr><td>ASSESSMENT</td><td>INTERVENTION</td></tr>
</table>

1. Assess and document signs and symptoms of respiratory and/or cardiac arrest:
   a. Level of consciousness
   b. Respiratory status:
      • Observe for chest movement.
      • Listen and feel for respiration.
   c. Circulatory status:
      • Check for carotid pulse for 5 to 10 seconds.

• Remain with patient in arrest. Call or send another person to contact life support team, responsible physician, and other appropriate assistants such as respiratory therapist, electrocardiogram technician, other physicians and nurses.
• Attempt to elicit response by verbal and tactile stimulation.
   • Call patient by name while shaking to arouse.
• Initiate respiratory support:
   a. Establish airway.
      • Hyperextend neck except for: infant and patient with suspected neck injury.
      • Perform triple airway maneuver:
         Thrust mandible forward.
         Seal nose with own cheek.
         Begin ventilation.
      • Give 4 quick breaths to check for obstruction and to expand lungs.
      • Sustain ventilation (maintain 1 respiration every 5 seconds)
      • Monitor central pulse.
• Initiate circulatory support for patient without carotid pulse.
   a. Begin external cardiac compression.
      • Ratio of compression to respirations:
         Infant: 5 compressions to 1 respiration maintains heart beat of 60 to 100 per minute
         Adult: If resuscitation is by one person, 15 compressions to 2 respirations maintains heart beat of 60 per minute. If resuscitation is by 2 persons, 5 compressions to 1 respiration maintains heart beat of 60 per minute.

2. Assess adequacy of perfusion after 4 cycles or 3 minutes and at frequent intervals thereafter.
   a. Check carotid (or femoral) pulses.
   b. Monitor ventilation continuously.
      • Observe for chest expansion on inspiration and sound or feel of exhaled air.
      • Abdominal distention
      • Emesis
   c. Check pupillary response (Note this is not a consistently valid sign).

   b. Take action based on assessment:
      • Spontaneous pulses: Discontinue external cardiac compression.
      • No pulse with compression: Check correct hand position and force on chest.
      • Spontaneous respirations: Discontinue artificial ventilation.
      • Inadequate chest expansion and/or air movement: Re-evaluate airway.
      • Abdominal distention:
         Do not attempt to expel air or stomach contents.
         Re-evaluate airway.
      • Emesis: Turn patient on side; wipe out mouth; and re-establish airway.
   c. Continue basic life support in absence of spontaneous pulses and respirations until supportive personnel and equipment arrive to initiate advanced life support.

3. Assist physician and life support team to assess priorities for advanced life support.
   • Check presence of necessary equipment for use when support personnel arrive.

Patient Outcome

Process

ASSESSMENT	INTERVENTION
• Defibrillator • Cardiopulmonary resuscitation cart • Medications • Equipment for intubation (including suction and oxygen) • Pacemaker • EKG machine • IV equipment	

4. Assess adequacy of ventilation
  a. Check patency and position of endotracheal airway.
  b. Look for symmetrical bilateral chest expansion.
  c. Auscultate for bilateral breath sounds.
  d. Obtain chest radiograph as soon as possible.
	• Utilize adjunctive measures for respiratory support.
	  a. Respiratory therapist introduces endotracheal or nasopharyngeal airway.
	  b. Use Laerdol or Ambu bag for ventilation via endotracheal tube.
	  c. Administer 100 per cent oxygen via Laerdol bag.
	  d. Suction trachea.
	  e. Introduce nasogastric tube and aspirate with bulb syringe, intermittent suction or gravity drainage.

5. Assess endotracheal (ET) aspirate for apparent stomach contents indicative of aspiration.
  a. Color
  b. Consistency
  c. Quantity
	f. Introduce oral airway if necessary to prevent occlusion of oral-tracheal tube or to stabilize ET tube.

6. Assess EKG for cardiac arrhythmias.
  a. Assess carotid pulses if ventricular tachycardia or coarse ventricular fibrillation occurs.
  b. Determine underlying cause as soon as possible.
    • Acid-base imbalance
    • Electrolyte imbalance
    • Cardiac tamponade
    • Cardiac arrhythmia
	• Utilize adjunctive measures for circulatory support:
	  a. Place cardiac board under patient's thorax.
	  b. Establish EKG monitoring via defibrillator monitor.
	  c. Start or insure patency of intravenous infusion.
	  d. Anticipate insertion of central venous line, pulmonary artery catheter, and/or arterial line for invasive monitoring.
	  e. Administer first series of medications as ordered:
	    • Sodium bicarbonate
	    • Calcium chloride or calcium gluconate
	    • Epinephrine
	    • Atropine
	    • Lidocaine
	  f. Have other emergency drugs available:
	    • Isoproterenol (Isuprel)
	    • Phenytoin (Dilantin)
	    • Procainamide (Pronestyl)
	    • Methoxamine (Vasoxyl)
	    • Propranolol (Inderal)
	    • Glucagon
	    • Edrophonium (Tensilon)
	    • Dopamine (Intropin)
	    • Levarterenal (Levophed Bitartrate)
	  g. Assist with defibrillation
	    • Have defibrillator ready for use.
	      Plugged in
	      Charged as ordered
	      Paddles lubricated
	      Physician or learned nurse will defibrillate.

Patient Outcome	Process	
	ASSESSMENT	INTERVENTION
		h. Assist with temporary pacemaker insertion.
		• Have pacemaker available.
		• Have equipment for transvenous or transmediastinal insertion.
		i. Send blood for appropriate laboratory analyses as soon as possible:
		• Arterial blood gases
		• Electrolytes
		• Other chemistries
		j. Send for 12-lead EKG machine.
		k. May need to initiate continuous medication support through IV drip of drugs, *e.g.,* (Intropin) dopamine, isoproterenol (Isuprel), lidocaine (xylocaine), levarterenol (Levophed Bitartrate), epinephrine (Adrenaline)
		l. Consider repeating first series of drugs.
		m. Consider internal massage, intra-aortic ballon pumping, membrane oxygenator, if cardiac perfusion continues to be inadequate.
	6. Assess need for psychosocial support for patient/family.	• Provide appropriate psychosocial support for patient and family.
	7. Assess need for transfer to speciality care area.	• Stabilize patient for transfer.

Critical care general guidelines—musculoskeletal

Patient Outcome	Process	
	ASSESSMENT	INTERVENTION
The patient attains optimal musculoskeletal function	1. Assess and document signs and symptoms of abnormal musculoskeletal functioning. Include preadmission problems and methods of relief.	• Provide preventive measures for all patients in critical care setting: a. Exercise program to include range of motion b.i.d. b. Special skin and bowel care programs • Adjust care accordingly for patient with pre-existing conditions, *e.g.,* rheumatoid arthritis. Use range of motion, medications, positioning, and assistive equipment such as splint, bed board.

	2. Assess musculoskeletal function.
	a. General:
	• Vascular
	  Pulse: strong, weak, absent
	  Temperature: warm, cool, cold
	  Color: red, pink, pale, blue
	  Pain due to ischemia
	  Capillary filling: rapid, slow, absent
	  Evidence of bleeding, ecchymosis, hematoma
	• Nerves
	  Sensation of each extremity and digit
	  Motion
	  Pain
	• Muscle
	  Motion
	  Size, atrophy
	  Pain
	  Strength.
		• Document baseline data and any significant changes.
		
		• Compress tips of fingers, toes, nail beds in affected extremity briefly and release quickly to check capillary filling: if normal, blanching and rapid return of pink color occurs.
		• Compare response with unaffected extremity.
		• Recognize the following as potential causes of peripheral nerve trauma.
		a. Prolonged pressure or traction, compression on nerves in arm, leg
		b. Inadvertent damage to radial nerve by injections, catheters; to sciatic nerve by injections
		• Report patient complaints of numbness, tingling, or inability to move fingers.

	• Bone
	  Deformity
	  Crepitus (grating sensation heard or felt as bone ends rub together)
	  Pain.
	• Joint
	  Active range of motion (do not encourage motion beyond patient's tolerance until radiograph, orthopaedic assessment confirms regimen)
	  Swelling
	  Redness
	  Pain
	  Heat
		• For any suspected fracture, splint (armboard) to immobilize and notify physician.
		
		• Check with physician for application of heat, cold and analgesics.

	b. Head/Face:
	• Change in level of consciousness
	• Ocular/orbital injury, *e.g.,* vision, eye movements, pupillary response, exudate, swelling
	• Asymmetry of facial structures
	• Impaired movement of jaw
	• Impaired upper airway; swelling due to facial trauma.
		• For patient with ocular/orbital injuries:
		a. Consult physician for ophthalmology evaluation and appropriate protection of eye.
		  • Cover eye with sterile patch until otherwise ordered.
		• For patient with facial or nasal fracture:
		a. Have suction and tracheostomy tray available.
		b. For wired jaws:
		  • Have wire cutters available.

353

Patient Outcome

Process

ASSESSMENT	INTERVENTION
	• Antiemetics to prevent vomiting/aspiration • Alternative means of communication (pad/pencil). c. Consider location of fracture when taping indwelling tubes. d. Special attention to mouth care, nutrition.
c. Neck: • Weakness in upper or lower extremity function • Anterior soft tissue swelling which could cause airway obstruction. • Intact trachea in midline • Signs: stridor, sternal and intercostal retractions • Cervical pain • Limited range of motion • Abnormal posture	• For patient with suspected cervical injury: a. Maintain neutral position of neck (no hyperextension or flexion); use sandbags, collar. b. Palpate cervical spine to determine areas of deformity, tenderness. c. Avoid lateral rotation of neck. Keep chin in line with sternum. d. No log-rolling until order written by physician. e. Have tracheostomy and suction tray available. f. Do not administer strong narcotic because of depressant effect: codeine is acceptable. g. Call physician to supervise positioning for cervical spine radiography unless otherwise ordered.
d. Ribs: • Flail chest: Paroxysmal movement on inspiration and expiration • Symptoms of pneumothorax: dyspnea, chest pain, absence of breath sounds	• For patient with severe flail chest: a. Anticipate intubation and ventilation. b. Provide positive pressure respiratory support. c. Encourage patient to voluntarily splint rib cage in response to pain. Provide other support or taping, elastic bandage, pain medications. d. Anticipate need for repeat chest radiograms. • For patient with 1 to 2 broken ribs: a. Provide rigorous pulmonary care to prevent atelectasis, pneumonia. b. Observe for signs of pneumothorax.
e. Pelvis: If severe fracture due to trauma, monitor for signs of internal bleeding: • Vital signs indicating shock • Oliguria • Hematuria • Rectal bleeding • Abdominal distention	• For patient with pelvic fracture: a. Discuss with physician appropriate turning activity regimen. b. Plan for position changes, use of bedpan depending on status of fracture, pain level. c. Provide good skin care to prevent breakdown. d. Check girth if abdomen distended. e. Check for symptoms of skin breakdown (especially patient using pelvic sling; those not permitted to turn; obese; and poor skin condition). f. Provide bowel routine to prevent constipation. g. Give frequent perineal care.
f. Arms, legs: • Voluntary motion	• Do not manipulate affected limb prior to orthopaedic assessment/recommendation.

Patient Outcome	Process	
	ASSESSMENT	INTERVENTION

<table>
<tr><td></td><td></td><td>• Begin assessment distally (farthest from trunk) and move proximally (closest to trunk). Move arms and legs by:
  a. Abduction (away from midline or axis of body or limb)
  b. Adduction (toward midline or axis of body or limb)
  c. Flexion (bending)
  d. Extension (straightening)
  e. Ballottement for a floating patella.</td></tr>
</table>

g. Upper extremities: Include fingers, wrist, elbow, shoulder.
   • Voluntary motion
   • Radial and ulnar pulses
   • Abnormal sensation, *e.g.,* numbness, tingling in fingers

• Move wrist by:
  a. Pronation (palm faces downward or backward)
  b. Supination (palm upward)
  c. Test range of motion of fingers and wrist.

h. Lower extremities: Include toes, ankle, knee, hip.
   • Voluntary motion

• Move lower extremities by:
  a. Internal rotation of leg
  b. External rotation of leg
  c. Plantar flexion (extension of foot: toes toward foot of bed)
  d. Dorsiflexion (flexion of foot: toes toward nose)

• Note inability to fully extend extremity. For patient with fractured extremity:
  a. Maintain elevation as positioned by physician to decrease pain and swelling.
  b. For wet new casts (less than 24 to 48 hours)
    • Leave cast uncovered 24 to 48 hours to dry completely.
    • Neurovascular checks to affected extremity q 1 to 2 hours × 24 hours then q 4 hours
    • Explain sensations of cast drying to patient. It is wet, hot, cold and damp for 24 hours.
    • Check edges of cast for pressure q 4 hours.
    • Listen to patient complaints of burning, pressure.
    • Note any odor in cast and report to physician.
    • Mark (circle and date) drainage on cast.

• For patient in traction
  a. Do not add or remove weights without physician order.
  b. Determine from physician the correct patient alignment for each traction setup.
  c. Attempt to maintain patient in this position with use of shock blocks as needed.
  d. Reinforce permitted and restricted activities and motions with patient.
  e. Raise head of bed intermittently unless otherwise ordered except for cervical and side arm traction.
  f. Check ropes for fraying.
  g. Consider bed height and elevator before transporting patient. Secure weights.

Patient Outcome

Process

ASSESSMENT	INTERVENTION
	h. Tighten knobs q 8 hours. i. Have trapeze to aid patient in moving unless contraindicated.

3. Assess for compartment syndrome: Be aware that ischemia may result from compression of blood vessels in the muscle due to:
  a. Swelling from trauma or to a cast that is too tight
  b. Crush injury
  c. Burns
  d. Anticoagluation therapy
  e. After continuous arterial (femoral, brachial) cannulation. Irreversible damage to muscle group and nerves may occur after six hours and may result in amputation of limb.
	• For patient with symptoms of compartment syndrome of arm or leg:
	  a. Call physician for immediate surgical intervention—fasciotomy (incision in fascia over involved compartment to allow muscle to swell freely).
	  b. Withhold pain medication until physician assesses.
	  c. Elevate extremity.
	  d. Remove constricting dressing and observe closely for progressive swelling.
	  e. May use wick catheter in muscle monitoring (greater than 30 mm Hg. abnormal).

4. Assess for swelling in forearm fracture or supracondylar fracture in elbow or fractured forearm (Volkmann's ischemia).
  a. Symptoms:
    • Pain on passive extension of fingers
    • Increased pain in forearm and hand and unrelieved by pain medications
    • Tight, swollen forearm
    • Numbness and burning in fingers	

5. Assess vascular compression with a proximal fracture in tibia. Symptoms: pain, burning in foot	

6. Assess need for active and passive range of motion, especially:
  a. Knee
  b. Hip
  c. Ankle
  d. Elbow
  e. Hand
  f. Shoulder
	• Prevent deformity due to immobilization.
	  a. Provide active or passive range of motion during bath.
	    • Report limited range of motion.
	    • Consider physical therapy consult.
	  b. Do not let patient lie with pillow under knee.
	  c. Do not have head of bed elevated continuously; have patient flat at least one hour b.i.d.

7. Assess pain as a result of immobility and stiffness of muscles and joints.	d. Provide proper position to maintain joints in functional position; use assistive devices, *e.g.*, towel roll, foot support. e. Assist patient to change positions as frequently as possible; offer comfort measures, *e.g.*, heat, cold. f. Provide exercises specifically designed to prevent contractures, *e.g.*, heel cord stretching.
8. Assess potential for and signs of muscle atrophy.	g. Instruct patient in isometric exercises: • Quadriceps setting—tighten kneecap, anterior thigh muscle. h. Consider trapeze so patient can lift torso, if appropriate. i. Supervise range of motion. j. Apply heat or cold if indicated.

9. Assess for symptoms of fat embolism which may occur 12 to 72 hours after fracture of long bones, major trauma to lower extremity, or multiple fracture.	• For patient with suspected fat embolism:
	  a. Call physician.
	  b. Prepare to draw arterial blood gases (ABG).

Patient Outcome

Process

ASSESSMENT	INTERVENTION

Symptoms:
a. Mental confusion, restlessness, belligerence
b. Low pO_2, low platelet count, increased lipase.
c. Fever, tachycardia, tachypnea, dyspnea
d. Petechiae on conjunctiva, soft palate, anterior chest
	c. Prepare to administer O_2 after ABG.
	d. Medical management may include:
	  • Administration of blood products
	  • Dextran
	  • Steroids
	e. Prepare for intubation and ventilation.

10. Assess for signs and symptoms of pulmonary embolus: a. Substernal pain, low pO_2 b. Dyspnea c. Rapid, weak pulse d. EKG changes e. Hemoptysis	• For patient with suspected pulmonary embolus: a. Call physician. b. Obtain ABG. c. Administer O_2. d. Anticipate lung scan, arteriogram. e. Medical management: anticoagulation f. Obtain EKG. g. Place head of patient's bed in upright position.

11. Assess for signs and symptoms of thrombophlebitis:
a. Homan's sign: pain on dorsiflexion of foot. Differentiate between this and pain from tight heel cord.
b. Warm, swollen, tender, red calf
	• For patient who is at risk for thrombophlebitis:
	a. Elevate foot of bed with legs higher than heart to promote venous drainage. Change positions back to sides frequently.
	b. Instruct and supervise patient in ankle circle exercises, or provide passive range of motion q 4 hours.
	c. Antiembolic hose
	d. Medical management may include:
	  • Heparin
	  • Dextran
	  • Aspirin

12. Assess for signs of peroneal nerve palsy (foot drop). Cause: pressure on nerve over head of fibula on lateral side of leg, approximately three inches below knee. May occur as a complication of long operative procedure. a. Inability to dorsiflex foot. b. Differentiate between this and tight heel cord.	• For patient with documented thrombophlebitis: a. Bedrest b. Avoid massage and excessive movement of affected extremity. Careful administration of heparin with microdrip intravenous equipment.

Patient Outcome	Process	
	ASSESSMENT	INTERVENTION

The patient attains optimal neurological functions	1. Assess neurological function.
	  a. Level of consciousness:
	    • Degree of responsiveness to verbal and tactile stimuli
	  b. Pupillary response:
	    • Size
	    • Reactivity to light
	  c. Motor and sensory function:
	    • Spontaneous or elicited to command or pain
	  d. Seizure activity:
	    • Onset
	    • Generalized or focal
	    • Progression
	    • Duration
	  e. Vital signs trends:
	    • Elevation of blood pressure
	    • Widening pulse pressure
	    • Change in respirations pattern, *e.g.,* bradycardia, sinus arrhythmia
	    • Rapid change in temperature
		• Perform initial essential neurological check. Document baseline data and significant change.
		• Anticipate needs if patient becomes unresponsive:
		  a. Check airway, breathing, circulation
		  b. Notify physician
		  c. Prepare for:
		    • Respiratory arrest
		    • Arrhythmia
		    • Cardiac arrest
		  d. Prepare equipment for:
		    • Patent IV
		    • Respiratory support
		• For changes indicating deterioration (decreased level of consciousness, pupil changes, motor weakness, increased blood pressure, widening pulse pressure, changes in respirations, subjective symptoms)
		  a. Notify physician.
		  b. Anticipate possible respiratory arrest.
		• For high temperature elevations:
		  a. Watch for possible seizure activity especially in children three years and under.
		• For seizure activity:
		  a. Support and turn head to side. Do not attempt to force mouth open with tongue blade; may result in broken teeth.
		  b. If patient is on respirator, disconnect from tubing if displacement of endotracheal tube or trauma is likely during major motor seizure. Reconnect tubing after seizure and hyperoxygenate patient.
		  c. Pad siderails and have airways and suction available to protect patient with generalized major motor seizure.
		  d. Always contact physician for first seizure activity.
		  e. Call physician and prepare for IV drug therapy if seizure persists more than five minutes.
		  f. Observe and document the following: Onset, duration, parts of body involved, neurological and respiratory status during and after seizure.

	2. Evaluate the measurement of intracranial pressure (ICP): (See Fig. 9-1, p. 360).
	  a. Greater than 200 mm of H_2O or greater than 15 mm of Hg is abnormal.
	    • Pressures are measured routinely during a lumbar puncture (LP) but an LP is often contraindicated for patient with known elevated ICP.
	  b. Indications for continuous monitoring of ICP: patient with head trauma, subarachnoid hemorrhage, postoperative craniotomy patient with massive swelling, child with Reye's syndrome.
		• For patient with increased intracranial pressure, management may include:
		  a. Maintain head of bed elevation as ordered (usually 30°).
		  b. Steroids (IM or IV)
		    Watch for GI bleeding.
		    Monitor urines per diabetes routine.
		    Administer anticholinergics and antacids as ordered.
		    Monitor BP if drugs given IM.
		  c. Mannitol/urea:
		    Maintain patent urinary catheter.
		    Monitor electrolyes, intake and output.

Patient Outcome

Process

ASSESSMENT	INTERVENTION
c. Types of continuous monitoring	d. Controlled hyperventilation.
• Transducer in epidural space with digital readout	e. Treatment for suddent severe increased ICP, e.g., due to shunt failure
• Richmond screw in subarachnoid space with wave form printout	Prepare for ventricular tap. Obtain twist drill set and ventricular tray.
• Intraventricular catheter in lateral ventricle with wave form printout	Anticipate respiratory arrest.
d. Transient elevations of pressure may be due to Valsalva's maneuver, coughing, neck flexion, restlessness, head of bed changed from upright to flat.	
3. Assess the level of consciousness (LOC).	• Consider essential aspects of thorough evaluation of LOC.
a. Normal: Alert; awake; oriented to time, place, person, self; appropriate response to environment	a. Know name patient is called.
b. Usual progression of deteriorating LOC:	b. Identify any difficulty in communication.
• Behaves and responds inappropriately to questions, situations	c. Stimulate vigorously—verbal first and then tactile.
• Increasingly irritable to environment	d. Observe subtle, gradual changes and compare with baseline data.
• Drowsy, lethargic, decreased responsiveness to stimuli	• Consider contributing factors affecting level of consciousness:
• Able to follow simple commands only	a. Systemic—respiratory, cardiovascular, fluid and electrolytes, metabolic. Discuss with physician.
• Responds to name verbally or nonverbally	
• Pushes away or withdraws from painful stimulus	b. Critical care environment: sensory overload, monotony, sleep deprivation
• Responds to pain or environment stimulus by abnormal posturing: decorticate, decerebrate	c. Affective reaction to stress and pain
• No observable response to stimuli including loss of gag, cough reflexes	• Institute measures for patients with moderate to severe decreased LOC, especially for patients in prolonged coma:
	a. Be aware that patient may hear; continue to communicate and give explanations.
	b. Encourage family to continue to talk to patient and provide stimulation.
	c. Be realistic with family about patient's status, *e.g.,* meaning of patient's motor response.

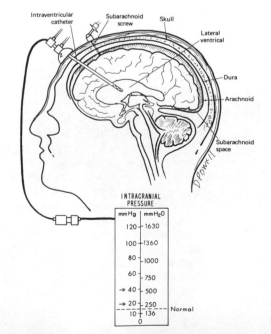

Fig. 9-1. Intracranial pressure monitoring.

Patient Outcome	Process

ASSESSMENT	INTERVENTION
	d. Provide eye, nose, mouth care frequently.
	e. Give range of motion exercises q 8 hours to prevent joint, muscle, and vascular complications.
	f. Check for symptoms of thrombophlebitis. Use antiembolic hose or elastic wraps.
	g. Collaborate with physician to initiate tube feedings as soon as it is apparent that patient will not be able to take p.o. feedings for a prolonged time.
	h. Give special attention to skin to prevent breakdown; frequent checks of pressure areas.
	i. Monitor bowel status; try to prevent problems; treat if they occur.
4. Evaluate dysfunction in communication.	• For patients with dysphasia:
a. Describe how patient communicates, *e.g.,* slurred speech, confused content, no speech.	a. Speak slowly, clearly.
b. Dysphasia:	b. Use simple content.
• Expressive dysphasia: appears to comprehend but cannot verbalize thoughts (nonfluent aphasia)	c. Use gestures and encourage patient's gestures.
• Receptive dysphasia: is inappropriate due to lack of ability to understand communication (fluent aphasia).	d. Consider use of pictures for patients who have difficulty with words.
• May have subtle combinations of both	e. Encourage early speech therapy consult.
c. Global aphasia: total inability to receive communication or express thoughts	f. Be aware that complex environment of intensive care unit is particularly confusing to patient with dysphasia.
5. Assess pupil reactions.	• Perform pupil check:
a. Compare right pupil to left pupil in size, shape, and reactivity to light.	a. Darken room.
b. Normal: PERRL (pupils equal, round react to light)	b. Use penlight or central beam flash light.
• Size 3 to 5 mm	c. Consider old trauma, blindness, drugs, alcohol, pain, emotions, cataracts, room light intensity, prosthesis when assessing pupillary activity.
• Bilateral brisk reaction to direct light, consensual response in both pupils (pupil reacts when beam directed to opposite pupil)	• Notify physician when pupil size and/or reaction to light changes, especially in combination with deterioration of LOC.
• Constricted (miotic): less than 3 mm	• Consider a fixed dilated pupil in combination with decreasing level of consciousness as a neurosurgical emergency for patient with head trauma.
• Dilated (mydriatic): greater than 5 mm	
c. Abnormal:	
• Anisocoria: one pupil larger than the other (normal finding in some individuals)	
• Sluggish or nonreactive pupils	
6. Evaluate abnormal eye signs:	• Provide measures for patient with special eye care needs:
a. Ptosis (dropping eyelid) cranial nerve c.n. III	a. Protect cornea by using artificial tears, ointment, plastic eye cover for patient with loss of corneal reflex (blink).
b. Extraocular movement (EOM) palsies (loss of eye movements within orbit); c.n. III, IV, VI.	b. Patch one eye for patient with diplopia.
	c. Instill artificial tears at least q 2 hours for comatose patient. Cleanse secretions as needed and tape eyes closed.
c. Loss of corneal reflex, c.n. V	• Provide care for patient with visual deficit.
d. Diplopia (double vision)	a. Provide input according to individual's present abilities.
e. Blurred vision	b. Give careful verbal explanations if patient is blind or eyes are bandaged.
f. Decreasing visual activity	

Patient Outcome	Process
	ASSESSMENT **INTERVENTION**

ASSESSMENT

g. Photophobia (increased sensitivity to light)

h. Nystagmus (oscillating movement of eye)
  - Rapid eye movements similar to nystagmus often observed until patient completely reactive postanesthesia.
  - Nystagmus may be due to cerebellar dysfunction.

i. Field cut (loss of peripheral vision)

j. In coma, physician tests brain stem function by:
  - Doll's eye maneuver and calorics: Normal findings in coma. Absence may indicate brain stem involvement.
      Doll's eye maneuver—head turned to left, both eyes roll to right; head turned to right, both eyes roll to left.
      Calorics—after administration of iced saline in ear canal, rapid nystagmus and eye deviation toward opposite ear
      Roving eye movements

7. Determine motor function:

a. Test upper, lower extremities for strength and movement, tone.
  - Compare right to left.
  - Use simple commands.
  - Observe patient's spontaneous movements.

b. Normal: moves all extremities well (MAEW)

c. Abnormal: Loss of upper, lower extremity function
  - Paresis (weakness)
  - Plegia (paralysis)
  - Strength:
      Upper extremities:
        Weak grip
        Drift (inability to hold arms out equally when raised above body)
        Cupping, reflex grip
      Lower extremities:
        Unable to dorsiflex foot or lift leg off bed
  - Movement of all extremities:
      Loss of voluntary, purposeful movements
      Loss of spontaneous movements
  - Posturing: may be unilateral or bilateral, spontaneous or in response to stimulus.
      Decorticate: upper extremity flexed; lower extremity extended
      Decerebrate: upper extremity extended and hyperpronated; lower extremity extended

INTERVENTION

- Consider the effect on motor checks of:
  a. Ability of patient to comprehend commands
  b. Restriction of movements due to IV or other lines
  c. Pain
- Provide careful positioning and exercise for deficit; coordinate with physical therapy.

- Provide care for patient with decorticate, decerebrate posturing:
  a. Avoid restraints.
  b. Do not try to "break" posture.
  c. Reposition q 2 hours. Consider effect of posturing when choosing sites for invasive lines.
- For patient in coma, interpret the following signs realistically to family. (They do not represent a return to normal neurological function).
  a. Cupping, reflex grips (will not let go on command)

Patient Outcome	Process	
	ASSESSMENT	INTERVENTION

ASSESSMENT

- Tone: flaccid (decreased tone)
  spastic (increased tone)
- Cranial nerve deficits:
  Facial palsies and inability to show teeth, c.n. VIII
  Difficulty swallowing (dysphagia) and/or loss of gag reflex
  Poor or absent cough, c.n. IX, X
- Elicited reflexes:
  Babinski (extensor fanning of toes to stimulation), present or absent.
  Deep tendon reflexes (DTR)
  greater than 3 hyperactive
  less than 1 hypoactive

8. Appraise cerebellar dysfunction:
   a. Incoordination
   b. Scanning speech
   c. Ataxia
   d. Nystagmus
   e. Tremor
9. Evaluate spinal cord dysfunction:
   a. Patent airway
   b. Respiratory status, *e.g.*, diaphragmatic breathing, loss of intercostals
   c. Neurological status (essential neurological check) to include:
      • Motor strength of upper and lower extremities
      • Sensory level
   d. Signs and symptoms of systemic shock, especially with multiple trauma patient
   e. Signs and symptoms of "spinal shock" such as loss of motor, reflex, sensory, and autonomic activity below level of spinal lesion
   f. Temperature (initially, perspiration may not occur below level of cord injury)
   g. Bladder (may be distended)
   h. Bowel sounds (paralytic ileus is common in acute phase)
   i. Subjective reports of pain, paresthesia. Palpate spines for tenderness and deformity.
   j. Skin condition and any abnormalities, *e.g.*, lacerations

INTERVENTION

b. Return of sleep, waking cycle; roving eye movements
- Provide care for patient with facial palsies
  a. Use caution in offering anything by mouth.
  b. Offer food and fluids on side in which swallowing is intact.

- Provide early physical therapy consult for evaluation of patient with cerebellar dysfunction.
- For patient with scanning speech, encourage patient to speak slowly.
- For patient with tremor, simplify environment for activities for daily living.
- Provide measures for patient with cervical spine trauma:
  a. Provide support to maintain cervical spine in neutral position (cervical, collar, spine board, sand bags).
  b. Monitor neurological status q 15 minutes until stable, then q 1 hour. Follow routine for essential neurological check.
     • Mark sensory level on patient's skin for later comparison.
  c. Be aware of possible deterioration of pulmonary status.
     • Check minute volumes hourly during acute phase (most essential for cervical high thoracic lesions).
     • Anticipate need for intubation, and/or ventilation and have available:
       Suction
       Tracheostomy tray
       Resuscitation equipment
       Nasogastric tube
  d. Anticipate medical management for spinal stabilization to include:
     • Application of tongs, and/or halo (obtain seven-foot bed, double mattress)
     • Administration of steroids
     • Surgical intervention, especially for ascending loss of function
     • Turning frame
- Provide measures common to all spinal cord dysfunction.
  a. Prepare bed prior to patient's arrival with skin protective devices (alternating pressure mattress, water bed).
  b. Begin log rolling patient as soon as ordered by physician.
  c. Maintain patient in good spinal alignment to prevent further cord damage. Use restraints as necessary.

Patient Outcome

Process

ASSESSMENT	INTERVENTION
	d. Provide preventive pulmonary routine appropriate to level of injury.
	e. Provide early attention to nutritional needs.
	f. Plan bladder management which may include:
	• Foley catheter routine until stable
	• Intermittent catheter routine
	• Spontaneous voiding
	• Residual urine checks
	g. Provide preventive bowel routine.
	h. Provide careful attention to back, and skin care.
	i. Be present during physician's explanation to patient/family.
	j. Note patient/family response to situation.
	k. Provide emotional support for what the patient hears and the needs being expressed through behavior.
	l. Contact nurse member of spinal cord injury team for evaluation and care, as needed.
	• Provide emergency measures needed based on assessment of signs and symptoms.
	m. Obtain physical therapy and occupational therapy consults.

Patient Outcome

Process

ASSESSMENT

INTERVENTION

PREFACE: A nosocomial infection is defined as infection that was not present or was not incubating at the time of admission; a hospital-acquired infection. Sources may be endogenous or exogenous Patients may be colonized with bacteria without being infected clinically. Evidence of infection with normal flora must be correlated with significant clinical observations.

The patient is free of or has minimal complications associated with infection

1. Identify high risk patients.
   a. Any patient in critical care unit
   b. Any patient who remains in hospital longer than three weeks
   c. Any patient with diagnosis of:
      • Blood dyscrasias
      • Collagen-vascular diseases
      • Diabetes
      • Burns
      • Severe nutritional impairment
      • Open skin lesions, widespread dermatoses
      • Frequent respiratory diseases and/or systemic infections

   d. Therapy/procedures:
      • Multiple blood transfusions
      • Multiple indwelling lines (arterial, central venous, pulmonary artery line)
      • Total parenteral nutrition
      • Indwelling bladder catheter
      • Respiratory support (endotracheal tubes, tracheostomy, ventilators)
      • Multiple antibiotic therapy
      • Surgical procedures lasting longer than three hours.

   e. Patients who are immunosuppressed because of disease or treatment.

2. Assess and document general signs and symptoms that may be present with infection
   a. Character of fever
   b. Lassitude, weakness, irritability
   c. Chills
   d. Anorexia
   e. Change in blood pressure, pulse, respiration
   f. Increased white blood count
   g. Pain

• Provide general preventive measures:
   a. Wash hands thoroughly before and after patient contact.
   b. Use aseptic technique.
   c. Maintain clean environment.
   d. Provide adequate nutrition.
   e. Prevent cross contamination.
   f. Isolate sources of infection.
   g. Minimize traffic in and out of patient area.
   h. Carry out procedures safely. Examples:
      • Foley catheter care
      • Pulmonary care
      • Mouth care
      • Suctioning
      • Care of specific indwelling lines, *e.g.*, monitoring line, infusion of blood or IV fluids, peritoneal dialysis
   i. Prevent contamination of lines, wounds and direct trauma by confused or uninformed patient, family, or staff.
   j. Minimize chance of infection via central and peripheral venous lines.
      • Remove indwelling lines as soon as possible.
      • Eliminate stopcocks when possible; cap all stopcocks.
      • Use povidone-iodine as antiseptic of choice for skin preps and dressing change.
      • Change dressing and tubing per hospital policy.
      • Cover line insertion site with sterile dressing and seal with water resistant tape. Put date change on tape.

• For patients who are immunosuppressed or lack antibody protection:
   a. Monitor white blood count.
   b. Eliminate unnecessary invasive techniques.
   c. Give good mouth care to prevent fungal infections.

• For patients who are suspected of having infection:
   a. Collect and send specimens to specific laboratory.
   b. Collect specimens prior to initiation of antibiotic therapy.
   c. Monitor culture reports of sensitivity studies.
      • Institute measures based on presenting signs and symptoms of infection.
      • Monitor temperature more frequently.

365

Patient Outcome   Process

	ASSESSMENT	INTERVENTION

	h. Abnormal character of wound: induration, inflammation, fluctuation, increasing size
	i. Abnormal character of body fluids, *e.g.*, color, clarity
	3. Assess for specific nosocomial infections:
	  a. Urinary tract infection/bacteriuria
	  b. Pulmonary/pneumonia
	  c. Bacteremia/septicemia
	  d. Wounds/abscess
	  e. Skin
	  f. Meningitis
	  g. Gastrointestinal
	    • Hepatitis
	    • Gastroenteritis/enteritis.	

Patient Outcome	Process

PREFACE: The patient and family should be prepared before and assisted throughout the critical care experience. This assistance includes meeting physical, emotional, and informational needs.

It is especially important to be alert to patients and families who have not had prior preparation and who may need special attention to their needs.

A. *The patient and family have sufficient information and emotional reassurance to achieve a realistic level of preparedness and understanding for the critical care experience*

1. Collect available data (from records, staff) if possible before approaching patient/family.
2. Initiate contacts as soon as possible.
   a. Begin to establish rapport through introduction of self and purpose of preparation.
   b. Determine priority needs of patient/family for:
      • Support
      • Information
      • Immediate physical needs
   c. Respond to needs and individualize approach.
3. Assess patient/family for factors affecting receptivity for preparation; document.
   a. Physical status, mental status (level of consciousness, pain, immediate needs, etc.)
   b. Duration and onset of critical care problem (new, pre-existing)
   c. Previous experience with and responses to illness, hospitalization, critical care
   d. Expectations of patient/family; (what, why, etc.)
   e. Emotional status: behaviors indicating anxiety level; support systems available (previous history/therapy/medications, tranquilizers)
   f. Cultural factors: socio-economic status, educational level, religious beliefs
   g. Characteristics of the setting and personnel; presence of interfering factors
   h. Specific fears, concerns (death, severe disability, unnecessary life prolongation)
4. Be aware continuously of changes in above factors which may alter patient/family needs.
5. Assist patient/family to cope with critical care experience on continuing basis.

B. *The patient and family maintain feelings of worth, personal identity and dignity*

   a. Demonstrate caring and compassion through expressions of concerns such as touching, eye contact, active listening, sitting with patient/family which reflects humanistic sensitivity to the issues with which patient and family are dealing.
   b. Determine with patient/family their perception of own needs and questions—if possible resolve these first.
   c. Identify:
      • Inherent support systems, such as family members, friends, significant others, faith
      • Available resources: health team members, hospital chaplain, personal minister.
   d. Assess and document patient/family understanding of illness and treatment plan; correct misconceptions and reinforce accurate perceptions.
   e. Give certain essential information, individualizing according to procedure and patient/family concerns and document.
      • Assure provision of consistent care by specially skilled personnel.
      • Describe critical care environment.
      • Progress to progressive care area as soon as condition permits.
      • Permit family visitors according to policy and care being given.
      • Explain care measures and rationale for them, including sensations patient will experience:
         Preoperative preparation
         Anesthesia
         Postoperative expectations (location postanesthesia, supplies, equipment commonly in place before waking)
         Position and activity
         Communication
         Incisions, bandages
         Ways nutritional needs are met
         Ways elimination needs are met
   f. Provide for privacy, dignity and personal space.
      • Use patient's preferred name.
      • Avoid body exposure as much as possible.
      • Assure privacy during personal time with family, examinations, and certain physical care.
      • Include patient in conversations within his hearing.
      • Avoid staff personal conversations while working near patient.

Patient Outcome	Process
	• Return important personal items as soon as possible, *e.g.*, dentures, glasses, rings, security objects. • Provide for visiting time between patient and family (or significant others). • Remain with family as appropriate when they are visiting patient to offer support, information. Respect their wishes to be alone. g. Anticipate and prepare patient/family for transfer as soon as physiological stability is achieved. h. Allow patient to help plan care as appropriate.

C. *The patient and family display behaviors which reflect met physiological and emotional needs and are conducive to recovery*	6. Recognize that basic human needs are often threatened throughout the critical care experience. Consider common fears which may threaten these needs:
	a. Death
	b. Long-term disability (change in body image, life-style)
	c. Loss of control
	d. Equipment
	e. Lack of confidence in personnel or or therapy
	f. Pain
	g. Loss of dignity
	7. Observe behaviors that reflect patient's physiological and emotional needs. Support those behaviors which are meeting current needs and are conducive to recovery.
	a. ''Moving toward'' behaviors (reflecting dependency needs):
	• Affection
	• Questioning
	• Seeking reassurance
	• Crying
	• Whining
	• Clinging
	• Demanding
	b. ''Moving away'' behaviors (reflecting safety and security needs):
	• Quietness
	• Shyness
	• Rituals
	• Denial
	• Withdrawal
	• Hallucinations
	• Failure to respond (no eye contact, verbal)
	c. ''Moving against'' behaviors (reflecting independence, control needs):
	• Assertiveness
	• Complaints
	• Criticism
	• Sarcasm
	• Displays of anger (verbal or physical attack)
	8. Identify patient behavior in order to determine what is being expressed. Differentiate between patient's feelings and needs. Institute actions based on findings.
	a. ''Moving toward'' behaviors (reflecting dependency needs):
	• Provide for dependency needs to be met.
	• Gradually progress towards independence.
	• Continually assess patient's ability to move to higher level of independence.
	b. ''Moving away'' behaviors (reflecting safety and security needs):
	• Allow patient to have support objects.
	• Establish trust relationship through:
	    Limited number of personnel
	    Consistent nurse-patient assignment
	    Structured environment
	    Preplanned daily schedule
	    Follow-through with promises
	c. ''Moving against'' behaviors (reflecting independence, control needs):
	• Allow patient to control environment as much as possible.
	• Limit frustrating elements in the environment.
	• Accept nonjudgmentally expressions of anger and criticism.

Patient Outcome	Process

	9. Assess possible contributing factors for behaviors:
	  a. Dysfunction of any organ or system which affects metabolic needs of the brain
	  b. Effects of medication
	  c. Degree of physiologic stress, including pain
	  d. Length of hospitalization
	  e. Environmental stresses
	    • Sleep deprivation
	    • Unit (noise, light, constant stimulation)
	    • Personnel, other patients
	    • Personal space
	  f. Immobilization
	  g. Developmental needs and place in life cycle
	  h. Behaviors previously used in crisis situations
	  i. Presence/absence of support objects and people
	10. Collect other data regarding behavior observed:
	  a. Identify precipitating event(s).
	  b. Duration—intermittent versus continuous
	11. Design plan of care which reflects anticipation of and responsiveness to patient's feelings.
	  a. Create an environment conducive to expression of feelings through verbal and nonverbal communication.
	  b. Utilize resource people in developing plan which is realistic and achievable.
	  c. Incorporate nursing approaches which support principles of consistency of intervention and continuity of personnel.
	  d. Assure that staff, patient and family are well informed regarding plan.
	  e. Reevaluate plan of care and revise as needed.

Patient Outcome	Process	
	ASSESSMENT	INTERVENTION

Patient Outcome	ASSESSMENT	INTERVENTION
The patient attains optimal renal function	**PREFACE:** Acute renal failure (ARF) is defined as the inability of the kidneys to maintain integrity of the internal environment. A hallmark sign is oliguria (less than 400 cc urine/day).	**PREFACE:** Be aware that acute renal failure is reversible but may take as long as six weeks for recovery. Prevention of ARF includes: a. Maintaining renal function: • Provide adequate fluid intake. • Monitor urinary output and daily weight. • Monitor cardiac output (BP, CVP). b. Awareness of nephrotoxic drugs. c. Awareness that prerenal problems can lead to renal parenchymal damage if untreated.
	1. Assess causative pathophysiologic factors for acute renal failure. a. Prerenal: decreased perfusion to kidneys leading to maximal sodium reabsorption and a small volume of urine with high concentration of urea and creatinine. Examples: • Burns • Hemorrhage • Shock • Dehydration • Cardiac failure • Sepsis • Cross clamping aorta during surgery • Hepatorenal syndrome b. Renal parenchymal disease: Direct damage to kidney impairs function. Examples: • Acute tubular necrosis • Acute cortical necrosis • Mechanical damage • Nephrotoxic drugs, *e.g.,* gentamicin, iodine based contrast agent • Glomerulonephritis • Hemolysis resulting from drugs, blood transfusions • Acute poststreptococcal infection. c. Postrenal: obstructive problems Examples: • Tumors • Calculi • Prostatic hypertrophy	• Document baseline and significant changes for all patients with ARF.
	2. Observe for signs and symptoms of ARF: a. Skin, pallor, decreased turgor, easily bruised b. Edema c. Inadequate nutritional status resulting from nausea, vomiting, diarrhea d. Dyspnea e. Neurological manifestations: sensorium changes, twitching, irritability, jerking, seizures f. Decreased salivary flow, ulcerations of mucous membranes	• Institute general nursing measures: a. Provide good skin and mouth care. b. Maintain seizure precautions. c. Keep side rails up. d. Initiate O_2 therapy if indicated and notify physician. e. Maintain patent urinary catheter; (if bladder distended obtain physician order and catheterize). f. Check with physician for altered dosages of essential drugs.
	3. Establish or compare with baseline renal data: a. History of renal or blood pressure problems, urinary obstruction, blood dyscrasias	• Document baseline assessment and significant changes.

Patient Outcome

Process

ASSESSMENT	INTERVENTION
b. Fluid intake and output c. Usual weight d. Normal voiding pattern e. Current drugs, *e.g.*, digitalis, diuretics	
4. Determine significance of other findings such as	• Document and report significant changes in vital signs and laboratory values to physician.

a. BP, T, P, R, CVP, pulmonary artery pressure
   b. Intake and output
   c. Weight
   d. Specific gravity
   e. Laboratory studies:
     • Urinalysis
     • Blood area nitrogen (BUN)
     • Serum and urine creatinine
     • Serum and urine electrolytes
     • Blood gases
     • Calcium and phosphorus
     • Total protein and albumin
     • Osmolalities
     • CBC
     • Urine culture
     • Blood culture
   f. Radiology studies
     • KUB (kidneys, ureters, bladder)
     • Chest
     • IVP
     • Retrograde studies	

5. Assess fluid status continuously.	• For patients with ARF, management may include severe fluid restriction, dialysis.

a. Accurate intake includes oral, IV fluids, blood products, tube feedings, and medications.
   b. Accurate output includes urine, emesis, drainage via tubes, and dressings.
   c. Be aware of insensible fluid loss.
   d. Observe for signs of fluid overload:
     • Dyspnea
     • Frothy, bloody sputum
     • Edema
     • Coughing
     • Hypertension
   e. Consider dialysate fluid balance.
	a. Indications for peritoneal or hemodialysis:
	     • Fluid overload
	     • Hyperkalemia
	     • Azotemia
	   b. Support respiratory status.
	   c. Treat thirst with appropriate mouth care, sourballs, etc.
	   d. Prepare patient/family for dialysis.

6. Inspect dialysis access sites for patency, signs and symptoms of complications.	• For patients receiving dialysis therapy, provide care to protect and maintain access sites: (Fig. 9-2)

a. Peritoneal dialysis catheter (Tenckhoff) site:
     • Bleeding, inflammation
     • Leaking of fluid, swelling, purulent drainage
	a. Daily Tenckhoff catheter care.
	   b. Allow no venipunctures or blood pressures in vascular access arm.

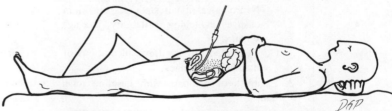

Fig. 9-2. Peritoneal dialysis catheter placement.

Patient Outcome	Process

ASSESSMENT	INTERVENTION

b. Arteriovenous shunt:
- Patency
- Bleeding, swelling, inflammation

c. Arteriovenous fistula:
- Patency
- Bleeding, swelling, inflammation

7. Assess chemical status continuously: Hyperkalemia:
a. Normal potassium 3.6 to 4.8 meg per l (values may differ according to laboratories.)
b. Signs and symptoms:
- Arrhythmias
- Nausea and vomiting
- Weakness
- Cramping
- Flaccid paralysis.

Hyponatremia (may be associated with fluid overload)
a. Normal sodium 135 to 145 meg per l.
b. Signs and symptoms:
- Weakness
- Increasing lethargy progressing to coma
- Seizures

Azotemia (uremic syndrome)
a. Normal BUN 8 to 25 mg per 100 ml
b. Normal creatinine 0.7 to 1.2 adult; under 5 years less than 0.5 mg per 100 ml.
c. Signs and symptoms (affects all systems):
- Nausea and vomiting
- Uremic fetor
- Sleep reversal
- Headache
- Somnolence progressing to coma
- Confusion, disorientation
- Seizures
- Dry, itching skin
- Platelet dysfunction—associated with GI bleeding, easy bruising, oozing from gums, puncture sites, wounds
- Diarrhea
- Stomatitis
- Lowered resistance to infection
- Delayed healing
- Thirst

INTERVENTION

c. Dry heat and elevation may be applied to vascular access arm.
d. Document and report any changes.
e. Limited and careful use of restraints.

- For patients with altered chemical status:
Hyperkalemia:
a. Monitor pulse and EKG.
b. Call physician for PVCs, peaking T waves, or widened QRS on electrocardiogram.
c. Restrict potassium intake (p.o. and IV) including drugs.
d. Provide symptomatic relief of cramping, *e.g.*, respositioning, passive range of motion.
e. Possible medications include:
- Sodium bicarbonate
- Intravenous combination:
Insulin, hypertonic glucose, calcium gluconate
- Sodium polystyrene sulfonate (Kayexalate), per rectum, nasogastric tube, with sorbitol (if given per rectum, follow by tap water enema.)

Hyponatremia
a. Restrict fluids.
b. Provide seizure precautions.
c. Possible medications include normal or hypertonic saline.

Azotemia
a. Document and report any significant changes.
b. Be alert to signs, symptoms, and potential problems of infection.
- Provide meticulous wound care.
- Remove urinary and other catheters or access lines as soon as possible.
- Carry out all aseptic procedures strictly.
- Give thorough pulmonary toilet.
- Provide good skin care and mouth care. Keep trauma to a minimum.
c. Provide special skin care.
- Use as little tape as possible.
- Apply skin oils and lotions.
- Clip fingernails to prevent scratching.
d. Give special attention to nutritional needs:
- Obtain appropriate diet order and dietary supplements, *e.g.*, vitamins, calorie count, tube feedings.
- Usual uremic diet: low protein, high caloric, low sodium, low potassium.
- Initiate dietary consult as needed.
e. Consider drug dosage modifications and contraindications.

Patient Outcome	Process
	ASSESSMENT / **INTERVENTION**

ASSESSMENT

Hypocalcemia
a. Normal calcium 8.5 to 10.5 mg per 100 ml
b. Signs and Symptoms:
    • Twitching or jerking
    • Tetany
    • Positive Chvostek's sign (a contraction or spasm of facial muscles resulting from tapping the facial nerves against the bone just anterior to the ear; seen in tetany)
    • Positive Trousseau's sign (carpal spasm induced by occluding the brachial artery for three minutes with an inflated blood pressure cuff; seen in tetany)
    • Numbness and tingling
    • Seizures.

Metabolic acidosis
a. Note recent blood gas and serum electrolyte reports.
b. Signs and symptoms:
    • Kussmaul's respirations
    • Somnolence

Hyperphosphatemia (often associated with low calcium level)
a. Normal phosphorus 4.5 to 6.5 mg per 100 ml
b. Signs and symptoms:
    • Itching
    • Constipation

8. Assess signs and symptoms of cardiovascular complications.
    a. Hypertension:
        • Increased BP, vital signs changes
        • Altered mental status, headache
    b. Pericarditis:
        • Pericardial friction rub

INTERVENTION

f. Be alert to signs, symptoms, and potential problems of bleeding.
    • May bleed from any site.
    • Guaiac test all drainage and stools.
    • Reduce stress as much as possible.
    • Hourly antacid regimen may be ordered. Consider constipating effects of antacids. Aluminum hydroxide (Amphojel) preferred because of low sodium content.
    • Minimize invasive procedures as much as possible.
    • Give special care to venipuncture sites to prevent oozing and infection.
    • Provide safety precautions to prevent accidental injuries, *e.g.*, hitting side rails.

Hypocalcemia
a. Medical management may include: IV calcium (contraindicated in patients with bradycardia).
b. Be aware that multiple blood transfusions and alkalosis may cause hypocalcemia.
c. Provide seizure precautions.
d. Decrease patient stimulation.

Metabolic acidosis
a. Medical management may include:
    • IV sodium bicarbonate
b. Be aware of potassium and calcium levels.
c. Be aware of respiratory compensatory mechanisms.

Hyperphosphatemia
a. Medical management may include: phosphorus binder, *e.g.*, aluminum hydroxide (Amphojel) preferred.
b. Consider stool softeners for constipation.
c. Use skin care lotions.
d. Itching may be controlled by medications, *e.g.*, trimeprazine (Temaril), diphenhydramine (Benadryl Hydrochloride).

• For patients with altered cardiovascular status:
a. Be aware that symptoms may be masked depending upon clinical condition, *e.g.*, hypovolemic shock. Document and report to physician any significant changes.
b. Hypertension:
    • Diet and fluids may be restricted.

Patient Outcome   **Process**

ASSESSMENT	INTERVENTION
• Pain	• Control environmental and emotional stresses to reduce anxiety levels.
c. Pericardial effusion:	• A combination of parental antihypertensives may be used:
• Respiratory distress	Hydralazine hydrochloride (Apresoline)
• Chest radiograph findings abnormal	Propranolol (Inderal)
• Breath sounds abnormal	Nitroprusside (Nipride)
• Paradoxic pulse	Tranquilizers, *e.g.*, diazepam (Valium).
d. Cardiac tamponade:	c. Cardiac tamponade. Possible interventions:
• Increased CVP	• Pericardiocentesis
• Increasing paradox	• Preparation of patient (and family) for operative procedure.
• Decreasing pulse pressure	
9. Assess patient/family response to situation.	• Remain realistically encouraging without conveying false hopes.

Patient Outcome	Process	
	ASSESSMENT	INTERVENTION

Patient Outcome: *The patient attains optimal respiratory function.*

Process

ASSESSMENT

1. Assess signs and symptoms of respiratory function abnormalities by inspection and determine significance.
   a. General body size—cachectic, normal, obese
   b. Body position—can lie flat or head must be elevated to breathe
   c. Mental status—alert progressing to comatose
      • Both hypoxia and hypercapnia can cause confusion, agitation, stupor and coma as they worsen.
      • Neurological disease can affect both ability to breathe and rhythm of breathing.
   d. Skin
      • Color
         Pallor—may be due to anemia, hypotension
         Cyanosis of lips and mucous membranes is central cyanosis. Note hypoxia.
         Cyanosis of tip of nose, extremities is peripheral cyanosis. Note decreased circulation.
         Flushing—may be due to CO_2 retention
      • Temperature and turgor very dry, tenting may be due to dehydration.
         Periorbital edema may be due to fluid overload.
      • Nasal flaring—may be due to respiratory distress
      • Lips
         Color
         Pursed lip breathing
   e. Neck
      • Retraction of accessory muscles may be due to respiratory distress.
      • Position of trachea—trachea shifts away from affected side may be due to tension pneumothorax or large pleural effusion. Trachea shifts toward affected side may be due to atelectasis.
      • Jugular venous distention may be due to increased pressure in right ventricle.
   f. Arms and hands
      • Compare capillary filling, color; and temperature of fingers of both hands, especially in presence of radial arterial line.
      • Asterixis (flapping of middle fingers when hand pulled back toward elbow) may be due to CO_2 narcosis and hepatic failure.
   g. Legs
      • Reddened, swollen calves or positive Homan's sign may be due to thrombophletitis or be a source of pulmonary emboli.

INTERVENTION

• Document baseline data and significant changes.
• Identify respiratory function by inspection. Notify physician and respiratory therapist as appropriate.
• Provide patent airway and proceed with ventilation and/or oxygenation.
   a. Hyperextend neck (Exception: In a suspected cervical neck injury, immobilize neck first).
   b. Remove obvious obstruction.
   c. Suction (oropharyngeal or endotracheal)
   d. Perform triple airway maneuver:
      • Thrust mandible forward.
      • Seal nose with own cheek.
      • Begin ventilation.
   e. Insert oral or nasal airway.
   f. Assist physician and therapist in intubation:
      • Assemble intubation and suction equipment.
      • Position patient with pillow under head and hyperextend neck.
      • Check breath sounds after intubation.
      • Secure tube.
      • Obtain arterial blood gases and chest radiograph
   g. Assist physician in tracheostomy if needed.
      • Assemble appropriate equipment.
      • Position and restrain patient.
      • Follow procedure and post-procedure care to include suctioning, cleaning, cuff care and placing identical tube at head of bed.
• Maintain adequate ventilation/oxygenation.
   a. Provide effective oxygen therapy through use of selected equipment as:
      • Oxygen mask and cannula
      • Tracheostomy collar aero-flo unit
      • Resuscitation bag
      • Respirator
      • Intermittent manditory ventilation
   b. Assure that patient is receiving prescribed concentration of oxygen.
      • Check flow meter for appropriate settings.
      • Check proper tube connections.
      • Call respiratory therapist to analyze oxygen concentration.
      • Call respiratory therapist to assist with transport of patient as needed.
      • Be aware of possible complications of oxygen for extended periods such as O_2 toxicity, depressed respiratory drive in patients with chronic obstructive disease.

Patient Outcome

Process

ASSESSMENT

h. Chest
- Shape and symmetry—
  Scoliosis—lateral curvature of spine
  Kyphosis—posterior curvature of spine
  } can cause restriction of lung expansion

  AP diameter of chest—if increased (barrel chest), can indicate normality in elderly or disease.
- Retraction of intercostal spaces on inspiration with respiratory distress may be due to chronic obstructive disease, asthma, foreign body aspiration.
- Movement
  Both sides should expand equally. If one area does not move consider pneumothorax, malpositioned endotracheal tube, pleural effusion.
  Flail chest—if chest falls on inspiration and bulges on expiration, may be due to traumatic separation from ribs.

i. Quality of respiration
- Rate
  Normal: 12 to 20 per minute in adults
  Abnormal: 30 to 60 per minute rapid, shallow. Consider hypoxia, pain
- Hyperventialtion: rapid, deep
  May be due to anxiety, acidosis, central nervous system disease
  Central neurogenic hyperventilation
  Kussmaul's—normal or fast, deep, sighing
- Ease of respiration
  Dyspnea—difficulty breathing at rest or on exertion
  Orthopnea—must elevate head to breathe easily
- Ratio of inspiration to expiration
  Normal—1:2
  Prolonged—1:3; may indicate chronic obstructive disease, asthma, airway obstruction.
- Rhythm
  Normal—inspiration of equal depth and length followed by expirations of equal depth and length with sigh 6 to 10 times/hour.
  Abnormal—
  Cheyne-Stokes—apneic periods alternating with periods of hyperventilation with increase of rapidity and depth.
  Biot's—apneic periods with irregular episodes of breaths of equal depth may indicate meningitis.

INTERVENTION

c. Artificial resuscitation
- Mouth-to-mouth breathing
- Bag to mask (with O_2)
- Bag to tracheostomy or endotracheal tube

d. Mechanical ventilation
- Constant surveillance of patient on ventilator to guard against hypo- and hyperventilation.
- Check ventilator hourly for:
  Inspiratory pressure
  Expired tidal volume
  Inspired oxygen concentration
  Rate
  Temperature of inspired air
  Compliance.
- Collaborate with respiratory therapist in maintaining clean equipment for patient to prevent infection.
- Prepare for and assist physician with insertion of chest tubes.
a. Assemble equipment.
b. Position and restrain patient.
c. Follow preprocedure and postprocedure care.

Patient Outcome	Process

ASSESSMENT	INTERVENTION

Agonal—irregular, gasping, slow breaths. Indicates impending death
Apnea—indicates respiratory arrest.
j. Tracheobronchial secretions
  • Color—clear, purulent, yellow, green, bloody, rusty.
  • Consistency—thin to tenacious, foamy
  • Amount—scant to copious
	• Send initial sputum for culture and sensitivity before antibiotics begin. Also send sputum when it changes.

2. Assess respiratory status by: palpation of:
  a. Tender areas
  b. Symmetry and degree of expansion of chest. Size of chest should increase about three inches on deep inspiration and be equal on both sides of chest.
  c. Fremitus—vibration from lungs to palm of hand.
    • Vocal fremitus
      Normal—slight vibration equal on each side of chest
      Consolidated area—will vibrate more than other side
      Pneumothorax, pleural effusion, atelectasis, decreased or absent vibration
    • Rhonchial fremitus—bubbling feeling under hand as patient breathes, caused by air moving through secretions in large airways.
    • Pleural friction rub—grating sensation under hand as patient breathes from inflamed pleura
    • Subcutaneous emphysema—crepitant feeling under skin due to leakage of air from pleura to soft tissues
	• Determine respiratory status by palpation.
	• Check for vocal fremitus by instructing patient to say "99" and comparing vibrations on each side of chest starting at apices and then the bases.

3. Assess respiratory status by percussion.
  a. Resonance—faintly hollow sound that is normal throughout the chest.
  b. Hyperresonance—more hollow, louder sound, heard when there is a greater than normal ratio of air to tissue, *e.g.* pneumothorax, chronic obstructive disease
  c. Tympany—very drum like, high sound, from air enclosed in a sac
  d. Dull—muffled short sound where tissue replaces air; (normal at the fifth right intercostal space over liver and third to fifth left intercostal space over heart) may be sign of atelectasis, consolidation, pleural effusion
  e. Flat—dead, short sound—no air at all. May indicate massive pleural effusion.
	• Percuss intercostal spaces, and compare sounds on both sides of chest.

4. Assess respiratory status by breath sounds.
  a. Normal breath sounds
    • Vesicular—soft rush of air on inspiration, little or no sound on expiration. Normal sound over periphery of lungs.
	• Auscultate chest.
	  a. Place warm diaphragm of stethoscope over lung area.
	  b. Listen to chest sounds in a quiet environment.

Patient Outcome

Process

ASSESSMENT	INTERVENTION

- Bronchovesicular—blowing, louder rush of air heard equally on inspiration and expiration.

  Normal only in apices near sternum or above scapula in back because of closeness of mainstem bronchi to chest wall.

  If heard over periphery, may indicate beginning pneumonia.
- Bronchial or tubular—loud, harsh, rush of air heard longer on expiration. If heard in periphery of lung, may indicate consolidated area or pleural effusion compressing lung.
- Diminished or absent breath sounds are normal in obese or muscular patient, or in chronic obstructive disease (bilateral finding).

  If heard in one area only may indicate mal-position of endotracheal tube, atelectasis, pneumothorax, large pleural effusion.

b. Adventitious or abnormal breath sounds.
- Râles—fine, crackling sounds heard on inspiration due to direct air moving through fluid in alveoli or terminal airways. If widespread usually indicates pulmonary edema; if localized, usually pneumonia.
- Rhonchi—low, rumbling, bubbling, sound usually on expiration (if on inspiration, called coarse râle), caused by air moving through larger airways narrowed by mucus. Usually heard in pneumonia.
- Wheeze—high pitched, musical, whistling sound caused by air moving through airways narrowed by edema or bronchoconstriction. Heard on inspiration or expiration. Usually heard in asthma, pulmonary emboli, chronic obstructive disease.
- Pleural friction rub—grating, leathery sound heard on inspiration and expiration due to inflamed pleura rubbing together. Disappears if effusion occurs.

c. Audible sounds
- Gurgling—on inspiration due to collection of secretions in trachea or in pharynx
- Snoring—tongue blocking airway on inspiration
- Crowing—high pitched sound caused by laryngeal edema
- Stridor—wheezing on inspiration due to foreign body in trachea

c. Instruct patient to breathe deeply through mouth.
d. Note that breath sounds are louder when patient is on a respirator.
e. Compare left side to the right.

Patient Outcome	Process

ASSESSMENT	INTERVENTION

ASSESSMENT

• Wheezing—high pitched sound on inspiration or expiration due to bronchospasm

5. Assess other parameter of respiratory function. (Values may differ according to laboratories).

   a. Arterial blood gases. Normal/abnormal values:

     • Normal: PaO_2 85–100 mm Hg
            $PaCO_2$ 35–40 mm Hg
            pH   7.35–7.47
            Bicarbonate 19–30 meq

     • Index to respiratory failure:
            PaO_2 ↓ 60 mm. Hg

     • Acidosis:

Primary		Compensation
Respiratory	↑ CO_2	↑ HCO_3
Metabolic	↓ HCO_3	↓ CO_2

     • Alkalosis:

Primary		Compensation
Respiratory	↓ CO_2	↓ HCO_3
Metabolic	↑ HCO_3	↑ CO_2

   b. History

     • Chronic illness, especially cardiac, obstructive pulmonary disease, cancer.

     • Acute respiratory infection in last two weeks or exposure to tuberculosis, influenza.

     • Occupational exposure to coal dust, asbestos, cotton fibers or hay

     • Smoking

     • Exposure to endemic disease through recent travel

   c. Allergies and home medicines

INTERVENTION

• Consider with the physician the identified imbalance to determine course of therapy. Initiate intervention and re-evaluate.

   a. Respiratory acidosis in the nonintubated patient:

     • Administer basic therapy modes to the patient in the following order—may omit certain modes for a particular patient.

       Positioning
       IPPB
       Ultrasonic nebulization
       Postural drainage with percussion
       Incentive spirometry
       Deep breathing, coughing, endotracheal suction
       Breathing exercises

   b. Respiratory acidosis in the intubated patient on a respirator:

     • Correct underventilation by increasing minute ventilation.
       Increase tidal volume.
       Increase rate.
       Increase both.

     • Consider treatment modes of pulmonary care.
       Positioning
       Bronchodilator therapy
       Lavage
       Postural drainage with percussion
       Sigh volumes
       Suctioning
       Humidification

   c. Respiratory alkalosis in the nonintubated patient:

     • Rebreathe using bag or rebreathing mask.

   d. Respiratory alkalosis in the intubated patient:

     • Decrease minute volume, decrease tidal volume, decrease rate or both.

Patient Outcome	Process	
	ASSESSMENT	INTERVENTION

The patient maintains optimal skin integrity	1. Assess present skin condition.
	  a. Color
	  b. Temperature
	  c. Laceration
	  d. Abrasion
	  e. Hematoma
	  f. Contusion
	  g. Local edema
	  h. Pressure area, decubitus
	  i. Rash
	  j. Ulcer, open wound
	  k. Burn
	  l. Drainage
	  m. Dryness, oiliness
	  n. Hair, condition and distribution
	  o. Condition of fingernails, toenails
		• Examine all skin surfaces thoroughly.
		• Document baseline data and significant changes in skin condition.

	2. Consider medical history, past skin disorder and current status.
	  a. Altered level of consciousness
	  b. Motor/sensory deficit
	  c. Elderly, debilitated
	  d. State of hydration and nutrition
	  e. Obese
	  f. Decreased peripheral circulation
	  g. Allergies
	  h. Decubitus, skin disorders
	  i. Hypersensitive skin
	  j. Diarrhea
	  k. Stoma
		• Initiate preventive skin care program which may include:
		  a. Frequent turning, progress to out of bed if possible
		    • Use of trapeze for self-help
		    • Use of turning sheet
		  b. Positioning
		  c. Use of assistive devices in preventing pressure areas
		  d. Special care of skin around tube sites
		  e. Bathing considerations:
		    • Dry skin: mild soap to axilla, feet, perineum, oil in bath water, lotion
		    • Oily skin: frequent washing; follow patient preference in treatment
		    • Dry scaly feet: soak in warm, soapy water q.o.d.; apply emollient
		    • Keep hair free of tangles and matting.

	3. Assess patient's sensitivity to tapes, dressing materials, solutions, soaps.
	4. Assess patients with special needs for care.
	  a. Decubiti
	  b. Fistula
	  c. Draining wound
		f. Avoid using solutions, types of tape, or other material which may be irritating.
		    • Document special needs.
		• Establish plan of care for patients with:
		  a. Decubitus
		  b. Fistula
		  c. Draining wound
		  d. Condom catheter/Foley catheter
		• Institute routine for dressing change on patient with incision:
		  a. Check need for dressing change.
		  b. Insure that orders are written to clarify physician/nurse responsibility for dressing changes and exact procedure to be followed.
		  c. Date and initial dressing after dressing change.

CHAPTER X
Guidelines for the rehabilitation patient

INTRODUCTION: These guidelines describe desirable patient care outcomes and associated nursing process for the patient who has rehabilitation care needs. Consideration is given to physical, psychological and socioeconomic components of care essential to achieve the degree of independence the patient is able or motivated to achieve.

Each guideline identifies nursing intervention to facilitate the expectation of the patient's fullest participation in care within limits of disabilities. There is emphasis on specific nursing skills to support, teach and supervise the patient and family in achieving restoration of functional ability in a purposeful manner.

Cerebrovascular accident, head injury, and other cerebral deficits—rehabilitation

Patient Outcome	Process

The patient functions at maximum ability in all aspects of daily living. This includes:

DESCRIPTION: Patients with brain damage from cerebrovascular disease, trauma, tumor, or other disease processes may have the following alterations depending on location and extent of lesion and degree of spontaneous recovery.

Alteration	*Example*
Motor	Hemiparesis/plegia, dysarthria
Sensory	Touch, visual field cut
Mental	Disorientation, memory loss, emotional lability
Language	Aphasia
Emotional	Depression
Bowel, bladder	Incontinence

NURSING ASSESSMENT: In addition to the general admission assessment, the following information is especially important.

1. Assess and document sensory/motor alterations.
   a. Area of paresis/paralysis
   b. Presence of contracture/subluxation/spasticity
   c. Presence of dysarthria/dysphasia
   d. Area of sensory loss/impairment including visual field cut
   e. Level of activity; transfers, wheelchair sitting, endurance
   f. Self-care skills including activities of daily living
2. Assess and document physiological factors which may affect rehabilitation.
   a. Skin
   b. Cardiovascular, *e.g.*, swelling of extremities
   c. Respiratory, *e.g.*, endurance, shortness of breath, ability to cough effectively
   d. Gastrointestinal, *e.g.*, current bowel program, bowel history
   e. Genitourinary, *e.g.*, current bladder care program
   f. Pathophysiological states, *e.g.*, obesity, diabetes, hypertension
3. Assess and document psychological/intellectual status.
   a. Language ability, *e.g.*, receptive/expressive aphasia
   b. Perceptual status, *e.g.*, one-sided neglect, disorientation
   c. Understanding of disability
   d. Psychological reactions to disability, *e.g.*, grief
   e. Emotional status, *e.g.*, lability, impulsiveness
   f. Personality/body image/self-concept
   g. Current coping strategy and resources
   h. Knowledge base and motivation for learning
   i. Learning impairments, *e.g.*, memory loss
4. Assess and document socioeconomic status.
   a. Funding sources for equipment
   b. Vocation/avocation
   c. Family role
   d. Home evaluation, *e.g.*, architectural barriers

INTERVENTION:

A. *Is free of or has minimal effects or complications*

1. Maintain skin care program.
   a. Provide and teach patient/family care for maintenance of intact skin.
      • Inspect skin daily. Teach use of mirror.
      • Bathe daily and after each incontinence.
      • Apply lotion to dry skin.
      • Do not use powder on skin.
      • Lift to turn q 2 hours and reposition to prevent shearing.
   b. Teach cause of pressure sores, prevention and care of ischemic areas.
   c. Provide appropriate equipment, *e.g.*, seat cushion.
   d. Give therapeutic skin care if breakdown present.
   e. Teach safety measures to prevent trauma, especially affected side.

• *Skin*

• *Bowel*

2. Facilitate regular bowel habits for the patient.
   a. Establish communication system for patient to make needs known, *e.g.*, signal for bathroom.

Patient Outcome	Process
	b. Obtain bowel history.
	c. Discuss program goals and routine with patient.
	d. Assure empty bowel at onset.
	e. Give glycerin suppository to patient with irregularity or incontinence. Schedule insertion of suppository q.o.d. within 30 minutes after evening meal. Alternative routines are daily or before morning meal.
	f. Assist patient to toilet or bedside commode.
	g. Use stimulus that has helped in past, *e.g.,* cup of coffee.
	h. Give stool softener/laxative/bulk agent as ordered.
	i. Provide balanced diet to include fruits, vegetable, bran cereal, wheat bread.
	j. Provide at least 2500 cc per day fluid intake which may include prune juice.
	k. Maintain bowel record.
	l. Have perseverence; anticipate relapses in the first one to two weeks. Expect that patient may have lapses of memory or attention.
	m. Give praise for small gains; do not criticize relapse.
	n. Teach patient/family all aspects of bowel care including medications.
	o. Continue training program as long as necessary; may be four to six weeks.
	p. Prepare patient to modify plan independently including medications.
• *Bladder*	3. Establish bladder program if patient is incontinent.
	a. Obtain bladder history.
	b. Obtain urinalysis/culture and sensitivity.
	c. Establish communication system for patient to make needs known, *e.g.,* signal for bathroom.
	d. Remove indwelling catheter if present.
	e. Provide adequate fluids at regular time intervals; decrease or discontinue fluids after evening meal until morning.
	f. Provide commode/bedpan/urinal q 2 hours without fail.
	g. Provide condom catheter/protective padding as appropriate.
	h. Expect nighttime incontinence to endure after daytime continence is established.
	i. Initiate intermittent catheterization program if urinary retention occurs.
	j. Teach patient and family all aspects of bladder care program.
• *Orientation*	4. Facilitate orientation.
	a. Reorient to physical and social environment frequently.
	b. Provide environmental stimuli, *e.g.,* radio, clock, TV, visitors.
	c. Provide light for nighttime disorientation.
	d. Provide safety measures, *e.g.,* side rails.
	e. Structure the routine of daily activities, *e.g.,* consistent time of bathing.
	f. Identify for the patient inappropriate/disoriented perception, *e.g.,* "This is not Tuesday."
	g. Reinforce appropriate perception.
	h. Teach/involve family in reorientation.
• *Visual*	5. Provide and teach measures to minimize effects of visual disturbances.
	a. Encourage patient with pre-existing visual problems to wear glasses. (Bifocals may interfere with ambulation.)
	b. For patient with diplopia:
	• Cover eye; alternate eye patched daily.
	• Explain loss of depth perception when only one eye used, need to gauge space and distance.
	c. For patient with field cut (hemianopia):
	• Place necessary objects within remaining field of vision and approach from visually intact side until patient is visually accommodated to surroundings; then place necessary objects to side of deficit to further facilitate compensation.
	• Instruct patient to compensate by turning head to scan defective visual field.
	• Use color cues to help establish habit of scanning, *e.g.,* line down margins of page for reading.
	d. Teach family and observe participation.
• *Communication*	6. Facilitate communication.
	a. Confirm the problem in communicating and provide reassurance about plans for care.
	b. Relate to patient in respectful and sympathetic manner without condescension.
	c. Provide quiet environment, *e.g.,* decrease noise from TV.

Patient Outcome	Process
	d. Avoid placing patient in social isolation. • Encourage staff/visitors to talk *to* the patient. e. Speak slowly and distinctly without overarticulating or shouting. f. Use level of communication patient can understand, *e.g.,* simple sentences, phrases, single words, gestures. g. Allow ample response time before interrupting or moving on to new idea. h. Establish reliability of patient's verbal or gestured yes-no responses. i. Encourage speech attempts without pushing patient to the point of frustration, severe anxiety. j. Use writing, alphabet/word, or picture boards as alternate means of communication if needed. k. Explain patient's communication needs to family and instruct in methods to stimulate speech improvement. l. Practice recommended speech therapy exercises with patient, *e.g.,* naming objects, sentence completion.
• *Eating*	7. Facilitate chewing and swallowing. a. Request dental consult if dentures fit poorly. b. Progress diet as tolerated from soft foods to regular consistency. c. Use stimulation techniques and lip and tongue exercises recommended by occupational therapist. d. Teach patient to put small amounts of food in unaffected side of mouth, use of mirror/finger to position food in mouth; check for food pooled in weak side of mouth. e. Use straight, upright, sitting position during eating/drinking. f. Supervise eating for safety, *e.g.,* choking/aspiration. g. Give thick fluids such as milkshakes rather than watery fluids to patient who tends to aspirate. Provide utensil with which patient can best manage drinking, *e.g.,* either cup or straw. h. Provide protection for clothing. i. Remind patient to correct for drooling, *e.g.,* use tissues to wipe mouth. j. Encourage patient to eat in dining room with others. k. Demonstrate acceptance of patient's eating efforts. l. Teach family and supervise participation.
• *Musculoskeletal*	8. Maintain normal joint range of motion. a. Give range of motion exercise b.i.d. Teach and supervise patient in doing range of motion exercises by self. b. Position/turn to maintain alignment and inhibit spasticity. Example: When in bed, position affected upper extremity in extension and abduction with thumb out of palm; position affected lower extremity in slight flexion with trunk straight. Use segmental-turning rather than log-rolling method. c. Use hand positioning device if necessary, *e.g.,* hard cone shape in palm, splint. d. Use lapboard to support arm in wheelchair. e. Use sling during ambulation if upper extremity is flaccid. f. Teach patient to observe affected arm frequently during activities to prevent injury/dislocation. g. Use lower extremity positioning device/splint to maintain neutral position/dorsiflexion of foot if necessary, *e.g.,* bootie. h. Facilitate use of weak extremity for functional activities, *e.g.,* affected hand as "helper" during bathing. i. Reinforce techniques used to decrease spasticity taught by physical and occupational therapists. j. Give medication as ordered to lessen spasticity/pain; teach about medications. k. Teach the cause of painful shoulder syndrome and exercises which control pain.
• *Circulatory*	9. Promote adequate peripheral circulation. a. Provide and teach passive and active range of motion exercises. b. Use elastic stockings/isotoner glove as indicated. c. Avoid prolonged position with legs crossed. d. Give anticoagulant as ordered; teach about medication.

Patient Outcome	Process
	e. Observe for edema, redness, changes in skin temperature. f. Relieve/prevent dependent edema by elevating extremity. g. Avoid external constriction, *e.g.,* tight clothing.

• *Compensation*	10. Assist patient to compensate for one-sided neglect.
	    a. Arrange environment to facilitate compensation.
	       • Structure environment on neglected side.
	       • Structure environment on unaffected side if neglect is severe and persistent.
	    b. Orient patient repeatedly to entire environment of room, unit and therapy areas including landmarks to the right and left in hallways.
	    c. Provide sensory input for neglected side, *e.g.,* touch affected arm during activities, speak from neglected side.
	    d. Give information/feedback repeatedly about neglected side, techniques for use in activities of daily living, and visual scanning toward neglected side to teach compensation for deficit.
	    e. Use calm, informative approach to intervene in neglect rather than condescending, nagging approach.

• *Learning*	11. Facilitate learning.
	    a. Memory loss
	       • Explain cause of memory loss to patient/family.
	       • Repeat information/instruction.
	    b. Short attention span/easy distractability.
	       • Provide consistent, explicit, and short instructions.
	       • Give information one step at a time.
	       • Provide climate conducive to learning, *e.g.,* quiet, privacy.
	       • Provide opportunity to rest frequently during activities.
	       • Redirect into desired activity if patient becomes distracted.
	    c. Inability to abstract/transfer learning.
	       • Structure consistent approach, *e.g.,* use same dressing routine in occupational therapy and nursing unit.
	       • Repeat teaching frequently.
	       • Explain and assist family to participate in approach.
	       • Provide positive feedback for successful learning.

• *Behavior*	12. Assist patient to achieve appropriate behavior.
	    a. Demonstrate acceptance of patient's feelings.
	    b. Teach patient/family cause of altered behavior and impaired intellect.
	    c. For patient with emotional lability:
	       • Provide diversional activities; involve patient in tasks to distract from lability.
	       • Approach patient calmly during crying/laughing episodes without directly focusing on lability, *e.g.,* when crying occurs, attempt to involve in other activity without asking reason for crying.
	    d. For patient with loss of self-control/regression:
	       • Ignore regressed behavior; reinforce appropriate behavior.
	       • Provide safety measures if impulsiveness causes risk or injury, *e.g.,* seatbelt.
	    e. For patient with personality change:
	       • Provide and teach participation in activities within limits, *e.g.,* family outing, household chores.
	       • Use behavior modification program if indicated.
	    f. For patient with decreased tolerance for stress.
	       • Establish consistent routine for care.
	       • Maintain quiet organized environment, especially for teaching.
	       • Explain all procedures before doing them.
	       • Introduce new ideas/tasks one at a time.
	       • Reduce stress if it occurs, *e.g.,* give rest period from stressful activity.
	       • Expect episodes of increased stress to impair patient's self-care and learning.

B. *Is coping with disability*	13. Assist patient to cope with disability.
	    a. Help patient/family to accept self by demonstrating acceptance.
	    b. Give repeated, specific, accurate information about abilities, strengths, and potentials.
	    c. Use terms "weak", "affected", or "right-left" to refer to hemiplegic side. Do not say "bad" and "good" side.
	    d. Give patient/family opportunities to participate in planning and implementing care.

Patient Outcome	Process
	e. Provide opportunity for patient/family to express feelings about disability and resulting limitation, *e. g.,* how this will affect life-style and future plans. f. Identify patient's grieving process and intervene appropriately. g. Give verbal recognition for successful coping strategy. h. Identify with patient resource persons for assistance in counseling, *e.g.,* social worker, chaplain. i. Provide opportunities for patient to make decision about environment, *e.g.,* arrangement of belongings in room. Identify things patient can control and areas of independence. j. Provide a variety of experiences for patient to learn about body and develop positive self-concept, *e.g.,* trips outside rehabilitation center, therapeutic home visit, recreational activities. k. Consider psychiatric referral when grief becomes maladaptive. 14. Counsel and teach patient and partner about sexual functioning. a. Teach about effects of related physical alterations if present, *e.g.,* aging, hypertension. b. Reassure about sexual ability/potential/alternatives. c. Identify resource persons for patient, *e.g.,* social worker. d. Counsel patient/family if lack of inhibition/hypersexuality present. Set limits, and give feedback about inappropriate behavior with nonjudgmental approach. e. Provide genitourinary/gynecological consult and information about contraception, if appropriate. 15. Assist patient to cope with headache if present. a. Monitor frequency and characteristics of headaches; monitor neurological signs if indicated. b. Provide comfort measures, *e.g.,* assist to lie down if headache severe. c. Teach relationship of headache to brain insult and expect decrease of headache over time. d. Give medication as ordered. e. Expect participation in rehabiliatation program unless headache severe.

C. *Is knowledgeable about nature of illness, self-care, and resources for continuity of care*	16. Teach patient and family about
	a. Structure and function of brain
	b. Effects of cerebrovascular accident/head injury/disease process
	c. Medications, *e.g.,* anticoagulant, anticonvulsive
	
	17. Teach patient and family activities of daily living (ADL).
	a. General
	  • Incorporate specific interventions related to impairments.
	  • Use demonstrations for patient with aphasia; use verbal instructions for patient with visual perceptual deficits.
	  • Provide positive feedback for accomplishments; correct errors without criticism.
	  • Give repeated instructions daily at patient's pace; expect relapses.
	  • Teach family about techniques for ADL and patient's ability to perform.
	  • Give progress reports to family and assure continuity of ADL function on therapeutic home visits; obtain feedback from patient and family concerning function on visit.
	b. Feeding
	  • Teach one-handed techniques for buttering bread, cutting meat, opening cartons.
	  • Provide special equipment if needed, *e.g.,* rocker knife.
	c. Bathing
	  • Teach hemi techniques for bathing in bed when limitations in movement *e.g.,* place unaffected leg under affected leg for position. Advance to shampoo, tub and shower when appropriate.
	  • Provide special equipment if needed, *e.g.,* long-handled sponge.
	  • Observe and correct for perseveration if it occurs, *e.g.,* repeated bathing of one body part.
	  • Observe and correct bathing errors due to impaired mental status, *e.g.,* not rinsing off soap.
	  • Use consistent, systematic order for bathing, *e.g.,* head to toes with affected side first.
	d. Dressing and undressing
	  • Teach hemi techniques when limitations in movement, *e.g.,* dress affected side first, undress affected side last, over the head method for shirts/blouses.
	  • Teach dressing and undressing in bed before progressing to other positions.

Patient Outcome	Process

	• Begin with basic skills before progressing to buttons, tying shoes.
	• Use patient's clothing from home. Avoid confusing colors, *e.g.,* white shirt when patient lies on white sheet to dress.
	• Observe and correct perseveration if present, *e.g.,* repeated buttoning of the same button.
	• Observe and correct dressing errors due to impaired mental status if present, *e.g.,* dressing with clothing inside out.
	• Use consistent order for dressing process.
	  e. Grooming
	• Promote patient's usual grooming habits, *e.g.,* use of cosmetics.
	• Encourage grooming at sink as soon as possible.
	• Supervise and assure safety, *e.g.,* shaving.
	  f. Transfers
	• Teach hemi techniques for transfers when limitations in movement, *e.g.,* wheelchair placement, visual check for placement of affected foot and arm, lead with unaffected side, stand upright before pivoting.
	• Emphasize safety factors, *e.g.,* lock wheelchair brakes.
	• Include car, tub, and commode transfers
	  g. Community skills, *e.g.,* use of telephone, elevator
	  h. Care of belongings and environment, *e.g.,* dentures, laundry
	  i. Home making
	  j. Use of adaptive equipment for activities of daily living
	18. Reinforce physical therapy and occupational therapy teaching to include:
	  a. Wheelchair manipulation, safety, and maintenance
	  b. Use of devices, if appropriate
	• Handsplint
	• Brace application
	• Brace/crutch/cane ambulation
	19. Counsel patient and family about:
	  a. Understanding of disability/ability
	  b. Realistic expectations of rehabilitation
	  c. Altered family roles, *e.g.,* vocational, educational, financial; consult Vocational Rehabilitation as needed.
	  d. Identify other resource persons and contact as needed.
	20. Plan home care with patient and family.
	  a. Teach all aspects of care for therapeutic leave from rehabilitation center.
	• Assure care will be adequate before allowing leave; review care and problem solve after patient returns.
	  b. Provide comprehensive teaching with written materials. Document learning and motivation status.
	  c. Collaborate with public health nurse and other health team members in evaluation of home environment.
	• Assist in making decision about home modifications if needed.
	  d. Discuss with family feasibility of home care and alternatives.
	  e. Share decision made by Physical and Occupational Therapy for needed equipment with patient and family.
	  f. Arrange for clinic follow-up.
	  g. Initiate interagency referral. Include discharge summary and projected plans.
	  h. Discuss community resources, activities, and barriers.
	• Attitudinal, social barriers/resources/supports
	• Architectural barriers/accessibility
	• Transportation, *e.g.,* wheelchair, taxi, airlines
	• Current legislation concerning disabled
	• Organizations, *e.g.,* American Heart Association, Senior Citizens Council

Patient Outcome	Process
The patient functions at maximum ability in all aspects of daily living. This includes:	**DESCRIPTION:** Patients with lower extremity amputation in need of prosthesis fitting and gait training may have the following characteristics: (1) recent amputation for any reason or long-term amputation without a rehabilitation program; (2) unilateral or bilateral amputation; (3) level of amputation may be Syme's (ankle), below knee, knee disarticulation, above knee, hip disarticulation, or hemipelvectomy; and (4) have immediate postoperative fitting or preparing for prosthetic fitting and gait training. Many patients are adults or elderly with long-term health problems causing or contributing to amputation.

NURSING ASSESSMENT: In addition to the general admission assessment, the following information is especially important.

1. Assess and document sensory/motor alterations
   a. Dysesthesia/pain
   b. Movement and positioning of involved extremity/contractures
   c. Level of activity, transfers, ambulation
   d. Self-care skills including stump care, activities of daily living
2. Assess and document physiological factors which might affect rehabilitation.
   a. Condition of stump
      • Skin
      • Swelling
      • Peripheral pulses
      • Shape
      • Suture line
      • Potential pressure areas
   b. Condition of other lower extremity
   c. Pathophysiological states as obesity, diabetes, peripheral vascular disease
3. Assess and document psychological/intellectual status.
   a. Psychological reactions to amputation
   b. Patient's self-concept and body image. Consider how patient touches self, body language, language patient uses to refer to stump, and how patient relates to others.
   c. Current coping strategy and resources
   d. Knowledge base and motivation for learning
4. Assess and document socioeconomic status.
   a. Funding sources for prosthesis and equipment
   b. Occupation
   c. Family role
   d. Home evaluation, *e.g.,* architectural barriers

INTERVENTION:

A. *Is free of or has minimal effects or complications*

1. Provide stump care to develop cone shape.
   a. Use figure-of-eight elastic wrapping and rewrap q 8 hours.
   b. Teach skill to patient and family.
2. Maintain mobility.
   a. Encourage active range of motion to affected extremity t.i.d.
   b. Provide quadriceps setting exercises t.i.d.
   c. Get patient out of bed and into wheelchair or ambulating at least b.i.d.
3. Maintain range of motion.
   a. Prevent contractures.
      • Position to maintain functional extension and flexion of hip and knee joints. Prone position 20 minutes t.i.d. and/or sleep in prone position.
      • Teach positioning and purpose to patient and family.
   b. Use measures to correct contractures if needed, such as
      • Positioning
      • Traction
      • Weights
      • Teaching patient exercises
4. Establish skin care program. See Chapter 2 Skin Care Guidelines, p. 31.
   a. Prevent stump/skin breakdown.
      • Observe for pressure areas.
      • Preventive skin care
   b. Give therapeutic skin care if skin breakdown on stump. Discontinue physical therapy unless continuation desired by physician.

Patient Outcome	Process

B. *Is coping with disability*	5. Assist patient to cope with disability.
	  a. Exhibit therapeutically accepting attitude and behaviors toward the patient and family.
	  b. Give repeated, specific, accurate information about abilities, strengths and potentials.
	  c. Give patient/family opportunities to participate in planning and implementing care.
	  d. Provide opportunity for patient/family to express feelings about disability and resulting limitation, *e.g.,* how this will affect life-style and future plans.
	  e. Give verbal recognition for successful coping strategy.
	  f. Identify with patient appropriate resource persons for assistance in counseling.
	  g. Use other amputee individuals as role models.
	  h. Provide a variety of experiences for patient to learn about body and self-concept, *e.g.,* recreation activities, therapeutic home visits.

C. *Is knowledgeable about nature of illness, care, and resources for continuity of care*	6. Decrease or minimize effects of phantom pain.
	  a. Explain cause of pain and expect decrease with time.
	  b. Minimize edema in stump by elastic wrap.
	  c. Teach patient to avoid guarding stump, *e.g.,* keeping leg flexed and elevated on pillow.
	  d. Expect participation in rehabilitation program in spite of pain.
	  e. Give mild pain relief medication as ordered but avoid long-term use.
	7. Teach/counsel patient to:
	  a. Assume responsibility for stump care and prosthesis
	  b. Practice ambulation
	  c. Perform activities of daily living
	8. Counsel with patient/family and use resource persons as appropriate.
	  a. Understanding of disability
	  b. Realistic expectations of rehabilitation
	  c. Altered family roles: vocational, financial, educational
	9. Plan discharge with patient and family.
	  a. Assess continuously the need for teaching and teach skill/knowledge as needed.
	  b. Reinforce physical therapist's instructions regarding exercises and ambulation.
	  c. Assess current needs of patient and family for assistance.
	    • Initiate home health agency, public health agency, or vocational rehabilitation agency referral as needed.
	  d. Arrange for follow-up health care in outpatient clinics. Communicate with those involved in follow-up care.
	  e. Provide information about community programs, *e.g.,* handicapped basketball program.

Spinal cord injury or deficit–rehabilitation

Patient Outcome	Process

The patient functions at maximum ability in all aspects of daily living. This includes:

DESCRIPTION: Rehabilitation patients with spinal cord deficit from trauma or disease may have the following characteristics: (1) recent complete or incomplete cord damage or long term deficit without a rehabilitation program, (2) medically stable to be out of bed, and (3) experiencing psychosocial crisis.

Quadriplegic patients have cervical spinal cord deficit, lower and upper extremity paralysis or paresis and at least some movement of shoulders, arms, or legs.

Paraplegic patients have thoracic, lumbar, or sacral spinal cord deficit and lower extremity paralysis or paresis.

NURSING ASSESSMENT: In addition to the general admission assessment, the following information is especially important.

1. Assess and document sensory/motor alterations.
   a. Level/location of paresis/plegia
   b. Level/location of sensory alteration
   c. Contractures/spasticity
   d. Level of activity, *e.g.,* transfers, sitting
   e. Self-care skills including activities of daily living (ADL)
2. Assess and document physiological factors which may affect rehabilitation.
   a. Skin condition
   b. Cardiovascular status, *e.g.,* swelling
   c. Respiratory status, *e.g.,* coughing and deep breathing ability, current respiratory care program
   d. Gastrointestinal status, *e.g.,* diet history, current diet, bowel history, current bowel program
   e. Genitourinary status, *e.g.,* urine characteristics, current bladder care program. For females: last menstrual period, method of contraception. For males: epididymitis.
   f. Occurrence/history of autonomic dysreflexia
3. Assess and document psychological/intellectual status.
   a. Current understanding of disability
   b. Psychological reaction to spinal cord injury
   c. Self-concept and body image
   d. Current coping strategy and resources
   e. Knowledge base and motivation for learning
4. Assess and document socioeconomic status.
   a. Funding sources for equipment and training
   b. Occupation/vocation
   c. Family role
   d. Home evaluation, *e.g.,* architectural barriers

A. *Is free of or has minimal effects or complications*

INTERVENTION:

1. Provide and teach prevention of stress to vertebral fracture or cord damage area through:
   a. Immobilization of area with prescribed brace, corset, cervical collar or halo
   b. Proper methods of movement and transfers; activity restrictions
   c. Early activity, *e.g.,* up in wheelchair
   d. Reassurance that patient can function safely within prescribed restrictions

• *Skin*

2. Maintain skin care program. See Chapter 2 Skin Care Guidelines, p. 31.
   a. Provide and teach patient/family preventive skin care.
      • Inspect skin morning and night. Teach to use skin inspection mirror.
      • Give gentle circular massage to any reddened or ischemic areas.
      • Bathe daily—if dry skin, every other day may be enough.
      • Apply lotion to dry skin. Use foot soaks or moist wraps daily until dry skin removed.
      • Do not use powder on skin.
      • Lift to turn q 2 hours or prone as tolerated.
      • Tilt back/lift up or lean/push up every 15 minutes while sitting in wheelchair.
      • Reposition p.r.n. to prevent shearing.
      • Take safety precautions during activities, *e.g.,* transfers.
      • Avoid tight clothing and inspect potentially constrictive devices frequently, *e.g.,* leg bag straps, splints, elastic stockings, condom catheter.
      • Use footwear for protection.
      • Avoid exposure to extremes of temperature, *e.g.,* hot water, heating pad, freezing weather.
      • Maintain well-balanced high-protein diet with 2500 cc intake daily minimum.

Patient Outcome	Process
	b. Teach cause of pressure sores, prevention and care of ischemic areas.
	c. Provide appropriate equipment, *e.g.*, seat cushion, air mattress, booties.
	d. Give therapeutic skin care if breakdown is present.
	e. Eliminate all pressure on any red area or breakdown area for 24 to 48 hours.
• *Bowel*	3. Establish bowel care routine.
	a. Take bowel history.
	b. Discuss program goals and routine with patient.
	c. Assure empty bowel at onset of program.
	d. Give suppository q.o.d. within 30 minutes after evening meal. Alternate routines are daily or every third day or after breakfast.
	e. Give stool softeners and laxative as ordered by physician. Time effect of oral medications to coincide with anal stimulation. May use tracer substance (iron dye, etc.) to determine time oral medication eliminated.
	f. Provide well-balanced diet to include fruits, vegetables, whole grains.
	g. Provide adequate fluid intake of 2500 cc daily.
	h. Use digital stimulation as indicated to initiate or complete bowel evacuation.
	i. Assist patient to use commode instead of bedpan as soon as able.
	j. Keep bowel record.
	k. Teach patient and family:
	• How spinal cord injury affects bowel emptying
	• Bowel routine most effective for patient
	• How to carry out bowel routine
	• Medications
	• Treatment for occasional diarrhea or constipation
	• How to modify routine to meet needs at home
• *Urinary*	4. Establish bladder care routine.
	a. Provide indwelling catheter care. See Chapter 2 Bladder Care Guidelines, p. 23.
	b. Institute program of intermittent catheterization.
	• Check urological evaluation.
	• Maintain intake and output program.
	• Discuss program goals and routines with patient and family.
	• Trigger voiding prior to catheterization.
	• Measure post-voiding residual.
	• Determine patient's emotional and physical ability to catheterize self.
	• Demonstrate catheterization until patient is capable of performing independently.
	• Provide protective pants and/or absorbent pad p.r.n. for female patient to wear between catheterizations.
	c. Assist patient to void.
	• Stimulate reflex voiding, *e.g.*, tapping abdomen.
	• Use Credés method for patient with lower motor neuron bladder.
	d. Give condom catheter care if needed. See Chapter 2 Bladder Care Guidelines, p. 23.
	• Remove condom daily for skin care.
	• Attach condom to leg bag when patient is mobile and attach to large drainage bag for bed use.
	• Tape condom to leg to prevent pulling or to abdomen when patient is prone.
	e. Teach patient/family:
	• Urinary tract structure and function
	• How spinal cord injury affects micturition
	• Routine diagnostic tests, *e.g.*, IVP, urodynamics
	• Medications
	5. Provide and teach care related to prevention of urinary tract infection.
	a. Routine Foley catheter care; remove catheter as soon as possible.
	b. Cap and cleanse tip of catheter and tubing when connecting to bedside drainage bag/leg bag.
	c. Change drainage bags weekly; clean bags daily.
	d. Encourage fluid intake of 3000 cc daily with indwelling catheter; 2400 cc daily with intermittent catheterization program; at least 2000 cc daily when adequate bladder emptying without catheterization is achieved.

Patient Outcome	Process
	e. Provide acid ash diet with citrus fruit or juice three times weekly maximum; encourage cranberry juice; apple or grape juice acceptable.
	f. Ensure regular bladder emptying without overdistension.
	g. Observe urine characteristics at least q 8 hours.
	h. Teach signs and symptoms of urinary tract infection and its prevention.
	i. Measure pH of urine every morning.
	j. Send urine for culture and sensitivity weekly for patient with indwelling catheter or intermittent catheterization. Urinalysis monthly.
	k. Instruct regarding signs and symptoms requiring medical assistance.
	6. Provide and teach measures to prevent calculi formation.
	a. Limit calcium intake, especially dairy products to 1 to 2 daily until patient is up in the wheelchair regularly.
	b. Sit upright in wheelchair as soon as possible.
	c. Encourage adequate fluid intake of 2500 to 3000 cc daily.
	d. Ensure regular emptying of bladder.
	e. Remove Foley catheter as soon as possible.
	f. Observe urine characteristics, especially sediment or calculi.
	g. Report abdominal/flank pain or persistent autonomic dysreflexia.
	h. Send urine for analysis monthly and for serum calcium at least twice weekly if patient is hypercalcemic.
	i. Provide acid ash diet with limitation of citrus fruits and juices to three times weekly.
	j. Measure pH of urine every morning.
	k. Give urinary acidification medication.
• *Respiratory*	7. Provide preventive care for patients with high thoracic/cervical deficit to avoid respiratory complications. See Chapter 2 Pulmonary Care Guidelines, p. 29.
	a. Teach deep breathing and coughing exercises.
	b. Assist patient in use of respiratory aids b.i.d.
	c. Teach family coughing and percussion techniques.
	d. Teach signs and symptoms of respiratory complications. Discuss increased susceptibilities, *e.g.*, common cold, episode of prolonged immobility, general anesthesia.
• *Circulatory*	8. Promote adequate peripheral circulation.
	a. Provide and teach:
	• Range of motion exercises
	• Antiembolic hose as indicated
	• Avoidance of prolonged sitting with legs crossed
	• Avoidance of external constriction, *e.g.*, tight leg bag strap, tight clothing.
	• Medication
	• Observation for edema, redness, changes in skin temperature
	9. Provide and teach prevention of postural hypotension when getting out of bed.
	a. Gradually elevate head (may require 20 to 30 minutes prior to getting out of bed). Take blood pressure before and after getting out of bed for first time, then q 5 minutes until stable.
	b. Apply thigh-high pressure gradient hose or elastic wraps.
	c. Consider abdominal binder or corset (until not needed).
	d. Dangle (head of bed 90° with feet down) patient 30 minutes before first time out of bed.
	e. Tilt back in chair, use of reclining wheelchair, elevation of legs in wheelchair or lowering head in bed.
	f. Teach patient and family
	• What is postural hypotension, cause and symptoms
	• Possibility of recurrence if patient is on prolonged bed rest
	• Possible hypotensive effects of medication
• *Musculoskeletal*	10. Maintain normal joint range of motion.
	a. Position correctly to maintain body alignment.
	b. Give range of motion exercises.
	c. Use footboard to keep linens from pulling feet downward.
	d. Use prone position for sleeping for patients with adequate respiratory function.
	e. Apply positioning devices as prescribed.
	f. Teach patient to wear shoes.

Patient Outcome	Process

	11. Decrease/control spasticity.
	    a. Teach cause, benefits, and hazards of spasticity.
	    b. Reinforce techniques taught by physical and occupational therapists used to relieve spasticity.
	    c. Give medication as ordered. Teach about medication.
	    d. Encourage use of safety belt.

• *Sexual activity*	12. Counsel and teach patient/family about sexual functioning.
	    a. How spinal cord injury affects sexual function including fertility.
	    b. Available resources for sexual information and counseling for patient and partner, if desired.
	    c. Alternative sexual activities and physical care concerns related to sexual function, *e.g.,* managment of bladder function, positioning, spasms
	    d. Specific gynecological/genitourinary needs: (Provide assistance as necessary.)
	      • Female patient needs pelvic examination and Pap smear annually and appropriate contraception if desired. Discuss effects of spinal cord injury on pregnancy, labor, and delivery.
	      • Male patient with ejaculation needs sperm examination.

• *Pain control*	13. Provide and teach pain management.
	    a. Explain cause, commonality, and expected improvement for patient with dysesthesia, *e.g.,* severely heightened sensation and pain in finger tips or burning in legs.
	    b. Discuss frequent short-term occurrence of pain related to increased activity following immobilization, *e.g.,* neck muscle pain for first week after halo brace is removed.
	    c. Wean patient from immobilizing device (collar, brace) while adjusting to increased activity.
	    d. Discuss disadvantages of surgical or pharmacologic treatment of dysesthesia or pain related to disuse.
	    e. Continue rehabilitation program in spite of dysesthesia and pain related to disuse unless otherwise ordered by physician.
	    f. Consider use of relief measures such as transcutaneous nerve stimulators, application of heat.

• *Skeletal*	14. Provide and teach measures to minimize effects of osteoporosis.
	    a. Get out of bed as soon as possible.
	    b. Provide safe activity and exercise to prevent fractures.
	
	15. Teach patient and family about loss of calcium from bone.

• *Dysreflexia*	16. Provide and teach intervention for autonomic dysreflexia for patients injured above T_5.
	    a. Recognize signs and symptoms.
	      • Elevated BP
	      • Slow heart rate
	      • Throbbing headache
	      • Flushing, blotching, or pallid above level of injury (may be asymmetrical)-
	      • Chills (usually without fever)
	      • Stuffy nose
	      • ''Goose bumps''
	      • Sweating above level of injury
	    b. Treat signs and symptoms.
	      • Sit patient up or raise head of bed.
	      • Check BP and P. Monitor until returned to normal.
	      • Observe urine output and check for bladder distension: irrigate catheter.
	      • Empty bladder by changing occluded catheter or catheterizing as needed.
	      • Check for fecal impaction; if present, insert anesthetic ointment and remove impaction.
	      • Get medical assistance as needed.
	    c. Teach patient and family:
	      • What is autonomic dysreflexia and causes
	      • Signs and symptoms
	      • Prevention
	      • Plan for treatment at home

Patient Outcome	Process

• *Temperature control*	17. Prevent/control hypo-/hyperthermia for patients with deficit above T_5:
	   a. Teach patient and family:
	     • Mechanism of body temperature regulation and effects of spinal cord injury on regulation
	     • Reason for occurrence only above the level of the deficit and that it is different from diaphoresis secondary to autonomic dysreflexia
	     • Need for increased fluid intake during hot weather or fever to replace fluid loss
	     • Control of environmental temperature, *e.g.,* avoidance of prolonged exposure to freezing or hot weather, proper room temperature.
	     • Proper hygiene and sponging dry if diaphoresis occurs.

B. *Is coping with disability*	18. Assist patient to cope with disability.
	   a. Help patient/family to accept self by demonstrating acceptance.
	   b. Give repeated, specific, accurate information about abilities, strengths, and potentials.
	   c. Give patient/family opportunities to participate in planning and implementing care.
	   d. Provide opportunity for patient/family to express feelings about disability and resulting limitation, *e.g.,* how this will affect life-style and future plans.
	   e. Identify patient's grieving process and intervene appropriately.
	   f. Give verbal recognition for successful coping strategy.
	   g. Identify with patient resource persons for assistance in counseling, *e.g.,* social worker, chaplain, psychologist.
	   h. Provide opportunities for patient to make decisions about environment, *e.g.,* arrangement of belongings in room, temperature, lighting. Identify with patient things he can control and areas of independence.
	   i. Utilize other spinal cord injury individuals as role models.
	   j. Provide a variety of experiences for patient to learn about body and develop positive self-concept, *e.g.,* trips outside rehabilitation center, therapeutic home visits, wheelchair athletics, and recreation activities.
	   k. Provide information and feedback about assertiveness. Assist patient to modify behavior that is too passive or too aggressive.

C. *Is knowledgeable about nature of disability, self-care and resources for continuity of care*	19. Teach patient and family about:
	   a. Structure and function of spinal cord
	   b. Effects of spinal cord injury
	   c. Area/level of patient's bone and nerve damage
	20. Teach patient and family activities of daily living which include:
	   a. Feeding
	   b. Bathing (include tub, shower, shampoo)
	   c. Dressing/undressing (include dressing in wheelchair)
	   d. Grooming
	   e. Transfers, *e.g.,* bed, car, commode
	   f. Community skills, *e.g.,* use of telephone, elevator
	   g. Care of belongings and environment, *e.g.,* washing clothes, making bed
	   h. Homemaking
	   i. Use of adaptive equipment for activities of daily living
	21. Reinforce Physical Therapy and Occupational Therapy teaching to include:
	   a. Wheelchair manipulation safety and maintenance
	   b. Use of handsplint for quadriplegics
	   c. Communication skills, *e.g.,* writing, typing
	   d. For paraplegics and incomplete quadriplegics:
	     • Brace applications
	     • Brace and crutch ambulation
	     • Skin observation
	22. Counsel with patient/family and use resource persons as appropriate, *e.g.,* vocational rehabilitation counselors.
	   a. Understanding of disability
	   b. Realistic expectations of rehabilitation
	   c. Altered family roles: financial, vocational, educational
	23. Plan home care with patient and family.
	   a. Teach all aspects of care for therapeutic leave from rehabilitation center.
	     • Assure care will be adequate before allowing leave; review care and problem solve after patient returns.

Patient Outcome	Process
	b. Provide comprehensive teaching with written materials. Document learning and motivation status.
	c. Collaborate with public health nurse and other health team members in evaluation of home environment.
	• Assist in making decisions about home modifications if needed.
	d. Discuss with family feasibility of home care and alternatives.
	e. Share decision made by Physical and Occupational Therapy for needed equipment with patient and family.
	f. Arrange for clinic follow-up and communicate with those involved in follow-up care.
	g. Initiate interagency referral.
	h. Discuss community resources, activities, and barriers.
	• Attitudinal, social barriers/resources/supports
	• Architectural barriers/accessibility
	• Driver evaluation/adaptive equipment
	• Transportation, *e.g.,* wheelchair, taxi, airlines
	• Current legislation concerning disabled persons
	• Literature, *e.g., Accent on Living, Paraplegia*

Total hip and knee replacements—rehabilitation

Patient Outcome	Process

The patient functions at maximum ability in all aspects of daily living. This includes:

DESCRIPTION: Patients needing rehabilitative care following total hip or knee joint replacement are often elderly. They may have a long history of degenerative joint disease (usually arthritis), causing pain and decreased mobility.

NURSING ASSESSMENT: In addition to the general admission assessment, the following information is especially important.
1. Assess and document physical and mental status.
   a. Ability to perform self-care skills
   b. Level of activity, *e.g.,* transfer
   c. Use of assistive devices
   d. Condition of surgical wound, *e.g.,* infection, hematoma
   e. Pain
   f. Peripheral circulation, *e.g.,* warmth, color, pulses, capillary refill
   g. Skin condition
   h. Functional limitations due to other involved joints
   i. Bowel and bladder habits
   j. Respiratory status
   k. Mental clarity
2. Assess and document patient's response to information about the disease process and treatment.
   a. Expectations regarding relief of pain and improvement in mobility
   b. Emotional readiness to participate in rehabilitation program
      • Family support
3. Assess and document patient's understanding of disease process and treatment.
4. Assess and document home environment.
   a. Need for assistive equipment, *e. g.,* walker, elevated commode
   b. Architectural barriers, *e.g.,* stairs
   c. Home supervision/support

INTERVENTION:

A. *Is gaining mobility*

• *Mobility*

1. Assist the patient to gain optimum mobility.
   a. Maintain body alignment. Refer to guidelines for Total Hip Replacement, p. 229, or Total Knee Replacement, p. 233 as needed for specific aspects of positioning.
   b. Teach aspects of positioning to patient/family, *e.g.,* no pillows under affected knee, thigh.
   c. Provide and teach range of motion exercises.
   d. Establish activity program with patient, physician and physical therapist.
      • Reinforce teaching by physical therapist in exercise program.
      • Supervise patient's participation providing assistance as indicated.
         Knee exercises, partial weight bearing with assistive devices, gait training
         Stress importance of following recommendations for weight bearing.
         Involve family as appropriate.
         Evaluate progress with patient.
   e. Observe for and teach signs and symptoms of dislocation of joint.
      • Pain in joint
      • May hear or feel "popping"
      • Change in leg length (shortening)

• *Comfort*

   f. Teach self-care skills related to activities of daily living.
   g. Establish pain control plan with physician and patient.
      • Emphasize to patient and family that it requires time to achieve the expected relief from pain and improvement in mobility.
      • Expect patient to participate in activities unless pain is severe.
      • Reposition limb for comfort.
      • Give medications for relief of pain as indicated.
      • Reassess with physician and patient as needed.

• *Wound*

2. Provide wound care.
   a. Observe and report to physician signs and symptoms of infection, hematoma.
   b. Change dressings as indicated.

• *Circulatory*

3. Promote adequate peripheral circulation. Document interventions.
   a. Give range of motion exercises.
   b. Apply antiembolic hose.
   c. Avoid position of prolonged sitting with legs down or crossed.

Patient Outcome	Process
	d. Check neurovascular status in extremities at least b.i.d. Include color, temperature, sensation, pulses, capillary refill and motion.
	e. Do not place pillow under knee.
	f. Place soft cushion under heel when knee immobilized or splint is in use.
B. *Is coping with limitations*	4. Assist patient to cope with limitations.
	a. Discuss goals of rehabilitation program with patient/family.
	b. Provide opportunity for patient/family to express fears, concerns, and questions about expectations and future plans.
	c. Give positive reinforcement throughout rehabilitative phase.
	d. Provide opportunities for patient to participate in planning care.
	e. Identify with patient resource persons, *e.g.,* social worker, vocational counselors.
	f. Explore with patient changes in daily living activities, *e.g.,* driving car.
	g. Help patient to set realistic goals, *e.g.,* job placement, recreational activities.
C. *Is knowledgeable about nature of illness, self-care, and resources for continuity of care*	5. Plan discharge with patient and family.
	a. Reinforce knowledge and skills related to self-care including:
	• Activity/exercise program
	• Use of assistive devices
	• Safety measures
	• Medications with written instructions
	b. Instruct patient to report to physician signs and symptoms of wound complications, dislocation of operative joint and infections such as sore throat, or urinary tract infection.
	c. Inform patient about community agencies which may assist in continuity of care.
	d. Initiate interagency referral as needed.
	e. Give return appointment.
	f. Communicate discharge status to staff involved in continuing care.

CHAPTER XI

Guidelines for the patient undergoing therapeutic procedures

INTRODUCTION: The plan of care for the hospitalized patient often includes therapeutic procedures and treatments of an invasive nature with significant implications for nursing care. Such procedures may be the primary responsibility of the nurse or they may take place away from the patient's room and require the specialized skill of a team of highly trained individuals. Nursing interventions are essential in providing continuity of care for these patients.

In these guidelines the patient's outcome of a comfortable, safe, and expedient treatment or procedure is promoted by the described critical elements of nursing care.

Patient Outcome

Process

The patient experiences a comfortable, safe, and expedient shunt procedure.
This includes:

A. *Is prepared for procedure*

1. Explain/answer questions and listen to concerns about preprocedure preparation, procedure and postprocedure care. Information may include:
   a. **Purpose:** To provide an immediate vascular access site for dialysis procedure. This access site is more commonly used for patients with acute renal failure.
   b. **Procedure:** A shunt can be created using an artery and a vein. The vessels most commonly used are the radial artery and the cephalic vein. The procedure is carried out in the operating room, under local anesthesia, unless the patient is unable to cooperate and requires general anesthesia. A routine surgical skin prep is carried out. After a small incision, the vessels are cannulated and connected by external silastic tubing (Fig. 11-1). The wound is sutured and a dressing applied to expose a portion of tubing so that blood flow can be observed.

A-V shunt

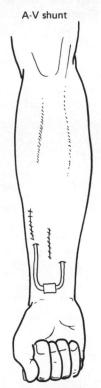

Fig. 11-1.   Arteriovenous shunt.

2. Institute immediate preparation of patient for procedure.
   a. Check for signed consent obtained by physician.
   b. Restrict diet and fluids as ordered.
   c. Apply local heat if ordered.
   d. Have patient void.
   e. Give preprocedure medication as ordered.

B. *Is free of or has minimal discomfort or complications following procedure*

3. Provide postprocedure care.
   a. Take no blood pressures, no blood samples or apply tourniquets in affected arm. Communicate importance of this to others including patient. Place sign to this effect above head of patient's bed if indicated.
   b. Observe insertion site and tubing at least q 30 minutes for first 24 hour period, then q 2 hours. Notify physician of any problems.
   c. Instruct patient/family capable of monitoring own shunt.
      • Check incision site for bleeding, swelling.
      • Auscultate cannula insertion site for bruit (buzzing sound caused by turbulent blood flow).
      • Palpate insertion site for thrill (slight vibratory sensation).
      • Observe regular light red appearance of arterial blood flowing through tubing. Darkened color and layering of cells and serum indicates clot formation.
   d. Have visible and available at bedside 2 clamps and scissors. In the event of tubing disconnection, both artery and vein must be clamped immediately.

Patient Outcome	Process

e. Use blood pressure cuff or tourniquet for hemostasis if massive hemorrhaging occurs or tubing disconnects.
f. Elevate arm on one pillow with shunt in place.
g. Avoid compression of affected arm *e.g.*, pressure created by patient lying on one side for an extended period of time and prolonged flexion of elbow.
h. Do not change dressings at site or clean or manipulate tubing. Dialysis staff will provide daily and p.r.n. dressing changes and declotting procedure.
i. Make sure patient and family have knowledge sufficient for self-care. This includes:
   • Dressing change and skin care
   • Monitoring of own shunt
   • Importance, use, and availability of clamp and scissors
   • Contacting physician immediately if any probelm occurs with shunt

| Patient Outcome | Process |

The patient experiences a comfortable, safe, and expedient blood transfusion. This includes:

A. *Is prepared for the therapy*

1. Explain/answer questions and listen to concerns about pretherapy preparation, procedure, and posttherapy care. Information may include:
   a. **Purpose:** To restore blood volume and blood counts by giving patient blood components in which he is deficient
   b. **Procedure:** Following typing and crossmatching the blood component(s) which have been collected from a compatible healthy donor are given intravenously at a slow rate. Multiple units may be given depending upon the condition and needs of the patient.
   c. **Possible reactions or complications:**
      • Chills and fever
      • Rash, hives
      • Pulmonary edema/congestive heart failure
      • Abdominal cramping (due to tetany)
      • Anaphylactic shock/reaction
          Respiratory distress, cyanosis
          Choking sensation
          Cold and clammy
          Decrease in blood pressure
          Elevation in pulse rate
          Edema
      • Serum sickness
      • Hepatitis
2. Institute preparation for therapy.
   a. Assure that typing and crossmatch have been done.
   b. Assure correct identification of blood and patient.
      • Check name, history number, blood type, blood number, and expiration date with another nurse or physician.
   c. Use appropriate infusion equipment.
      • Blood administration set with filter for whole blood, packed red cells, white cells, and plasma
      • Platelet administration set for platelets
      • Blood warmer if indicated by patient's condition
   d. Keep blood at appropriate temperature.
      • Do not refrigerate any blood components except in Blood Bank refrigerator. Remove one unit at a time from refrigerator.
      • Give fresh frozen plasma within two hours after thawing.
      • Do not refrigerate platelets or leukocytes.

B. *Is free of or has minimal discomfort or complications following therapy*

3. Provide care during transfusion.
   a. Position patient for comfort.
   b. Perform venipuncture. Refer to Intravenous Therapy guideline, p. 411 for nursing considerations relative to intravenous infusions.
   c. Check identification of blood and patient at bedside reading aloud with another nurse or physician.
   d. Observe closely for signs and symptoms of adverse reactions.
   e. Administer at slow rate as ordered.
   f. Initiate measures if reaction occurs:
      • Stop transfusion. Keep vein open with normal saline using new administration set.
      • Monitor vital signs.
      • Notify physician.
      • Monitor urinary output and characteristics.
      • Send to Blood Bank per hospital policy.
      • Sample of patient's blood
      • Remainder of transfusion and container
      • Urine specimen
      • Appropriate documentation of events
4. Provide posttherapy care.
   a. Continue to monitor for delayed reactions.
   b. Provide reassurance.

Electroconvulsant therapy (ECT)

Patient Outcome	Process

The patient experiences comfortable, safe, and expedient electro-convulsant therapy. This includes:	1. Explain/answer questions and listen to concerns about pretherapy preparation, therapy and posttherapy care. Correct misconceptions and allow opportunity to share feelings about treatment. Information may include:
	  a. *Purpose:* To interrupt the current maladaptive behaviors (symptoms) so as to facilitate the learning of new, adaptive behaviors.
	  b. *Procedure:* The patient is taken to a special treatment room which contains a stretcher and medical equipment. An anesthetist, a physician, and a nurse are present throughout the procedure. The patient is asked to lie supine on the stretcher. An IV needle is placed in the patient's arm to allow the giving of a sedative and muscle relaxant. After the patient is asleep a small amount of electrode paste and an electrode are placed on each temple. A calculated amount of electric current suited to the patient's age, sex, and physical status is allowed to pass through the electrodes. The anesthetist assists the patient to breathe using a bag and mask until the patient becomes responsive. After completion of the treatment the respiratory equipment and the IV are removed.
	    There should be no pain except for the brief discomfort of the IV injection. The treatment usually lasts about 10 minutes, after which the patient is assisted to a side-lying position and moved to a special room for the recovery period during which pulse and respirations are monitored frequently. Patients may feel sleepy and temporarily disoriented. Within a half hour, the patient should regain alertness and is then returned to the ward via wheelchair where he may wish to rest or resume activities.

	2. Assess and document baseline physical-mental status:
	  a. Level of orientation to person, place self, time
	  b. Current functional ability (include assistance needed in activities of daily living.)

A. *Is prepared for study*	3. Institute immediate preparation of patient:
	  a. Check for signed consent obtained by physician.
	  b. Check that medical workup, reports of CBC/urinalysis, EKG, blood chemistries, radiographs of chest and spine are in patient's chart.
	  c. Give n.p.o. after midnight.
	  d. Give premedication (atropine), a half hour before treatment.
	  e. Have patient void before leaving for treatment.
	  f. Check that clothing is loose fitting, *e.g.,* nightgown, open collar (to facilitate resuscitation).
	  g. Check that no socks or hose are worn. Slippers will be removed in treatment room.
	  h. Remove dentures, eye glasses, hearing aids, jewelry of any sort.
	  i. Check that patient has no chewing gum.
	  j. Remove makeup or nail polish if necessary.

	4. Prepare treatment room for patient and procedure.
	  a. Schedule patient for ECT according to priorities, including anxiety and physical status.
	  b. Check ECT machine for proper functioning.
	  c. Check that physical preparation of patient was completed.
	  d. Clean site of electrode placement.
	  e. Take vital signs and record.
	  f. Apply electrode paste to each of patient's temples.
	  g. Hold electrodes after placement by physician.
	  h. Assist as needed throughout the procedure to insure patient safety.
	  i. Remove intravenous infusion.
	  j. Assist in turning patient to side and transport to appropriate room for recovery.

B. *Is free of or has minimal discomfort or complications following therapy*	5. Provide posttherapy care.
	  a. Monitor and record physiologic response q 5 minutes during recovery phase.
	    • Color, pulse, respiration; compare with baseline vital signs.
	    • Level of consciousness
	  b. Provide comfort measures, as needed.
	  c. Transport patient via wheelchair to ward when responsive and able to sit unaided.
	  d. Report patient status to charge nurse if staff member has not been present during treatment.
	6. Encourage patient to resume his normal activities as soon as possible. Nursing activities include:
	  a. Assess level of orientation to place, self, time and level of functioning. Compare with baseline.
	  b. Assist patient according to lack of functions.

Patient Outcome	Process

	c. Intervene for patients who are confused during the first several hours post-ECT.
	   • Reorient patient to person delivering care; what is being done; give clear directions.
	   • Reassure that effects are temporary.
	   • Avoid unnecessary disturbances:
	     Visitors
	     Telephone
	d. Encourage patient to relax and stay in bed until he is capable of functioning without close surveillance/assistance.
	e. Offer comfort measures as appropriate for headache, muscle aches.

Patient Outcome	Process

PREFACE: This guideline is applicable to the patient receiving any intravenous therapy except total parenteral nutrition.

The patient experiences safe and comfortable intravenous therapy. This includes:

1. Institute preparation for therapy.
   a. Assure that patient is informed by physician or nurse that an intravenous (IV) is needed and reason(s).

A. *Is prepared for therapy*

   b. Ascertain patient's understanding and concerns about IV therapy. This includes:
      • What an IV is
      • Why it is important
      • Whether this IV will be short-term or long-term
      • Sensations patient will feel as needle is inserted
      • Procedures to be performed
   c. Answer patient's questions and obtain verbal agreement to accept therapy.
   d. Assess general condition of the patient as it relates to intravenous therapy. Considerations include:
      • Mental status
      • Illnesses such as seizure disorders, long-term illness requiring prolonged IV therapy
      • Presence of other invasive lines
      • Projected activity level
   e. Interview patient for:
      • Allergies, including povidone-iodine
      • Preference of IV site (patient request is granted when possible)
   f. Assist patient in becoming as comfortable as possible prior to venipuncture.

B. *Experiences maximum safety and comfort in initiation of therapy*

2. Identify correctly:
   a. The patient by nameband and calling name on approach.
   b. The IV fluid (with or without admixtures) using physician orders. Check container label.
3. Prepare equipment and work area:
   a. Wash hands before working with each patient.
   b. Examine fluid container for particles, leakage, cracks in glass, expiration date.
   c. Check administration set for defects such as missing sterile covers.
   d. Prepare administration set for use according to manufacturer's instructions.
4. Select venipuncture site and device by considering the following:
   a. Condition of the vein:
      • Geriatic patient with fragile veins:
         Consider not using tourniquet if vein is palpable or visible (prevents excessive bleeding when vein entered with needle).
      • Veins that ''roll'' or that are extremely elastic:
         Hold skin over venipuncture site securely.
         Loosen tourniquet after vein selected. Reapply only when ready to perform venipuncture.
         Use direct venipuncture method rather than indirect.
      • Forearm veins sclerosed with lower veins free of complications:
         Insert IV device in nonsclerosed vein area with end of device directed toward hand rather than toward body.
      • Veins that are difficult to palpate or visualize:
         Apply warm compresses to entire extremity for 20 minutes.
         Tap proposed venipuncture site gently.
         Moisten area with alcohol swab (shininess may make vein visible).
         Lower the extremity below heart level.
      • Veins into which catheters are not easily advanced:
         After tip of catheter has been inserted into vein begin the infusion of solution and advance catheter as solution flows.
      • Already impaired circulation which may be further impaired by tourniquet or IV.
   b. Areas to avoid: Inner aspect of wrist and lower extremities without physician's permission.
   c. Specific contraindication for use of certain sites. Signs should be posted at head of bed. Examples:
      • Traumatized extremities
      • Extremities with impaired circulation
      • Paralyzed extremities
      • Replants

Patient Outcome	Process

- Arteriovenous fistula or shunt
- Parathyroid transplant
- Radical mastectomy

d. Type of fluid, medications to be administered. Examples:
  - Routine: 20-gauge catheter
  - Blood, rapid infusions of large volumes of solutions: 18-gauge catheter
  - Amphotericin B: 23-gauge catheter
  - Paraldehyde: Any scalp vein needle

e. Duration of IV therapy: Scalp-vein needles are used for short-term therapy (12 hours or less).

f. Patient's preference

5. Consider using a local anesthetic according to hospital policy to make venipuncture less painful when large gauge catheter is used or when patient is especially apprehensive. *Check for allergy to medication* before administration.

6. Prepare venipuncture site:
   a. Shave hair if excessive and patient permits.
   b. Cleanse skin using povidone-iodine preparation for these reasons:
     - Bactericidal and fungicidal
     - Action more rapid than alcohol
     - Continued release of free iodine
   c. Use expanding circular motion when cleansing area to prevent carrying of bacteria over venipuncture site. Do not touch site after preparation.

7. Perform venipuncture according to established procedure in hospital.
   a. Discard each needle or catheter after one use.
   b. Maintain sterility of equipment.
   c. Apply sterile Band-Aid or 2 × 2 dressing at IV site. Secure with tape as needed.
   d. Apply covered armboard to prevent motion if IV crosses joint area.

8. Consider the use of restraints for patients unable to protect own IV site.

9. Provide routine maintenance to achieve goals of therapy.
   a. Periodic inspection of patient and IV devices:
     - Height of drip chamber: 30'' above level of heart
     - Solution: proper type, quantity, temperature (refrigerated solution may cause venous spasm), proper rate of flow
     - Tubing: closed system, free of kinks, excessive air, clotted blood
     - Control clamps: adjusted to allow proper flow
     - Needle/catheter: properly aligned with vein-check that bevel is not resting against wall of vein or valve.
     - Extremity: positioned so that blood circulation and flow of solution are unimpeded
     - IV site appropriate and clean
     - Dressing: clean and intact

C. *Experiences minimal or no complications related to therapy*

   b. Routine care:
     - Change infusion sites and tubing:
       Continuous peripheral infusion, q 48 hours
       Heparin lock and heparin drip infusion, q 4 days.
     - Change dressings using sterile technique at appropriate intervals: Central IV catheters (CVP, subclavian, jugular) three times a week.
       Heparin lock, heparin drip, q 48 hours
       Wet, soiled dressing: as needed
     - Change administration set any time site or dressing is changed.
     - Wash patient's hand and change armboard daily.

10. Take preventive measures to avoid complications of IV therapy. Provide treatment if complications occur.
    a. Infiltration:
      - *Symptoms:* Swelling over site (compare extremities)
      - *Prevention:* No impaired circulation in extremity used for IV therapy, *i.e.,* proper taping, no blood pressure cuffs, use of IV armboard, restraints properly applied
      - *Treatment:* Remove IV; apply warm compresses, elevate extremity.
    b. Phlebitis:
      - *Symptoms:* Red, warm, painful, hard cord-like vein

Patient Outcome	Process
	• *Prevention:* Use of armboards, proper administration rate and dilution of medications (as recommended by manufacturer), periodic site change
	• *Treatment:* Remove IV; apply warm compresses.
	c. Clotted needle and/or tubing:
	• *Symptoms:* Infusing slowly or stopped, possible traces of blood in tubing.
	• *Prevention:* Maintain fluid in container; keep air filter dry; keep in-line filter free from obstruction by particles or air.
	• *Treatment:* Change extension tubing if necessary; do not irrigate. If infusion does not resume, remove IV.
	d. Loose connection between parts of administration set:
	• *Symptoms:* IV site dressing wet or bloody
	• *Prevention:* Make connections secure by twisting 90° when attached.
	• *Treatment:* Change tubing.
	e. Local infection at site:
	• *Symptoms:* Purulent drainage from IV site, usually after IV removed.
	• *Prevention:* Proper skin preparation, maintain sterility of administration set, IV catheter or needle, and solution.
	f. Allergic reaction to IV infusion:
	• *Symptoms:* Rash, hives, headache, itching, chills, fever
	• *Prevention:* Obtain history of any previous allergic reactions.
	• *Treatment:* Discontinue infusion but keep IV open and notify physician.
	g. Fluid overload:
	• *Symptoms:* Dyspnea, frothy sputum
	• *Prevention:* Maintain ordered rate of infusion, assess patient's renal and cardiovascular status.
	• *Treatment:* Decrease rate of infusion to minimum to maintain patency of vein and notify physician.
	h. Septicemia:
	• *Symptoms:* Fever, symptoms of shock
	• *Prevention:* Maintain sterility of IV solution and supplies. Eliminate openings in the system.
	• *Treatment:* Start new IV in new site using sterile equipment and solution. Remove old IV and save for culture. Notify physician.

Iodine[131] *therapy for thyroid cancer*

Patient Outcome	Process
The patient experiences comfortable, safe, and expedient Iodine[131] *therapy. This includes:*	1. Explain/answer questions and listen to concerns about pretherapy preparation, procedure, and posttherapy care. Information may include:
	a. *Purpose:* To irradiate metastatic thyroid tissue.
	b. *Procedure:* The patient is given a large amount (based on extent of metastasis) of Iodine[131] by mouth in Nuclear Medicine. Following the dose the patient is monitored daily for radiation level.
A. *Is prepared for therapy*	2. Institute immediate preparation of patient for the therapy. Patient must be in private room until radiation level is safe.
B. *Is free of or has minimal discomfort or complications following therapy*	3. Provide posttherapy care.
	a. Maintain strict isolation until radiation level is safe in room as determined by Radiation Safety (usual time range is 12 hours to three days). See Isolation Manual for specifics of care.
	• Permit no visitors in room.
	• Notify Radiation Safety and Nuclear Medicine technologist immediately of any complication after dose administration.

NOTE: Restrict pregnant personnel from caring for patient.

Patient Outcome	Process

The patient experiences a comfortable, safe, and expedient leukapheresis. This includes:

1. Explain/answer questions and listen to concerns about pretherapy preparation, procedure, side effects, and posttherapy care. Information initially given by physician and oncology nurse clinician may include:

   a. *Definition:* Leukapheresis is a process by which blood is separated mechanically into its various components. Using peristaltic pumps, the desired component is collected and the remaining components are returned to the patient. The procedure may be repeated multiple times depending on the clinical circumstances.

   b. *Purposes:*
   - Therapeutic
     To collect white blood cells from healthy individuals for transfusion into leukopenic patients
     Removal of various blood components in a variety of patient populations, *i.e.,* leukemia, polycythemia, thrombocytosis, hyperviscosity
     Collection of lymphocytes to make a vaccine for immunotherapy
   - Research: To analyze blood components of healthy individuals and those with disease

   c. *Procedure:* The procedure takes place in the Leukapheresis Laboratory with the patient in a bed or chair. Using a #14 or #16 size needle, venipunctures are made in the antecubital fossa in one arm and in the lower arm in the other. These needles are attached to tubing that carries the blood to and from the machine. Prior to the procedure, the entire closed system is primed with heparinized saline and the patient receives intravenous heparin. The patient's blood is pumped into a bowl of the separator where, by centrifugal force, it is separated into its various components. Through a seal at the top of the bowl, various pumps pull off the individual components. The element to be collected is separated into blood transfer bags while the remaining blood is recombined and returned to the patient. Fluid balance is maintained by either saline, blood, or plasma. The system allows safe processing of 10 to 12 liters of patient's blood in three to four hours. After the procedure, the patient may receive protamine sulfate. Pressure dressings are applied to puncture sites.

   d. *Side effects:* Possible reactions that may occur during or after the procedure include:
   - Chills and fever may occur due to allergic response which usually responds quickly to treatment.
   - A temporary anemia may occur when some of the RBC are unavoidably collected with the white cells or plasma.
   - If a transfusion is given, there is a chance of serum hepatitis.
   - Hemolysis (breaking up of RBC) can occur, although it is extremely rare.
   - Temporary bruising may occur at needle sites.
   - Weakness, dizziness, tingling, pain, or nausea

A. *Is prepared for study*

2. Institute preparation of patient for procedure.

   a. Help patient to lower anxiety and fears; that is,
   - Give patient opportunity to see machine, meet staff who will attend him during procedure, and ask questions.
   - Have patient talk with another patient who has experienced procedure.
   - Encourage family to be present during procedure if this is a source of support to patient.
   - Inform patient of multiple safety measures to prevent any accidental problem during the procedure.

   b. Tell patient of his involvement in preparation and procedures.
   - Try to get a good night's rest so procedure won't be too tiring.
   - Eat a good breakfast but restrict fluids as this reduces the need to void during procedure.
   - Void just before the procedure is begun.
   - Remove constricting jewelry, since some edema may occur.
   - During the procedure, the patient:
     May move around in bed and have the head of the bed elevated
     Must keep the arms straight if the needles are in the anticubital fossa. The arms can be moved with caution.
     May eat or smoke
     May read or watch TV if desired
   - Should inform the staff immediately of any unusual feelings such as weakness, dizziness, numbness or tingling, pain, or nausea.

   c. Provide immediate preparation of patient for procedure.
   - Avoid venipunctures in antecubital fossae in both arms.

Patient Outcome	Process
	• Notify physician or oncology nurse clinician about patients who may require sedation during procedure.
	• Limit fluids on the morning of procedure.
	• Send blood slips with chart as all blood work for the day will be drawn during the procedure.
	• Check if patient is anemic, blood should be typed and crossmatched and blood ready at the blood bank.
	• Schedule no other studies on same day except for emergencies since procedure takes four to five hours.
B. *Is free of or has minimal discomfort or complications following therapy*	3. Provide comfort measures during procedure. (Procedure is not painful but length of time can result in patient being very tired and uncomfortable.) Staff in attendance will give:
	a. Assistance in changing positions
	b. Passive exercise of arms
	c. Back massage
	d. Heating pad
	e. Food/fluids
	f. Analgesics, p.r.n.
	4. Provide postprocedure care.
	a. Observe patient for allergic response of chills, fever, rash, bleeding under dressings. (If this occurs, it is during or soon after completion of procedure. If bleeding, apply pressure for 15 to 20 minutes. Notify physician of patient response.)
	b. Keep pressure bandages in place 8 to 10 hours.
	c. Omit taking blood pressures in either arm for 8 to 10 hours.
	d. Reassure patient that increase in thirst and decrease in urinary output as well as some edema in the hands are due to the saline used during procedure. The symptoms are only temporary.
	e. Provide food and fluids *ad lib,* unless restricted for other reasons.
	f. Provide for adequate rest.
	g. Check if patient is going home after the procedure and if from out of town that someone is available to drive patient home.
	h. Give instructions for patient to be discharged.
	• Do not shave with straight razor for 12 hours.
	• Apply ice to hematoma at needle sites for 24 hours, then warm compresses until hematoma resolves.

Patient Outcome	Process

The patient experiences a comfortable, safe, and expedient leukocyte transfusion. This includes:
 	
A. *Is prepared for therapy*
	1. Explain/answer questions and listen to concerns about pretherapy prepara[...] posttherapy care. Information may include:
	  a. ***Purpose:*** To help the leukopenic patient fight infection by transfusing le[...] from a healthy donor
	  b. ***Procedure:*** Following typing and crossmatching, the leukocytes which are collected by leukapheresis are given intravenously at a slow rate. The cells must be transfused immediately after collection.
	  c. ***Possible reactions or complications:***
	    • Chills and fever
	    • Rash, hives
	    • Pulmonary edema/congestive heart failure
	    • Anaphylactic shock/reaction
	      Respiratory distress, cyanosis
	      Choking sensation
	      Cold and clammy
	      Changes in vital signs
	2. Institute preparation for the therapy.
	  a. Assure that typing and crossmatch have been done.
	  b. Assure that CBC with differential and platelet count are done.
	  c. Have available at bedside:
	    • Oxygen equipment
	    • Ampules of Adrenalin, diphenhydramine (Benadryl), methylprednisolone (Solu-Medrol)
	    • Needles, syringes, tourniquet, alcohol sponge
	  d. Assure correct identification of patient and transfusion.
	    • Check patient's name, history number with label on transfusion container with the physician.
	  e. Use a blood administration set with a filter.
	  f. Administer transfusion as soon as leukocytes are available.

B. *Is free of or has minimal discomfort or complications following therapy*	3. Provide care during therapy.
	  a. Position patient for comfort.
	  b. Perform venipuncture. Refer to Intravenous Therapy Guidelines, p. 411.
	  c. Check identification of patient and transfusion label at bedside, reading aloud with the physician.
	  d. Administer at slow rate as ordered.
	  e. Monitor vital signs at start of transfusion and then q 15 minutes × 4, q 30 minutes × 4, and q 1 hour × 2.
	  f. Observe closely for signs and symptoms of adverse reactions and initiate measures if reaction occurs.
	    • Stop transfusion. Keep vein open with normal saline using new administration set.
	    • Monitor vital signs.
	    • Notify physician and administer medication and oxygen as ordered.
	    • Provide reassurance to patient.
	    • Document the events.
	4. Provide posttherapy care.
	  a. Continue to monitor for delayed reactions.
	  b. Relieve symptoms of reactions.
	  c. Obtain CBC with differential and platelet count one hour following transfusion and the following morning.

Patient Outcome	Process
The patient experiences a comfortable, safe, and expedient lung lavage. This includes	1. Explain/answer questions and listen to concerns about pretherapy preparation, therapy, and posttherapy care. Information may include:

The patient experiences a comfortable, safe, and expedient lung lavage. This includes

A. *Is prepared for therapy*

B. *Is free of or has minimal discomfort or complications following therapy*

1. Explain/answer questions and listen to concerns about pretherapy preparation, therapy, and posttherapy care. Information may include:
   a. *Purpose:* To remove secretions from the alveoli which may promote improvement of pulmonary function in patients with cystic fibrosis and alveolar proteinosis.
   b. *Procedure:* The patient is taken to the operating room (OR) and the procedure is carried out under general anesthesia. The patient is positioned on the side. Through an endotracheal tube, the dependent lung is infused and drained intermittently with large amounts of saline solution while the upper lung is ventilated. Repositioning may be indicated to facilitate drainage of the saline. Usually only one lung is lavaged during the procedure but some patients are able to tolerate bilateral lavage. The length of the procedure varies from 4 to 6 hours. The patient is transported to the Recovery Room to remain a few hours or overnight depending on response.
2. Institute immediate preparation of patient for the therapy.
   a. Check for signed consent obtained by physician.
   b. Assure that baseline studies are completed, *e.g.,* pulmonary function, blood gases, chest radiograph and sputum culture.
   c. Keep n.p.o. after midnight.
   d. Give care according to physician's orders and hospital routine in preparation for OR.
3. Provide posttherapy care.
   a. Maintain adequate respiratory function.
      • Give O_2 by mask following removal of endotracheal tube and stabilization of blood gases. Continue O_2 therapy usually overnight and p.r.n. thereafter.
      • Maintain arterial line for close monitoring of blood gases.
      • Observe for signs and symptoms of respiratory distress and report to physician.
      • Give IPPB t.i.d. until discharged.
      • Request physical therapy consult for chest percussion and postural drainage t.i.d.
      • Turn, cough and deep breathe q 2 hours.
      • Document amount and character of sputum daily.
      • Obtain chest radiograph immediately postlavage and p.r.n. as ordered by physician.
   b. Give full liquid diet the first night and progress diet as tolerated.
   c. Ambulate as tolerated.
   d. Provide supportive care, *e.g.,* mouth care, measures to soothe sore throat.
   e. Repeat baseline studies as ordered.
   f. Give medications as ordered, *e.g.,* antibiotics.

Patient Outcome	Process

The patient experiences a comfortable, safe, and expedient thoracentesis. This includes:

A. *Is prepared for study*

1. Explain/answer questions and listen to concerns about prestudy preparation, procedure, and poststudy care. Information may include:
   a. ***Purpose:*** (1) To detect inflammatory disease and tumors of the lung and pleura through analyzing fluid or biopsy specimen, and (2) To therapeutically relieve lung compression caused by an accumulation of air or fluid in the intrapleural space.
   b. ***Procedure:*** The procedure usually takes place in patient's room. The patient is asked to assume a sitting position, straddling a chair with the arms stretched forward resting on the back of the chair. A pillow may be used under the arm to increase the intercostal space. Alternate position: the patient sits on the bed, leaning forward with arms and head resting on an elevated overbed table.

      The patient's hospital gown is opened to expose the entire back. The physician percusses down the intercostal spaces until he identifies the fluid level indicated by a dull sound. The first interspace below the dull sound will be the puncture site.

      Antiseptic solution (feels cool to patient) is applied to skin and local anesthetic (stings) is injected. After being draped with sterile towels, the patient is instructed to hold his breath until needle insertion is completed. Since nerves and blood vessels, which supply the intercostal muscles, lie on the inferior surface of each rib, the needle will be inserted on the superior side of the rib to avoid injury to the nerves and vessels. The insertion will create a feeling of deep pressure but there should be no sharp pain.

      Fluid will be withdrawn by a syringe. Some fluid is saved and sent in specimen tubes for laboratory analyses. The remaining fluid is discarded after measurement of quantity and observation of characteristics, *e.g.*, ''600 cc of purulent, pink fluid''. Fluid removed may be serous, bloody, or purulent.

      If a biopsy is to be obtained, the needle is directed into the lung tissue. The obturator is removed and a cutting needle is inserted. The specimen is snipped and removed with the cutting needle. The obturator is replaced to facilitate removal of the needle sheath. Manual pressure is applied over the site for several minutes. A Band-Aid is applied and the patient is assisted to a reclining position.

2. Institute immediate preparation of the patient and equipment for the study.
   a. Obtain chest radiographs prior to study to determine fluid level and presence of pathology.
   b. Signed consent obtained by physician
   c. Baseline vital signs and auscultation of breath sounds
   d. Hospital gown with back opening
   e. Equipment needed for sterile procedure:
      - Thoracentesis tray
      - Antiseptic wash
      - Lidocaine (Xylocaine) anesthetic (1% or 2%)
      - Sterile gloves
      - Extra culture tubes and tape to identify tubes
      - Drainage bottle if large amount of fluid is anticipated

B. *Is free of or has minimal discomfort or complications following study*

3. Provide postprocedure care.
   a. Have patient lie on nonaffected side for one hour; then position for patient's comfort.
   b. Obtain chest radiograph within one hour following study.
   c. Check vital signs and breath sounds and compare with baseline: q 30 minutes × 3 or until stable.
   d. Observe puncture site for signs of bleeding when checking vital signs.

Patient Outcome	Process

The patient functions comfortably within limitations due to illness and therapy. This includes:

DESCRIPTION: Traction is a pulling force applied to some part of the body. The three types of traction are manual, skin, and skeletal. There are numerous reasons for the use of traction: to immobilize a body part; to reduce a fracture, dislocation or subluxation; and to maintain alignment. Other purposes include reduction of pain due to muscle spasm, nerve root compression, or prevention of contracture.

This guideline is applicable to any patient who has one or more of the following methods of traction: cervical (skin or skeletal), side arm, skin, lower extremity with special skin traction, or balanced skeletal. There may be modification of these techniques due to the available equipment and the physician's discretion.

NURSING ASSESSMENT: In addition to the general assessment, the following information is especially important.
Assess and document physical and mental status including age and related problems:
- a. General
  - Peripheral vascular status
  - Skin assessment, sensitivities to tape
  - Bowel and bladder habits
  - Smoking, drinking, drug history
  - Level of consciousness, orientation
- b. Specific body part to be immobilized:
  - Neurovascular status (color, temperature, capillary filling, sensation, motion, pulses)
  - Swelling
  - Skin condition (scars, lacerations, decubiti, skin disorders, poor hygiene)
  - Position of body part (abducted, adducted, flexed, extended, internally or externally rotated)
  - Pain (site and character)

INTERVENTION:

A. Is prepared for application of traction and immobilization

1. Explain all care related to traction application to patient and family to maximize cooperation and reduce anxiety. Prepare patient for restrictions in movement and allowed activities as appropriate.
2. Provide immediate care of area needing immobilization. Immobilize and/or elevate to reduce swelling, pain, prevent further injury. Apply ice packs as ordered.
3. Assemble equipment necessary for type of traction to be used. This may include:
   - a. Overhead frame, trapeze, side rails, bed board
   - b. Alternating pressure mattress and sheep skin to prevent skin breakdown
   - c. Weights, weight pan, rope, pulley bed attachment, spreader bar, sling, side bar, shock blocks

• Skin traction

4. Provide care for patient receiving skin traction:
   - a. Remove hair by razor or depilatory, if ordered.
   - b. Wash skin as appropriate to skin condition, pain level.
   - c. Apply skin adhesive, if ordered.
   - d. Apply straps to extremity; pad bony prominences and avoid superficial nerves and blood vessels.
   - e. Use bias cut wrap in spiral or figure of eight application. Avoid elastic bandages and circular application which can constrict nerves and blood vessels.
   - f. Never use more than 5 to 8 pounds of weight on traction because of damage to skin.
   - g. Remember that skin traction is generally not used for longer than a two week period.

• Skeletal traction

5. Prepare patient and equipment for skeletal traction.
   - a. Premedicate patient, as ordered.
   - b. Assemble tray to use in shaving area for traction. Include povidone-iodine, several sets of sterile gloves, lidocaine (Xylocaine).
   - c. Secure appropriate equipment for traction application.
     - Steinmann's pin tray and pin cutters
     - Crutchfield tongs
   - d. Remain with patient to provide emotional and physical support.
   - e. Explain procedure to patient: local anesthetic injection will sting and the purpose is to numb skin and the surface of the bone. There will be another person holding the body part steady. A small cut will be made in the skin and a sterile metal pin will be secured to the bone using a sterile surgical drill. The insertion causes a feeling of deep pressure. A pin bow, rope and

Patient Outcome	Process
	pulley system permits the proper amount of weight to be attached. As the local anesthetic wears off, the patient may experience a minor ache in the pin insertion site. This should diminish within 24 hours. Medication is available to relieve discomfort.

f. Make sure that pin corks are placed over the protruding ends of pins to protect them and the patient.

B. *Is benefiting from properly functioning traction*

6. Provide nursing care measures relevant to traction:
   a. Check traction equipment, q 8 hours and as needed.
      • Ropes should be unfrayed and in pulley tracks, not resting against pulley.
      • Knots should be secure and taped.
      • Weights should be in weight pan, suspended freely and not resting on floor or bed.
      • Vertical bar on balanced traction should not touch floor even when bed is in lowest position.
   b. Keep bed clothes and other objects away from rope and frame assembly.
   c. Do not alter or remove weights, *e.g.,* making beds, during transfer of patient, unless specifically ordered by physician. The exception is daily skin care for patients with Buck's traction.
   d. Guide weights rather than lifting during positioning of patient.
   e. Tighten knobs on frame assembly q 8 hours.
   f. Check patient's position in bed frequently. Consider the use of blocks under foot of bed to prevent patient from being pulled to end of bed.
   g. Use manual traction to hold body part if ropes break; notify physician and obtain more rope.
   h. Avoid bumping or jerking bed which may be painful to patient.
   i. Transport patient only with physician's order. Nurse or physician should accompany patient. In general, radiographs should be portable.
   j. Place head of bed away from all for cervical traction patient.

• *Buck's traction*

7. Provide care for patient with Buck's traction.
   (Purpose: Lower extremity immobilization using special skin traction.)
   a. Consider using foam "Buck's boot" for patients with fragile skin.
   b. Remove traction, inspect skin, give skin care, and reapply traction at least once daily.
   c. Tighten knobs on frame assembly q 8 hours.
   d. Prevent peroneal nerve damage:
      • Avoid wrapping over head of fibula.
      • Remove metal stay on "Buck's boot".
      • Avoid sand bags placed against lateral aspect of knee.
   e. Keep heels off bed; consider sheep skin and other skin protection under heels.
   f. Raise foot of bed 15° to prevent sliding down in bed. (Contraindicated in patients with knee problems).
   g. Assure that spreader bar does not touch skin and that rope is pulling in straight line from knee.

• *Head halter traction*

8. Provide care for patient with head halter traction.
   (Purpose: Immobilization for neck injury/pain using special skin traction)
   a. For patients with cervical instability due to trauma:
      • Have available suction and tracheostomy tray.
      • Maintain prescribed position. No pillows
   b. For patients using head halter for relief of pain:
      • May remove halter as prescribed
      • May raise and lower head of bed; use pillow for patient comfort
   c. For all patients with head halter:
      • Provide skin care under straps and inspect for reddened area q 8 hours. Halter may be slightly loosened to permit this, but maintain neck in prescribed position.
      • Prevent rope from rubbing on ears.

• *Balanced skeletal traction*

9. Provide care for patient with balanced skeletal traction.
   (Purpose: Immobilization for fractured femur.)
   a. Provide pin care once daily.
      • Remove existing 2 × 2 gauze dressing and gently remove old povidone-iodine.
      • Reapply povidone-iodine ointment to pin site and cover with new gauze dressing.
      • Report any sign of infection: redness, swelling, drainage around pin site.

Patient Outcome	Process

b. Check status of fractured leg q 8 hours.
  • Ability to dorsiflex foot
  • Numbness in foot
  • Presence of posterior tibial and dorsalis pedus pulses
c. Prevent damaging of sciatic nerve by checking thigh strap for tightness and pressure, q 8 hours.
d. Prevent peroneal nerve damage which may occur when patient rests lateral aspect of affected leg on splint for prolonged periods.
e. Check likely pressure points q 8 hours.
  • Under groin ring
  • Under popliteal fossa (knee)
  • Achilles tendon

• *Side arm traction*

10. Provide care for patient with side arm traction (Purpose: Immobilization for shoulder pain or fractured humerus). There are different techniques used in the application of side arm traction. The most common are:
  • Skin traction with shoulder externally rotated and abducted at a 90° angle and elbow flexed at 90°
  • Skeletal—skin traction with shoulder and elbow flexed as above; pin used at elbow.
a. Provide pin care once daily.
b. Rewrap skin traction once daily and p.r.n. Check skin condition.
c. Check for pain on *passive* extension of fingers which could indicate Volkmann's ischemia. Call physician immediately if indicated.
d. Assess neurovascular status q 4 hours until stable, then q 8 hours.
  • Radial nerve:
      Motor: wrist extension, abducting thumb
      Sensory: sensation in webspace between thumb space and index finger
  • Ulnar nerve:
      Motor: ability to abduct (separate) all fingers
      Sensory: sensation in little finger
  • Median nerve:
      Motor: ability to pinch thumb and little finger together
      Sensory: sensation in tip of index finger
  • Radial and ulnar pulses
e. Prevent damage to radial nerve which may occur by improper position of traction straps or pressure of arm resting on bed for prolonged periods.
f. Use techniques to keep patient positioned in middle of bed, *e.g.*, blocks under head and foot of bed on same side as traction and/or torso restraint.
g. Provide skin protection, *e.g.*, sheep skin, alternating pressure mattress.
h. Provide back care q 8 hours and as needed.
i. Prevent any alteration of traction equipment which could disrupt desired effect.
  • No movement of bed
  • All radiographs portable
  • Patient can turn toward affected side only.

• *Crutchfield tongs*

11. Provide specific equipment and care for patient with Crutchfield tongs.
  (Purpose: Immobilization of cervical fracture with special skeletal traction)
a. Have equipment available.
  • Suction
  • Tracheostomy tray
  • Head halter
  • Seven-foot bed, bed board, two bed mattresses, and one air mattress, or special frame as ordered
  • Equipment/supplies needed for preparation and insertion of tongs
b. Inspect insertion side q 8 hours for signs of inflammation, infection.
c. Provide pin care.
d. Maintain traction manually until head halter can be applied if tongs become dislodged.

• *Halo traction*

12. Provide specific equipment and care for patient with halo traction.
  (Purpose: Immobilization of cervical fracture with special skeletal traction)
a. Have equipment available:
  • Suction

Patient Outcome	Process

- Tracheostomy tray
- Equipment and supplies needed for preparation and insertion of halo

b. Inspect insertion site q 8 hours. Observe for skin folds above pins that indicate they have slipped out of bone. Check back of head for edema as result of dependent positioning.

c. Provide pin care b.i.d.; assure that physician tightens pins daily. Have two wrenches available. Be aware that patient may have sore jaws when chewing during first few days after application.

d. Alert patient to expect minimal discomfort after 24 hours. Pain is symptom of loose or infected pins.

• *Body jacket or cast*

13. Provide care for patient with body jacket or body cast.
    - Include aspects of care for patient with halo traction and in addition:
        - Keep wrenches taped to jacket/cast at all times.
        - Check skin under jacket/around edges of cast b.i.d. for redness or pressure area.
        - Observe for respiratory distress. Know how to remove jacket. Have cast saw available.
        - Take care not to get cast/jacket wet when washing patient's hair.
        - Check cast for rough edges, "petal" cast with soft material, *e.g.,* moleskin, adhesive tape.
        - Avoid placement of foreign objects down in cast which may erode skin.
        - Protect cast if needed when patient uses bedpan.

C. *Is free of or has minimal adverse effects related to immobility*

14. Promote optimal physiological functions.
    a. Check immobilized area and compare with baseline neurovascular data:
        - Color, temperature, capillary filling, motion, sensation and peripheral pulses q 1 to 2 hours × 24 hours; then q 4 hours for duration of traction. Report to physician as indicated.
    b. Provide attention to skin especially around traction site and bony prominences.
        - Check for signs and symptoms of infection around pin sites: redness, drainage, pain.
        - Provide pin care once daily:
            Wash gently with povidone-iodine.
            Apply 2 inch povidone-iodine gauze covering around pins.
        - Check skin condition at least q 8 hours especially at traction pressure points and body position pressure points (elbows, heels, sacrum, occiput).
        - Use pressure relieving equipment: fleece boots, air pressure mattress, sheepskin.
        - Provide good skin hygiene, especially in periurethral and sacral areas.
    c. Maintain peripheral circulation.
        - Check for calf redness, tenderness, swelling, warmth. Check for Homan's sign q 8 hours.
        - Teach patient and supervise performance of ankle circles q 4 hours with vital signs.
        - Apply antiembolic stockings to all patients on bedrest.
        - Institute medical management orders which may include heparin, warfarin (Coumadin), aspirin, dextran, application of heat, elevation of extremity.
    d. Provide thorough pulmonary toilet.
        - Check T, P, R, and breath sounds q 4 hours. Report signs and symptoms indicating pulmonary problems such as:
            Fat embolus: confusion, tachycardia, dyspnea, and petechiae, Usually occurs within three days after injury.
            Pulmonary embolus: dyspnea, chest pain, anxiety, tachycardia, low grade fever, low pO_2. Usually occurs within three weeks after injury.
        - Turn, cough, deep breathe, use incentive spirometry, q 2 hours × 24 hours, then q 4 hours × 48 hours, then q 8 hours for duration of traction.
        - Discourage or limit cigarette smoking.
        - Institute orders for medical management which may include ultrasonic nebulizer, humidification, IPPB treatments, chest physical therapy.
    e. Minimize muscle atrophy.
        - Provide for active and passive exercises to unaffected extremities, 2 to 4 times daily. Encourage patient to use trapeze.
        - Position patient using foot board or brace-boot. Check for proper positioning frequently.
    f. Assist patient to maintain normal bowel and bladder function.
        - Plan with patient for bowel and bladder regimen considering initial assessment, individual preferences and usual time schedule.
        - Assure adequate fluid intake: 2500 cc (unless fluid restricted) to prevent urinary calculi, stasis, dehydration.

Patient Outcome	Process

• Suggest use of fracture bedpan for patients whose restricted movements affect pelvic area.
• Check and notify physician for signs and symptoms of urinary tract infection: frequency, urgency, burning, retention. Consider color, clarity, odor and amount of urine. Send specimen for analysis, culture, and sensitivity if urinary tract infection suspected.
• Check and record bowel status, *i.e.*, amount and consistency of stools. Check for abdominal distention, absence of bowel sounds.
• Institute bowel program as needed. This may include: diet, fluids, stool softeners, laxatives.

D. *Is adjusting to immobility while achieving maximum independence*

15. Collaborate with patient to maximize independence considering current limitations. Considerations are:
    a. Need for maintenance of alignment of affected body parts
    b. Pain level and response to pain
    c. Emotional response to traction/immobility
    d. Mental status
    e. Preexisting physical limitations, *e.g.*, arthritis, other injuries.
16. Reinforce the rationale for the traction techniques being used and the patient's responsibility for maintaining the prescribed treatment.
17. Plan care and assist patient in meeting basic needs.
    a. Eating, drinking:
       • Monitor intake; encourage balanced diet to promote healing.
       • Request diet consult for patient with long-term traction or special dietary needs.
       • Assist patient to most comfortable position.
       • Place food within reach and prepare containers and food for ease of eating.
       • Offer variety of fluids to encourage intake of 2000 to 3000 cc per day.
       • For patients in supine position use straws; have suction available.
    b. Bathing:
       • Wash and gently massage back and sacrum at least once a day.
       • Cleanse body part in traction.
    c. Dressing:
       • Consider modification of undershorts, pajamas.
       • Ensure personal privacy through draping with sheets.
    d. Positioning:
       • Be aware that patient may be unwilling to turn because of fear of pain or injury to involved area.
       • Be positive and emphasize the importance of regular, careful turning.
       • Consider use of analgesics prior to turning.
    e. Comfort: Listen to patient's suggestions for comfort measures and incorporate into care plan.
18. Plan for patient's diversionary needs:
    a. Select from a variety of materials, *e.g.*, prism glasses, TV, tapes of music, literature or other narratives, written materials, contact with others, games.
    b. Consider importance of family and visitors to patient's emotional status.

F. *Is prepared for removal of traction, application of another means of immobilization, and eventual discharge*

19. Prepare patient for traction removal and application of another means of immobilization.
    a. For patient having pin removed:
       • Explain there may be momentary discomfort and a relief of pressure.
    b. For patient going to surgery:
       • Provide appropriate preoperative teaching.
       • Assure that traction site is clean.
       • Report signs of skin breakdown or infection.
    c. For patient having cast application:
       • Explain process of cast application and sensations patient will experience.
       • Transport to cast room in patient's bed.
    d. For patient having brace application:
       • Explain process of brace application. If moved to another area, transport in bed.
       • Anticipate need for post-application radiographs.
20. Obtain order for progressive mobilization beginning with tilt-table.
21. Teach appropriate discharge care.
    a. For patient using home traction:
       • Assure that patient has proper equipment or knows how to obtain it and has written instructions.

Patient Outcome	Process
	• Demonstrate traction application and care techniques. Supervise patient and/or family in technique.
	b. For patient in cast or brace.
	• Teach cast/brace and skin care, give written instructions. Supervise patient and/or family in care.
	• For patients who will have restricted mobility, suggest bowel routine to prevent constipation. See Chapter 2 Bowel Care Guidelines, p. 25.
	• Discuss activity restrictions as prescribed by physician.
	c. Emphasize the signs and symptoms to report immediately:
	• Change in neurovascular status, *i.e.,* numbness, tingling, decreased movement
	• Increased pain and swelling, foul odor, indicating infection
	• Damage of cast or brace.
	22. Consider interagency referral
	23. Assure that patient has been given return appointment for follow-up care.

APPENDIX
Evaluation Tools

INPATIENT GENERAL CARE GUIDELINES EVALUATION FORM (Patient interview/direct observation)

INSTRUCTIONS: Each item is related to one of the General Care Guidelines. Be sure that one block for each guideline has been checked. Write in patient responses on lines provided. *Always add a "Comment" when you check the "Partial" or "Not Met" blocks and when it will add meaning in understanding your answer.* Make your answers as complete and informative as possible.

INTERVIEW: Each interview item first lists the guideline to be met. Then questions are written that will help you to gather enough information to make a judgment about whether or not the guideline is met. *Do not read the guideline to the patient*; but generally ask questions as they are listed; add other questions if appropriate. If guideline is not applicable, write N/A under the blocks.

	GUIDELINE		
	MET	PARTIALLY MET	NOT MET

PATIENT'S RESPONSES

PATIENT'S OR REVIEWER'S COMMENTS

1. GUIDELINE: The patient knows about room and unit as he needs to use it ....
   QUESTIONS:
   a. Did someone explain your room and surroundings to you when you were admitted to this ward? (For instance: call system, bed, bathroom, privacy curtains, where to keep your belongings) ....
   b. When was it explained to you? ....

2. GUIDELINE: Room is arranged for patient's safe and efficient use ....
   QUESTION
   a. Are the things you need to use within reach? ....

3. GUIDELINE: Patient has had needed rest ....
   QUESTIONS:
   a. Have you been able to rest during the day and night? ....
   b. (If a. is "no") What is the reason you have not had enough rest? ....
   c. Can you think of ways that the nurses could help you to get more rest? (For instance: close the doors, adjust lighting) ....

4. GUIDELINE: Patient can describe, in general, type of diet he is receiving. ....
   QUESTIONS:
   a. What kind of diet are you receiving? ....
   b. (If it is a modified diet) Can you tell me why a special type of diet has been ordered for you? ....

5. GUIDELINE: The qualities (taste, quantity and temperature) of the food are acceptable to the patient ....
   QUESTIONS:
   a. How do you like the taste of the food? ....
   b. Is the food the right temperature when it comes to you? ....
   c. Do you get enough to eat and drink? (Note restrictions in fluid, food) ....

	GUIDELINE			
PATIENT'S RESPONSES	MET	PARTIALLY MET	NOT MET	PATIENT'S OR REVIEWER'S COMMENTS

6. GUIDELINE: Patient is prepared for and assisted with feeding as necessary ....
   QUESTIONS:
   a. Do you need any help getting ready to eat or with feeding yourself? ....
   b. Is help available when you need it? ....

7. GUIDELINE: Patient can describe, in general, the plan for dealing with his discomfort..........
   QUESTIONS:
   a. Have you been uncomfortable since being here? (pain, nausea, gas) ....
   b. Have the nurses discussed with you what can be done to help you get relief if you are uncomfortable? ....

8. GUIDELINE: The patient feels that his requests for relief of discomfort are responded to promptly ....
   QUESTIONS:
   a. When you reported your discomfort, how long did you wait before you received help? (estimate, if possible) ...
   b. Does this differ on various shifts? (explain) ....
   c. If you needed pain medication, did you receive it promptly? ....
   d. If you did not receive your medication promptly, was any reason given for the delay? ....

9. GUIDELINE: The measures for dealing with the patient's pain are effective ....
   (Check chart to identify patients with chronic pain syndrome).
   QUESTIONS:
   a. Is your pain medicine (or other measures) relieving your discomfort? ....
   b. (If a. is "no") Do the nurses assist you in other ways to deal with your discomfort? (Describe nursing measures taken). ....

10. GUIDELINE: Patient feels that his need for privacy has been respected ....
    QUESTIONS:
    a. Do you feel that the nurses have been aware of your need for privacy? ....
    b. What has been done to provide the privacy you would like? ....

11. GUIDELINE: Patient requests are responded to as promptly and completely as possible. ....
    QUESTIONS:
    a. When you have asked for something or someone to help you, how long have you had to wait? ....
    b. Is there anything that you have asked for that you were not able to get? ....
    c. (If b. is "yes") Have patient describe circumstance ....

12. GUIDELINE: Patient verbalizes that his nurses have demonstrated to him a sense of warmth, concern, and courtesy ......

QUESTIONS:

a. Do your nurses introduce themselves to you? ......
b. Do you feel you are included in conversation when nurses are in your room? ......
c. How would you describe the attitudes of the nursing staff toward you? ......

13. GUIDELINE: Patient and/or family has the opportunity to discuss worries, fears, anxieties ......

QUESTIONS:

a. Does a nurse spend time with you when you feel you would like to talk? ......

14. GUIDELINE: Patient knows about and participates in planning his/her individual care plan ......

QUESTIONS:

a. What are your daily care routines such as hygiene, activity, treatments? ......
b. Have you had a part in planning your daily care? ......
c. If you could, what changes would you make in your daily care? ......

15. GUIDELINE: Patient has received thorough information about diagnostic studies ......

QUESTIONS:

a. What tests have you had since you've been in the hospital? (Check chart for diagnostic studies) ......
b. Have you received enough information from the nurses before each test so that you felt well prepared for it? ...
   • Why you are having the test. ......
   • What would happen during the test. ......
   • Any special care required after the test ......

16. GUIDELINE: Patient/family member has knowledge of patient's health status ......

QUESTIONS:

a. Do you feel you have been kept informed about your progress? ......
b. Is there more you would like to know about your illness? ......
c. Have the nurses been helpful in answering your questions or have they tried to find answers? ......

17. GUIDELINE: Patient/family member has received thorough information regarding treatment, medications and care ......

QUESTIONS:

a. What have you been told about your treatments, medications and care?
   (Check chart to determine specific areas applicable to this patient). For example, patient should know purpose and when treatment is to be given. Describe patient's answer ......
   _____ Medications:
   _____ Activity permitted:
   _____ Treatment:
   _____ Diet:
   _____ Other care:
b. How have the nurses helped you to understand this information? ......

	GUIDELINE			
PATIENT'S RESPONSES	MET	PARTIALLY MET	NOT MET	PATIENT'S OR REVIEWER'S COMMENTS

18. GUIDELINE: Patient/Family member has knowledge of plan for continuing health care after discharge. (Check chart for discharge summary form) ....

QUESTIONS:

a. What health care will you or your family need to carry out after you leave the hospital? ....

b. How have the nurses helped you prepare for your discharge/home care? ....

OBSERVATION: Be sure to explain your answers when there is a "Partial" or "Not Met" check.

1. Patient is free of signs or symptoms requiring immediate attention (such as: pain, dyspnea).

2. Patient is identified by armband including name, history number and patient unit.

3. Patient's bed and room are free from hazards. Examples:
   a. Floor clean and dry
   b. No trash outside container, no needles left in room
   c. No electrical cords or other obstructions
   d. No medication left at bedside
   e. No unused equipment and supplies left in room

4. Patient's room and bath are clean.

5. Side rails are in place when needed by patient for turning or safety.

6. Level of bed is in low position when unattended.

7. The room is arranged to meet the patient's individual needs (right/left handed, equipment, call bell).

8. Drinking fresh, cool, and available water unless fluids are restricted

9. Patient's position is correct for proper body alignment and comfort.

10. Patient appears well-groomed and clean.

11. If patient has IV in place:
    a. Fluids are infusing.
    b. No signs of infiltration/inflammation
    c. Arm, armboard and tape clean
    d. Properly labeled

DIABETES MELLITUS EVALUATION FORM (Patient interview/direct observation)

This form is related to the patient outcomes described in the Diabetes mellitus guideline and may be used prior to and following patient teaching to measure outcomes.

DESIRED OUTCOME

MEASUREMENT CRITERIA/SOURCE	MET	NOT MET	ACCEPTABLE ANSWERS/TECHNIQUES
1. "Do you have diabetes?"			____ Yes
2. "Do you have diabetes identification?"			____ Yes ____ Wallet (minimum of one) ____ Necklace ____ Bracelet
3. "Can you tell me what you know about how long you will have diabetes?"			____ Chronic or lifelong

4. "How do you think you got your diabetes?"			____ Inherited tendency
			 ____ Precipitating factors including:
			    ____ Stress
			    ____ Obesity
			    ____ Pregnancy
			    ____ Other

5. "Tell me what your body lacks to cause diabetes?"			____ Body does not produce enough insulin
6. "What complications of diabetes are you trying to prevent?" a. Short-term b. Long-term			Short-term: (mentions one) ____ Hyperglycemia/ketoacidosis/coma ____ Hypoglycemia/insulin reaction Long-term: (mentions two) ____ Foot (or skin) ulcers (problems) ____ Loss of vision ____ Kidney failure ____ Cardiovascular
7. "What things help you control your sugar?"			____ Insulin/oral agent (consult written orders) ____ Diet ____ Exercise/activity

437

MEASUREMENT CRITERIA/SOURCE	DESIRED OUTCOME		ACCEPTABLE ANSWERS/TECHNIQUES
	MET	NOT MET	
8. "How will you collect a double void urine for testing?"			___ Need to empty bladder, wait 20 to 30 minutes, void again
9. "Why should you use this method?"			___ (Ideal) Gives more accurate reading ___ (Acceptable) Urine is "fresh" from the kidneys.
10. "How often and when do you collect and test your urine?"			___ (Ideal) Four times a day—Before meals and at bedtime ___ (Acceptable) Three times a day
11. "Show me how you test your urine." (Circle method used) • Two-drop method			*Two drop method:* ___ 2 drops urine in test tube ___ 10 drops water in test tube ___ 1 tablet in tube (without touching with fingers) ___ Recap bottle tightly. ___ Wait 15 seconds past bubbling. ___ Holding top of tube, shake it gently. ___ Accurately compare color with chart. ___ Accurately record results. ___ Rinse test tube and store upside down.
• Tes-tape method (Ginger ale may be used instead of urine to demonstrate positive test for glucose in urine.)			*Tes-tape method:* ___ Tear off 1½" of tape. ___ Close tes-tape package securely. ___ Do not touch end to be dipped in urine. ___ Wet with urine (from container or midstream or ginger ale). ___ Wait 60 seconds and read *darkest* part of tape (closest to fingers). ___ Indicate where results should be recorded (diabetes record).
• Acetest			*Acetest:* ___ Place 1 tablet on paper (without touching with fingers). ___ Recap bottle tightly. ___ Drop one drop of urine on tablet. ___ Wait 30 seconds. ___ Correctly interpret and state results (no color change indicates negative results). ___ Accurately record results.

Insulin, Medications
(correctly names strength and type(s))

12. "What kind of insulin (or pill) do you take?"

_____ U100, _____ type
_____ U100, _____ type
or
_____ Oral agent, _____

13. "How often and when will you take your insulin (or pill)?"

_____ ½ hour before breakfast, every day
_____ or prescribed time if more than once a day

14. "Point to the places where you give your insulin."
"Point to the places you will give your insulin five days in a row."

Check sites selected:
_____ left arm _____ right arm
_____ left thigh _____ right thigh
_____ abdomen
_____ left buttock _____ right buttock

15. "Within any one site, _e.g._, arm, how will you change the place of injection?"
"How far apart should the injections be?"

_____ Shows or tells about "grid" or using multiple sites within any area; about 1" apart.

Example . . . .
of "grid": . . . .
. . . .

16. "Why should you rotate your injection sites?"

_____ Skin will get tough/get "lumps"/poor absorption/lipoatrophy (fat wasting)

17. "Show me how how you give your insulin?" If documentation of injection technique unavailable:
1) Observe patient at time of actual insulin administration.
2) Observe entire procedure using normal saline.

_____ Roll insulin bottle to mix.
_____ Use aseptic technique throughout procedure (no contamination).
_____ Draw up proper amount of insulin.
_____ Injection technique acceptable

18. "Where do you store your insulin?"

_____ Cool place, _e.g._, refrigerator or cool room (Approximately 70° or below)

Diet

19. "What times will you be eating your meals each day?"

_____ Describe patient's response (times, regularity).
Times:

"What will happen if you don't eat at regular times?"

_____ Hypoglycemia/"low blood sugar"/symptoms of hypoglycemia

DESIRED OUTCOME

MEASUREMENT CRITERIA/SOURCE	MET	NOT MET	ACCEPTABLE ANSWERS/TECHNIQUES
20. "How do you feel when you have 'low blood sugar'/ hypoglycemia/insulin reaction?"			(Should name four) ___ Sweaty ___ Nervous ___ Shaky ___ Confused ___ Dizzy ___ Headache ___ Other _____, _____
21. "What would you do if you felt that way?"			___ (Ideal) ½ cup orange juice, 1 tablespoon jelly, honey, jam, or sugar ___ (Acceptable) Something sweet
22. "What might have made your blood sugar go low?"			___ Increased activity ___ Not eating on time ___ Not eating all the food ___ Taking too much insulin (if applicable)
23. "What would your family and friends do if they could not wake you up?"			___ Put something non-liquid and sweet inside cheek (avoid anything easily aspirated). ___ Call rescue squad.
24. "How do you feel if your sugar gets much too high?" "What happens to your body?"			(Should name three) ___ Frequent urination ___ Thirsty ___ Fatigue (drowsy) ___ Nausea and vomiting ___ Weight loss ___ Other _____, _____
25. "What would you do if that happened?"			___ Test your urine. ___ Drink warm liquids. ___ Take regular dose of insulin. ___ Call your doctor (essential).
26. "What might have made your blood sugar go too high?"			___ Eating too much ___ Eating wrong foods ___ Decreased activity ___ Not taking enough insulin ___ Illness or infection
27. "What do you do every day to protect your feet?" "Tell me how you take good care of your feet."			___ Inspect feet daily. ___ Wash feet daily and dry between toes.

	____ Apply lotion.
	____ Cut toenails straight across, above quick, or let someone else do it.
	____ Change hose daily.
	____ Wear proper fitting shoes
	____ Protect from corns, calluses (e.g., sheepskin).
	____ Don't use strong solutions (corn medicines, antiseptics).
	____ Don't let feet come in contact with hot objects (heaters, water, hot water bottles).
	____ Or very cold temperatures
	____ Don't go barefoot.
28. "What are you looking for when you check your feet daily?"	____ Sores, bruises, cracks, poor color
29. "What things do you avoid to help the circulation in your legs?"	____ Don't cross legs.
	____ Don't wear tight fitting garments, girdles, socks that are tight at the top, garters.
30. "How do you care for your teeth?"	____ Brush teeth every day.
	____ See dentist at least once a year.
31. "How many calories are you supposed to eat each day?"	____ Calories (check written order)
32. "When was the last time a dietician gave you a meal plan to follow?"	____ (If longer than six months ago, request dietician instruction.)

TOTAL HIP REPLACEMENT EVALUATION FORM (Patient interview/Direct observation)

Each item is related to a patient outcome described in the Total hip replacement guideline. Unless otherwise indicated, all responses in each block must be checked in order to consider the patient outcome met.

MEASUREMENT CRITERIA/SOURCE	DESIRED OUTCOME				COMMENTS
	MET	PARTIALLY MET	NOT MET	NOT APPLICABLE	
A. PATIENT OUTCOME: PREPARED FOR SURGERY. (evaluate postoperative day 3 to 4)					
1. "How did you find out information about your surgery?" (nurse, physician, booklet)					
2. "Before surgery did a nurse show you how to take deep breaths, cough and do leg exercises?"					
3. "How often do you do them?" Describe.					
4. "What other information would have been helpful to know before surgery?" Describe.					
B. PATIENT OUTCOME: FREE OF OR HAS MINIMAL POSTOPERATIVE DISCOMFORT OR COMPLICATIONS (evaluate postoperative day 3 to 5)					
5. "Does your pain medication (or other measures) relieve your pain?"					
6. "Does the nurse ask you when you need your pain medication?"					
7. "When you ask for something for pain how long do you wait before you receive it?" Describe answer.					
8. Patient Appearance: • No facial grimaces					
• Color of skin normal					
• No diaphoresis					
• Relaxed body position					
9. Spirometer within reach.					
10. "How often do you use your spirometer?"					
11. Patient demonstrates proper use of spirometer.					

443

MEASUREMENT CRITERIA/SOURCE

	DESIRED OUTCOME				COMMENTS
	MET	PARTIALLY MET	NOT MET	NOT APPLICABLE	

12. "How do you position your legs?" (abducted, neutral position of knees and toes)

13. "Show me how to do ankle exercises."

14. "Tell me how you turn in bed?"

15. Bed is in proper position per physician's order: _____

    Legs elevated 15°   No acute flexion of hips

16. Negative Homan's sign (no pain in calf on dorsiflexion of foot).

17. "Have you had any problems with bowel elimination?"

18. If 17 is yes—"What was done about this problem?"

19. "Are you having any problems with emptying your bladder?"

20. If 19 is yes—"What was done about this problem?"

21. Skin observation: note redness, blisters, other signs of impending breakdown. No skin problems with:
    _____ heels
    _____ elbows
    _____ sacrum (if position permits)

22. "Are your hose removed once each day and your legs washed?"

23. Knee exerciser correctly assembled and

24. Within patient's reach.

25. Observation of patient using knee exerciser independently.

    "Please show me how you use your knee exerciser." (Should demonstrate hip flexion, abduction, straight leg raising)

26. "How frequently do you use this?" (15 minutes, 2 times daily, dependent upon physical capabilities)

27. "What are you doing in physical therapy?"
   - Progressive ambulation as ordered: usually third to fifth day; begin physical therapy: begin ambulation with walker, progress toward independence in this area (in and out of bed, sit on toilet, etc.).

C. PATIENT OUTCOME: HAS KNOWLEDGE AND SKILLS RELATED TO SELF-CARE
   (evaluate day prior to discharge)

28. "Have you received written discharge instructions?"

29. "Has the nurse discussed these with you?"

30. "Will you have any help when you go home?"

31. "Do you have any stairs at home?"

32. If 31 is yes— "Have you practiced walking up stairs?"

33. "Have you discussed with anyone whether you need any household assistive devices?" e.g., toilet seat extender, hand bars for tub and toilet.

34. "Has anyone reviewed with you possible hazards within your home?", e.g., throw rugs, furniture arrangements, pets.

35. "How long will you be using crutches/walker?" (6 weeks)

36. "What activity limitations have been discussed with you?" (Describe answer)
   - No crossing legs or ankles
   - No acute hip flexion (> 90°, e.g., low chairs)
   - Driving

37. "What will you do to prevent your legs from swelling?"
   - Wear support hose
   - Elevate legs

38. "Can you show me the exercises you will do at home?"

39. Patient demonstrates:
   - Hip flexion

MEASUREMENT CRITERIA/SOURCE	MET	PARTIALLY MET	NOT MET	NOT APPLICABLE	COMMENTS
• Extension					
• Abduction					
• Straight leg raising					
40. "How often will you do them?"					
41. "What medications will you be taking when you are at home?" • Analgesic					
• Anticoagulant					
• Others: (for other medical conditions)					
42. "Have you received written instructions about the medicines?"					
43. "Has someone reviewed these with you?"					
44. "Could you tell me the precautions you will have to take while taking these drugs?"					
45. "Are there any drugs you were on when you were admitted that you need to resume?"					
46. "What are the signs of infection that you have been instructed to look for and report?" (redness, heat, swelling, drainage)					
47. "What other infections or symptoms would you be concerned about and report to your doctor in relation to your hip replacement?" *i.e.,* sore throat, urinary tract infection, dental.					
48. "Has anyone discussed with you about getting a medical identification card?"					
49. "Have you received a return medical appointment?"					

TOTAL HIP REPLACEMENT EVALUATION FORM (Chart review of documentation)

Each item is related to a patient outcome described in the Total hip replacement guideline. All responses in each block must be checked in order to consider the patient outcome met.

MEASUREMENT CRITERIA/SOURCE	MET	PARTIALLY MET	NOT MET	NOT APPLICABLE	COMMENTS
Documentation of ADMISSION NURSING ASSESSMENT (evaluate preoperatively)					
1. Baseline neurovascular status					
a. Pedal pulses					
b. Ability to dorsiflex ankle					
c. Lower extremity numbness					
d. History of phlebitis (positive or negative)					
2. Physical abilities/self-care/assistive devices					
3. Assessment of home environment					
4. Bowel history					
A. PATIENT OUTCOME: PREPARED FOR SURGERY (evaluate preoperatively)					
5. Has demonstrated coughing, deep breathing, ankle exercises					
6. a. Has received written information					
b. Has verbalized usual expectations of surgery: n.p.o., IV, probable time of surgery, recovery room care, availability of analgesics)					
c. Has verbalized specific expectations of hip surgery (ankle exercises, trapeze, abduction positioning, bedrest, turning)					
B. PATIENT OUTCOME: FREE OF OR HAS MINIMAL POSTOPERATIVE DISCOMFORT OR COMPLICATIONS (evaluate 3 to 5 days postoperative)					
7. a. Presence of pulmonary routine, q 2 hours first 24 hours, then q 4 hours until ambulatory					

MEASUREMENT CRITERIA/SOURCE	DESIRED OUTCOME				COMMENTS
	MET	PARTIALLY MET	NOT MET	NOT APPLICABLE	
b. In event of any of the following: Temperature: > 37.5° Pulse: > 100/minute Respirations: > 20/minute documentation of nursing action.					
8. a. Description of circulation, peripheral pulses, movement and sensation to toes, q 2 hours × 24 hours, then q 8 hours					
b. Presence of antiembolic hose (explain any exception)					
9. Presence/absence of pain in calf on ankle dorsiflexion (Homan's sign)					
10. Patient without catheter: a. Description of ability to void independently, first 8 hours postoperatively					
b. If voiding difficulty noted or dribbling of urine, describe nursing action.					
11. Urine output recorded q 8 hours as long as patient has urinary catheter or IV or voiding problems exist.					
12. Amount and tolerance for fluids and foods recorded q 8 hours for first 3 postoperative days.					
13. If greater than 20 per cent difference noted between ordered intake and actual intake, nursing action documented.					
14. a. Wound drainage recorded q 8 hours until drain removed.					
b. Time/date drain removed.					
15. Description of dressings checked q 30 minutes × 4, then q 4 hours × 24, then q 8 hours.					
16. a. Absence of presence of wound warmth, swelling, redness, q 24 hours					
b. Action is taken if signs of infection are present.					
17. Description of pain, type, site, severity q 24 hours					

18. a. Anticoagulants are administered as ordered.

    b. Any adverse reaction to anticoagulant is noted.

    c. Nursing action is taken in the case of b.

19. a. Any signs of impending or current skin breakdown are noted.

    b. Action is taken regarding any skin problems.

20. a. Description of amount, consistency of bowel movements

    b. Any bowel problem is noted and action is taken.

21. Description of activity status daily:
    a. Movement in bed (first 24 to 48 hours)

    b. Knee exerciser (72 hours +)

    c. Progress toward ambulation: (fourth to fifth day)

D. PATIENT OUTCOME: HAS KNOWLEDGE AND SKILLS RELATED TO SELF-CARE
   (evaluate day of transfer or discharge)

22. If *transferred*, summary of significant events during hospitalization.

23. Summary of teaching by nurse related to home care:
    a. Medications

    b. Avoiding infections

    c. Follow-up medical care

    d. Activity regimen

    e. Preventing accidental injury

    f. Written instructions given

24. Level of understanding of patient regarding above noted

25. Discharge summary:
    a. Teaching carried out (content of teaching may be in previous note).

    b. Verify patient's understanding of care.

    c. Verify that patient has or knows how to obtain equipment or supplies needed for home care.

QAPN Review Committee Meeting Report

Ward _____ Date Held _____

Number of reviews studied _____ Phase _____

Personnel attending Meeting   Name, Position   Name, Position
(should include as many QAPN
reviewers as possible and at   _____   _____
least 2 RNs and 2 LPNs)

_____   _____

_____   _____

_____   _____

Summary of meeting (use back of page for additional space)

1. Identified strengths:

2. Identified needs:

3. Trends noted in identified strengths and needs since previous reviews:

4. Chosen course(s) of action:

5. Resources identified to help with chosen course(s) of action.
   (*e.g.,* resource people, inservice programs, published materials, etc.)

_____
Signature

Copies are sent to: Representative, Unit for QAPN Manual, Supervisor, Inservice Instructor
                     and QAPN Office